Understanding Vulnerability

You must be the change you wish to see in the world.

Mahatma Ghandi

Understanding Vulnerability: A Nursing and Healthcare Approach

Edited by

Vanessa Heaslip

Bournemouth University, UK

Julie Ryden

Bournemouth University, UK

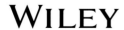

Library of Congress Cataloging-in-Publication Data

Understanding vulnerability : a nursing and healthcare approach / edited by Vanessa Heaslip and Julie Ryden.
    p. ; cm.
  Includes bibliographical references and index.
  ISBN 978-0-470-67136-8 (pbk.)
I. Heaslip, Vanessa, 1974–   II. Ryden, Julie, 1961–
[DNLM: 1. Ethics, Nursing–Great Britain.   2. Coercion–Great Britain.   3. Nurse-Patient Relations–ethics–Great Britain.   4. Quality of Health Care–ethics–Great Britain.   5. Vulnerable Populations–psychology–Great Britain. WY 85]
  RT82
  610.7306′9–dc23
                                    2013009647
A catalogue record for this book is available from the British Library.

Wiley also publishes its books in a variety of electronic formats. Some content that appears in print may not be available in electronic books.

Cover image: Photoscan/Shutterstock
Cover design by Design Deluxe

Set in 10/12.5pt Times by SPi Publisher Services, Pondicherry, India
Printed and bound in Singapore by Ho Printing Singapore Pte Ltd

1   2013

This book is dedicated to all of the people who shared their stories and experiences with us; we hope that by allowing us a window into their experiences it will enable each of us to reflect upon our practise and commit to 'making a difference', so that people's experiences of vulnerability are reduced.

We would like to express our thanks to our families for their ongoing support during this process, and Angela Warren who kindly undertook some proofreading for us.

Contents

Notes on contributors   viii

1   Introduction   1
Vanessa Heaslip and Julie Ryden

2   Understanding vulnerability   6
Vanessa Heaslip

3   Power, discrimination, and oppression   28
Julie Ryden and Chris Willetts

4   Processes of oppression   65
Julie Ryden

5   Professional culture and vulnerability   91
Karen Cooper and Janet Scammell

6   The social construction of vulnerability   111
Janet Scammell and Gill Calvin Thomas

7   Psychological perspectives of vulnerability   132
Nikki Glendening and Sid Carter

8   Psychosocial experiences and implications of vulnerability   154
Chris Willetts, Gill Calvin Thomas and Vanessa Heaslip

9   Working to reduce vulnerability   177
Chris Willetts, Julie Ryden and Gill Calvin Thomas

10   Conclusion   209
Julie Ryden and Vanessa Heaslip

Index   218

Notes on contributors

We are a group of experienced professionals, academics, and educationalists who have expertise in the exploration of vulnerability from both an educational as well as a research perspective. We have developed and run a variety of educational units at different educational levels for nurses, paramedics, and community workers. We believe that an understanding of vulnerability is essential in providing humanistic person-centred care.

Sid Carter, **PHD, MSc, BA, PGCEA, RNLD**, teaches and researches in the areas of learning disability and psychology at Bournemouth University. He is a learning disability nurse and thus has a long-term interest in the processes of discrimination and vulnerability. Sid's current research includes investigating methods to enhance the involvement of young people with learning disabilities in the services they use.

Karen Cooper, **MA (Health and Social Care Education), BNS (Hons), RGN, Dip NS**, has 30 years clinical experience within medicine and care of the older person and, ultimately as a Ward Manager in a rehabilitation setting. She moved into education in 2005 initially as a Practice Educator and is currently a lecturer in adult nursing. Areas of academic and research interests are in practice learning, assessment, and mentorship in relation to practitioners' personal and professional practice.

Nikki Glendening, **PGDip, BSc (Hons), RN, RHV, RNT**, is a senior lecturer in adult nursing at Bournemouth University. She is a qualified and registered nurse, health visitor, and nurse educator as well as a Specialist Public Health practitioner. Areas of academic and research interest include epistemological and psychological experiences of higher education among nursing students, including the experience of student vulnerability in both education and practice.

Vanessa Heaslip, **MSc (Health and Social Care Education), BSc (Community Nursing), DipHe Nursing**, is a Senior Lecturer in adult nursing; her clinical background was as a District Nurse and specialist practitioner for older people. She is aligned to the Society and Social Welfare Academic Community within Bournemouth University, due to her research interests regarding marginalised, minority groups whose voices are often not heard. Her current PhD study explores experiences of vulnerability from a gypsy/travelling perspective. Other research work has centred on vulnerability as well exploring the human dimension of care.

***Julie Ryden*, MSc (Psychotherapy), BSc (Hons) (Nursing), PGCEA, Dip DN, RGN,** is a Senior Lecturer at Bournemouth University with a nursing background as a District Nurse. Her academic and research interests have always focused upon the experiences of minority groups, anti-oppressive practice, and discursive constructions of vulnerability. Additionally, the interpersonal and human dimension of practice is a key interest.

***Janet Scammell*, DNSci, MSc (Nursing), BA (Social Science), Dip NEd (London), SRN, SCM**, is a registered nurse by background. She has over 20 years' experience as a lecturer and educational manager with under-graduate and post-graduate students in nursing. Janet also facilitates inter-professional education for health and social care students and has led research projects in this area. She is currently an associate professor in education within the School of Health and Social Care at Bournemouth University. Janet's research interests are two-fold: practice learning and ethnicity and health care practice, including workforce considerations.

***Gill Calvin Thomas*, MA Ed.**, is a qualified, registered social worker, who has worked with older adults, younger adults with physical disability and with adults living with HIV/AIDS within a local authority setting. She is a qualified practice educator and is a senior lecturer in practice learning for the BA social work programme in Bournemouth University. Areas of academic and research interests are in service user involvement within practice learning and the experience of BME students in their practice placements in a predominantly white, rural environment.

Chris Willetts lectures in the School of Health and Social Care at Bournemouth University, in subject areas such a Vulnerability, Social Exclusion and Discrimination, and Anti-Oppressive Practice to undergraduate nurses, social workers, and community development workers (amongst others). He also has professional experience in working with children and adults with learning difficulties in a range of health and social care settings.

Chapter 1

Introduction

Vanessa Heaslip and Julie Ryden

To be a nurse, midwife or care giver is an amazing role. There is hardly any intervention, treatment or care programme in which we do not play a significant part. …We support the people in our care and their families when they are at their most vulnerable and when clinical expertise, care and compassion matter most.

(DoH 2012a: 4)

Vulnerability is a key quality that all of us as health carers will encounter in the people we work with. To be a nurse, midwife, or carer working with such individuals is to have a privileged role within society, a role which demands that we exercise that privilege with responsibility, care, and compassion. We are aware that there are numerous examples of excellent care that people experience everyday within the National Health Service (NHS). It is our experience of working with colleagues and students that most people enter the profession with a desire to enhance the lives of individuals with whom they are working, to reduce their level of vulnerability, as well as an on-going commitment to enhancing the nursing profession and the NHS.

However, we are also aware that there are examples of poor quality care experienced. The recent Winterbourne View review (Flynn 2012) and Mid Staffordshire NHS Trust enquiry (Healthcare Commission 2009 and Francis 2010) have identified that some individuals who find themselves receiving care, can and have, received degrading, inhumane treatment by those paid to care for them. The highly publicised Winterbourne View review identified clear examples of horrific, abusive practices that appeared to be woven into the culture of the home. Whilst this case is a relatively rare occurrence in healthcare, there have been a number of recent examples highlighting the provision of poor quality care in health and social care settings (DoH 2008, Parliamentary and Health Service Ombudsman 2011, Commission on Dignity in Care for Older People 2012). In addition, the Mid staff NHS Trust review by Francis (2010) presented detailed accounts of poor quality care which were often linked to fundamental aspects of care such as nutrition and hydration, continence, privacy and dignity, personal care, and pressure area care. The findings are of great concern to anyone in a caring role and reflect a misuse and abuse of the privileged position we are given. As with the Winterbourne View review, it also transpired that the personal actions of practitioners were compounded by the culture of the organisation.

Understanding Vulnerability: A Nursing and Healthcare Approach, First Edition. Edited by Vanessa Heaslip and Julie Ryden.
© 2013 John Wiley & Sons, Ltd. Published 2013 by John Wiley & Sons, Ltd.

Therefore, when examining quality of care and the vulnerability of patients, clients, service users, or families, it is evident that we need to consider both the personal interactions between those individuals and healthcare practitioners as well as exploring the cultural aspects of the care environment. This book offers that breadth of examination of the topic, and also goes further by exploring some of the structural issues which affect vulnerability.

Nationally there are also structural factors that impact upon quality of care. There has been a drive within the NHS to provide evidence-based standardised care, and this has largely been achieved through the development of care pathways such as Liverpool Care Pathway (NICE 2004) and #Neck of Femur Care Pathway (National Clinical Guidelines Centre 2011). However, there is the possibility that by focusing upon 'standardised' approaches to care, it could be at the expense of personalised care – responding to the condition rather than the individual. In addition, there is also a focus nationally on meeting targets within the NHS (DoH 2011); this can result in people being thought of as a number within a service rather than as an individual who is unwell. This demonstrates how structural factors can also contribute to the care experienced by individuals within a service; indeed, this is one of the main criticisms of the Francis Review (2010), which highlighted that people must always come first:

> ... if there is one lesson to be learnt, I suggest it is that people must always come before numbers. It is the individual experience ... that really matters. (Francis 2010: 4)

Because of such high-profile cases identifying poor quality care in the NHS and private care organisations, there has been an increased focus nationally on identifying and promoting the core values of the NHS which were published as a part of the NHS Constitution (DoH 2012b). These core values include:

- *Respect and dignity* – Here a link between the constitution and human rights is established, clearly denoting a commitment to ensuring that people accessing services in the NHS are treated with dignity and respect as enshrined in the Human Rights Act. Specifically identified within this is the right not to be subjected to inhumane or degrading treatment as well as a right to respect for family life. This is central to providing high-quality care by ensuring that individuals are treated respectfully.
- *Commitment to quality of care* – The NHS is committed to providing high quality of care by suitably qualified and experienced staff. In addition to this, there is a clear commitment to monitor patients' experience of care and, where necessary, make changes.
- *Compassion* – Compassion is at the heart of the NHS. When people are unwell, they feel exposed and vulnerable, and the NHS has a responsibility to ensure that people receive compassionate care.
- *Improving lives* – The constitution highlights the responsibilities of the NHS as well as the wider public in working together to improve people's health by preventative measures, such as screening programmes, whilst also identifying that the public have a responsibility to proactively access health services.
- *Working together for patients* – This core value reflects how the NHS will work in partnership with individuals, highlighting that they are a central team member working

together with NHS staff. It also recognises people's autonomy acknowledging their right to refuse treatment and the importance of communication by individuals, having the right to have access to their own medical records as well as having sufficient information regarding any proposed treatment.
- *Everyone counts* – This last core value recognises that the NHS is a resource for all people within society. It reinforces that people have the right not to be discriminated against in the provision of NHS services on the grounds of gender, race, religion or belief, sexual orientation, disability (including mental illness and learning disability), or age.

We believe that this book has something to offer the reader in relation to each of these core values and can enhance the readers' depth of understanding of each value. A focus upon providing individualised, person-centred care is central to ensuring that the core values of the NHS are met within healthcare; this book will enable you to understand some of the factors that occur at the personal, cultural, and structural level which can inhibit the delivery of person-centred care. The last value 'everybody counts' reflects the fact that we live in a diverse society and healthcare practitioners must be equipped for this; yet numerous reports (Mencap 2007, DoH 2008, Michael 2008, Healthcare Commission 2009, Equalities and Human Rights Commission 2010) have highlighted that individuals from diverse backgrounds do not always experience high-quality care. However, professional codes of conduct assert that healthcare practitioners should provide anti-discriminatory practice (HCPC 2008, NMC 2008). Whilst educational preparation for the professional role will address such issues, there is also a potentially flawed assumption that individuals enter their preparation as 'an empty book, waiting to be writ-ten'. However, individuals enter their professional programme of training and practice having already been exposed to a wide variety of perceptions and having experienced a diversity of life experiences that may affect their ability to provide anti-discriminatory care without further time and attention to those perceptions. This book provides readers with the opportunity to critically question their individual and collective practices and beliefs and to do so at a time and place of their choosing. A key message of the book is that there should be no fear attached to such critical reflection; there are no recriminations. Indeed, it is the hallmark of a professional to be able to reflect and learn, rather than turning away from such opportunities.

Government strategy has traditionally considered vulnerability from the perspective that particular 'groups' of people who by reason of age, ethnicity, disability, and health status are deemed to be more vulnerable to harm than the rest of society. This book takes the view that such a perspective not only imposes vulnerability on members of these groups regardless of their individual situation and thus may deny their individual differ-ence and experience, but it also obscures the potential vulnerability of other individuals who do not fit within these traditional categories but may still be feeling vulnerable. It is our contention that vulnerability is a 'condition humana' (Kottow 2003: 461), which is a potential experience for *all* people. In this way, the book encourages its readers to see vulnerability in its widest sense, and thus enhances their ability to address and reduce vulnerability for *all* their clients, not just particular groups of clients. Equally it encourages readers not to assume that an individual is vulnerable just because they can be categorised in a 'vulnerable group'. This book aims to open the readers' eyes to the individuality of each client, seeing the person for who they are, rather than making false assumptions based on a tick box mentality. Thus, readers may expand their understanding of the concept of 'individualised, person-centred care'.

Another key difference in the book's underpinning philosophy comes from our belief that vulnerability is a socially constructed phenomenon, and that vulnerability is created not by the individual's personal qualities but by the world they inhabit. This follows the social model of disability (Oliver 1983), in seeing vulnerability as being the result of the environment the person lives in, consisting of attitudes, cultural beliefs, media images, power, strategy and policy, dominant discourses, and other factors. It is our contention that these factors create and construct the experience of vulnerability to an equal or greater extent than any condition or life experience. Through this text, these factors are explored in some depth, and their particular impact upon vulnerability is explored throughout the book.

This book is useful for all healthcare practitioners (students, qualified practitioners, and unqualified practitioners) that are committed to providing person-centred care from a variety of different professional specialties (nursing, physiotherapy, occupational therapy, paramedic science, operating department practitioners, and community workers). In addition, this book can also be used within the undergraduate nursing curriculum to support the essential care clusters identified in the Standards for Re-registration Nursing Education (NMC 2010). We believe that this book can assist practitioners in understanding the wider, human experience of vulnerability. A key strength of the book is its inclusion of people's voices, thus offering the lived experience of vulnerability which we feel is central to understanding how care is experienced by others. These lived experience accounts are from our personal and professional practice, together with experiences that have been shared by other colleagues. In order to protect the confidentiality and anonymity of the individuals, names and circumstances have been changed, and some accounts have even been constructed from collations of several stories. This provides both the foundation for a critical examination of the social construction of vulnerability as well as a constant sense of the 'real world' to illustrate and bring to life the theoretical issues under discussion.

This book, we hope, will assist you in developing your thinking and enhancing your practice. As such the book challenges you to reflect throughout on your own contribution to vulnerability and the impact of the healthcare environment in which you work. Just a note regarding terminology: within the book a variety of terms have been used to denote people who experience care (patient, service user, client, people, individual), likewise a variety of terms have been used to denote people who provide care (carer, practitioner, nurse, care giver, health carer), and this has occurred in order to reflect the widest diversity of care and care settings.

References

Commission on Dignity in Care for Older People (2012) *Delivering Dignity: Securing Dignity in Care for Older People in Hospitals and Care Homes*. Available from http://tinyurl.com/cque4ox [accessed on 31 July 2012].

Department of Health (DoH) (2008) *Confidence in Caring – A Framework for Best Practice.* Department of Health, London.

Department of Health (2010) *Equity and Excellence – Liberating the NHS.* Department of Health, London.

Department of Health (2011) *The NHS Outcomes Framework 2012/13.* Department of Health, London.

Department of Health (2012a) *Developing the Culture of Compassionate Care; Creating a New Vision for Nurses, Midwives and Care-Givers.* Department of Health, London.

Department of Health (2012b) *NHS Constitution.* Department of Health, London.

Equalities and Human Rights Commission (2010) *How Fair is Britain?* Available from http://www.equalityhumanrights.com/key-projects/triennial-review/full-report-and-evidence-downloads/#How_fair_is_Britain_Equality_Human_Rights_and_Good_Relations_in_2010_The_First_Triennial_Review [accessed on 20 October 2010].

Flynn, M. (2012) *Winterbourne View Hospital – A Serious Case Review.* South Gloucestershire Council. Available from http://hosted.southglos.gov.uk/wv/report.pdf [accessed on 31 October 2012].

Francis, R. (2010) *Independent Inquiry into Care Provided by Mid Staffordshire NHS Foundation Trust January 2005 – March 2009.* Stationary Office, London.

Health and Care Professions Council (HCPC) (2008) *Standards of Conduct, Performance and Ethics.* Available from http://www.hpc-uk.org/aboutregistration/standards/standardsofconduct performanceandethics/ [accessed on 31 October 2012].

Healthcare Commission (2009) *Investigation into Mid Staffordshire NHS Foundation Trust.* March 2009, Available from http://www.nmc-uk.org/Publications/Standards/The-code/Introduction/ [accessed on 24 September 2010].

Kottow, M. (2003) The vulnerable and the susceptible. *Bioethics*, 17, 5–6, 460–471.

Mencap (2007) *Death by Indifference.* Available from http://www.mencap.org.uk/campaigns/ take-action/death-indifference [accessed on 24 September 2010].

Michael, J. and the Independent Inquiry into Access to Healthcare for People with Learning Disabilities (2008). *Healthcare for All.* Available from http://www.dh.gov.uk/en/Publicationsandstatistics/ Publications/PublicationsPolicyAndGuidance/DH_099255 [accessed on 15 October 2010].

National Clinical Guidelines Centre (2011) *The Management of Hip Fracture in Adults; Methods, Evidence and Guidance.* National Clinical Guideline Centre, London.

National Institute for Clinical Excellence (NICE) (2004) *Guidance on Cancer Services Improving Supportive and Palliative Care for Adults with Cancer.* National Institute for Clinical Excellent, London.

Nursing and Midwifery Council (NMC) (2008) *The Code: Standards of Conduct, Performance and Ethics for Nurses and Midwives.* Available from http://www.nmc-uk.org/Publications/Standards/ The-code/Introduction/ [accessed on 8 July 2012].

Nursing and Midwifery Council (2010) *Standards for Pre-Reg Education.* Nursing and Midwifery Council, London.

Oliver, M. (1983) Social Work with Disabled People. Macmillan, Basingstoke.

Parliamentary and Health Service Ombudsman (2011) *Care and Compassion? Report of the Health Service Ombudsman on Ten Investigations into NHS Care of Older People.* Available from http://tinyurl.com/clmnu32 [accessed on 27 July 2012].

Chapter 2

Understanding vulnerability

Vanessa Heaslip

Introduction

This chapter will introduce the concept of vulnerability. It will begin by looking at dictionary definitions and develop to explore the link between vulnerability, health, and healthcare by presenting the different ways in which people are viewed as being vulnerable. The chapter will then continue by exploring the differing theoretical explanations of the concept of vulnerability as well as the implications for healthcare practice. Throughout the chapter, readers will be urged to recognise the importance of practitioners having an awareness of vulnerability, and how in their daily practice they can either contribute or reduce a person's experience of feeling vulnerable.

Defining vulnerability

Little *et al.* (2000) argue that vulnerability has been studied less than it merits considering the stories of patients and healthcare workers who often identify it as a central theme in the healthcare relationship. Few studies have explored the use of the term vulnerability in healthcare; one such study was by Appleton (1994) who explored health visitors' perceptions of vulnerability in relation to child protection and identified a lack of consensus and clear definition of the term.

Therefore, before we can explore this concept further, some clarification of the term is required. For example, dictionary definitions identify multiple perspectives:

- The *Oxford English Dictionary* defined vulnerable as being 'exposed to being attacked or harmed, either physically or emotionally' (Pearsall 2002: 1608).
- The *Concise Oxford Dictionary* defined it as 'that which maybe wounded, susceptible of injury, exposed to damage by a weapon, or criticism' (Sykes 1982: 1205).

A common factor in each of these definitions is the notion of harm which denotes a holistic experience as well as a danger or threat to the person. The Latin root of the term vulnerability is 'vuln' which means wound or 'vulnare' meaning to wound. This supports

Understanding Vulnerability: A Nursing and Healthcare Approach, First Edition. Edited by Vanessa Heaslip and Julie Ryden.

Box 2.1   Time for reflection

Using the dictionary definitions provided earlier, identify a time in which you felt vulnerable, for example, your first day at school or university, or starting a new job, or moving to a new area.

- How did this feel?
- What were the factors which contributed to you feeling vulnerable?
- Did anything make it worse?
- Did anything make it better?
- How did it affect you at that time?
- How did it affect you afterwards?

---

this sense of harm and wounding which is implied by the dictionary definitions. Now let us consider what this experience means in reality (Box 2.1)

You may have written about times in which you were frightened or felt a lack of control. Indeed, control is a theme that is closely linked to the experience of vulnerability, in that the less control we have over an experience the more vulnerable we may feel, and conversely the more in control we feel we are the less vulnerable we feel. When I think about my own experiences of feeling vulnerable, it is often in situations where I feel out of my depth, where I do not know what will happen, or where I feel isolated and alone.

Vulnerability and healthcare

If we think about times we have felt vulnerable, some of these may have been during periods of ill health or when we have been patients. The NMC (2002) identify that people can experience feeling vulnerable whenever their health or usual function is compromised; thus, vulnerability increases when they enter unfamiliar surroundings, situations, or relationships. Before we go on any further, please read the case study of Peter (Box 2.2).

Box 2.2   Case study of Peter

Peter is 74 years of age and during the night he had a fall at home, injuring his hip. Peter was brought to the hospital emergency department, where he had a variety of tests and x-rays and has been diagnosed with a fractured neck of femur. In the early hours of the morning, Peter was brought to the orthopaedic ward, as he will require surgery to repair the fracture.

Thinking about Peter,
- Do you think he could be feeling vulnerable?
- If so what are the factors which have contributed to him feeling vulnerable?

Often as practitioners, we can forget what it may feel like to be admitted to hospital or how strange this experience may be for someone. In some ways, an admission to a hospital or a care setting can appear to the individual as though they have been transported to an alien world. Thinking of Peter and his story, please read Peter's perspective (Box 2.3).

> **Box 2.3   Peter's perspective**
>
> 'It was dark and I woke up because I needed a wee, I tripped and fell. I cannot believe how stupid that was. My leg really hurts and I called to my wife, the next thing I remember is being greeted by the paramedics who rig me up to a heart monitor (is there something wrong with my heart??, now I'm frightened) they put a needle in my arm which hurts, then it's bright and I'm in the back of the ambulance. I cannot remember what he said as my leg really hurts. The next couple of hours go in a blur, I am given something for the pain, which has stopped the pain but I feel a bit woozy now, I keep hearing words but cannot really make sense of what people are saying. I've had a variety of tests and finally they have told me I have a bed…. I'm tired… it must be the early hours of the morning now. I arrive to the ward and it's dark, I am greeted by a nurse who is whispering and I hear the nurses talking about me, but I don't really understand what they say, the words they use, it's very medical. It's dark and I am being wheeled around, but I don't know where I am going or what's happening.'

Thinking about Peter's story from this perspective makes it easier to see why he may feel wounded or feel a fear of harm and especially points to a lack of control affecting his vulnerability. Often in doing our jobs, I think we forget about what the experience must feel like for the person at the receiving end of care. In hospitals and care environments, there are different smells and noises, and even the language that patients hear but maybe do not understand; this can be especially more challenging if English is not the patient's first language. In this alien world, patients have to share personal intimate experiences with a stranger, telling them about things they may never have shared with another human being before (such as their bowel habits). They have to remove their clothes and may even have to have a stranger touching them intimately, exposing their body. For the majority of patients, the only privacy they are afforded is a curtain, and how many times have healthcare practitioners entered a curtain that is closed without asking the patient if it is okay or warning them they are about to enter. It is perhaps unsurprising when considering this that patients may experience feeling vulnerable within a healthcare setting. This coupled with fear and maybe a lack of knowledge and understanding about their health issue can perpetuate the feelings of vulnerability.

There is evidence that unthinking and unquestioning practice does sometimes occur in healthcare which could increase an individual's propensity to experiencing vulnerability. For example, there is a tendency in healthcare to abbreviate and focus upon the illness or condition (e.g. #NOF, MI, dementia, acopic, Parkinson's, to name a few) which results in a person losing their identity, and this will be explored further in Chapters 4 and 6. We may question how this increases a person's likelihood of feeling vulnerable, yet the Confidence in Caring Report (DoH 2008) identified that patients were less confident about being cared about as individuals than concerns they had about their clinical care. There is further evidence of this lack of caring within the Health Ombudsman Report (Parliamentary and Health Service Ombudsman 2011) which included quotes from relatives such as:

> Our dad was not treated as a capable man in ill health, but as someone whom staff could not have cared less whether he lived or died (Parliamentary and Health Service Ombudsman 2011: 2)

> from the moment cancer was diagnosed my dad was completely ignored. It was as if he did not exist he was an old man and was dying (Parliamentary and Health Service Ombudsman 2011:16).

Box 2.4　Alice's case study

Alice was admitted to hospital in the early evening following a myocardial infarction. She was 75 years of age, and this was her first hospital admission since the birth of her children many years previously. It was suppertime and the dinners were being distributed. As Alice was not there in the morning, she was unable to order her choices for the evening meal. The nurses brought round the spare meals that were left which included a white ham sandwich and a brown cheese sandwich. Alice asked for a brown ham sandwich and was told that this was not possible; she had to make a choice from the sandwiches that were on offer. Alice declined to eat and went without supper.

Thinking about this case study,
• How do you think Alice may have felt?
• What could the nurses have done?

What these quotes demonstrate is how through unthinking practice staff actually increased the vulnerability of the clients and their families by not focusing upon the individual and their needs. These are extreme cases of how staff increase the vulnerability of clients within their care, but there are more subtle ways, see Alice's case study (Box 2.4).

As a practitioner working in a busy environment, this scenario may seem insignificant and that Alice could easily have chosen one of the sandwiches on offer. However, to Alice this was really important, as she had never eaten white bread in her life and to her, the fact that the staff did not appear to care about her and her choices may have led her to question what else she will have little control over in the care environment. In this case, a lack of choice increased Alice's experience of feeling vulnerable. It can be argued that in healthcare, choice is still largely limited as the health service remains predominately based around the needs and ease of the staff and organisation (service led) rather than the needs of the person (needs led). Indeed, if the service was truly needs led, then the nurses could have simply rung the catering department to ask for a brown ham sandwich.

Therefore, in the context of healthcare, vulnerability has to be viewed as an overarching concept which contributes to, and results from, a range of personal, family, societal, and political factors (Shepard and Mahon 2002). This identifies a much wider, more holistic perspective than the dictionary definitions, which tend to focus upon individual characteristics of being liable to harm. Appleton (1994) agrees and notes that vulnerability is caused by a combination of medical, psychological, social, and cultural factors. Thus, it can be argued that vulnerability has to be considered holistically and contextually.

There are health implications of vulnerability which can include both physiological and psychological implications for clients (Rogers 1997) (Table 2.1). Feeling vulnerable has a profound impact upon psychological well-being and can induce feelings of anxiety, helplessness, and loss of control. These psychological feelings impact upon the body physically, which can lead to both increased morbidity and mortality. It is therefore vital that we as practitioners understand how and why patients may experience feeling vulnerable, so that we can mitigate these experiences. By having an understanding

Table 2.1   Health implications of vulnerability (Rogers 1997).

Physiological effects of vulnerability	Psychological effects of vulnerability
• Fatigue	• Helplessness
• Muscular tension	• Loss of control
• Urinary frequency	• Lowered self-esteem
• Weight loss	• Fear
• Depression	• Embarrassment
• Anorexia	• Loss of self-worth
• Accident prone	• Desperation
• Acne	• Powerlessness
• Insomnia	• Inability to express feelings
• Back pain	• Anger
• GI distress	• Isolation
• Menstrual irregularities	• Uncertainty
	• Anxiety/worry
	• Inability to concentrate
	• Weakness

of vulnerability, it also enables us to ensure that we do not inadvertently create feelings of vulnerability in others or perpetuate their vulnerability through our daily practice.

Professional definitions of vulnerability

Whilst not written about extensively in the professional literature, there are some key definitions of vulnerability. Phillips (1992, cited in Rogers (1997: 65)) defines vulnerability as 'susceptibility to health problems, harm or neglect'. Let us just take a moment to unpick this definition in more detail. Susceptibility to health problems could either be caused by physical (genetic predisposition), psychological (mental illness, fear, or lack of control), or sociological (lack of access to healthcare or financial) factors, thus calling for a holistic interpretation of the danger or threat. Likewise, susceptibility to harm could also be influenced by physical, social, or psychological factors. It is also really important to remember that the threat may be real or perceived and both can contribute to an individual's experience of feeling vulnerable. For example, there may be two men living on the same street; one feels vulnerable due to a fear of crime and the other does not. The fact that only one of the two gentlemen feels vulnerable does not diminish his experience of it. Vulnerability therefore is similar to the experience of pain, in that it is exactly what the individual experiencing it says it is, and they experience it when they say they are (McCaffery 1968).

In addition, vulnerability is not a dichotomous experience, by that I mean you are either vulnerable or you are not, rather it is situational (Rogers 1997), in that a person who is not particularly vulnerable in one environment may feel highly vulnerable in another, and this could be linked to the amount of control one has over the situation. This situational perspective of vulnerability can help us to understand how individuals that

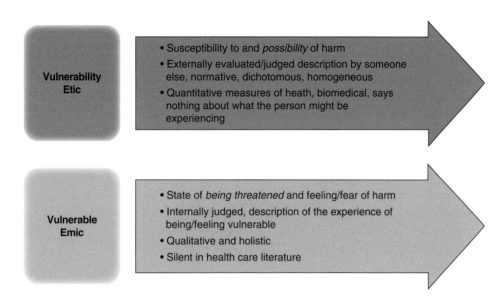

Vulnerability Etic
- Susceptibility to and *possibility* of harm
- Externally evaluated/judged description by someone else, normative, dichotomous, homogeneous
- Quantitative measures of heath, biomedical, says nothing about what the person might be experiencing

Vulnerable Emic
- State of *being threatened* and feeling/fear of harm
- Internally judged, description of the experience of being/feeling vulnerable
- Qualitative and holistic
- Silent in health care literature

Figure 2.1   Spiers (2000) etic and emic perspectives of vulnerability.

may not be vulnerable may experience feeling vulnerable when they enter healthcare, especially as the amount of control clients have in a healthcare situation is limited, as we explored earlier.

However, when we think of vulnerability in healthcare we most typically think of vulnerable groups in society (Box 2.5).

Within your list, you may have noted groups such as older people, children, people with a mental illness, individuals from ethnic minorities, people with disabilities, and people who are homeless. This is because in healthcare the term 'vulnerability' is often used as an external judgement to an individual or group that may be susceptible to ill health. The work by Spiers (2000: 716) can help us to understand this in more depth; Spiers makes a distinction between the 'etic' and 'emic' perspective (Figure 2.1).

The etic perspective of vulnerability relates to the 'susceptibility and possibility of harm'. This is externally evaluated or judged by others (e.g., healthcare practitioners) and reflects the normative or professional perspective. This approach focuses upon groups of people and identifies that vulnerability is dichotomous (you are either vulnerable or you are not) and that everyone in that group is the same (homogenous); these judgements are often based upon quantitative measures of health. Many of the clients you identified in Box 2.5 (where you had to list vulnerable groups) would be based upon this normative etic perspective of vulnerability, which focuses upon groups in society with poorer health outcomes. Older people are often identified by practitioners as a vulnerable group due to the increased likelihood of ill health and mortality, yet it has to be questioned whether vulnerability is an inevitable consequence of ageing. It can be argued that ageing is not a dichotomous experience (e.g. that all older people have the same experience) but an individual one; for example, would Queen Elizabeth identify herself as a vulnerable person automatically because she happens to be in the older age group?

In contrast, Spiers (2000) also identified the emic perspective which relates to the 'state of being threatened and a feeling of fear of harm'. This perspective is identified by the individual actually experiencing feeling vulnerable; therefore, it is an individual interpretation of the experience. In this perspective, vulnerability is exactly what the person experiencing it says it is; therefore, if they say they are experiencing feeling vulnerable, then they are. Under this perspective, any individual can experience feeling vulnerable regardless of age, gender, ability, etc. This way of seeing vulnerability is more silent within the professional literature. For example, have you ever considered that every client you have worked with could have experienced feeling vulnerable, and indeed you yourself could also experience feeling vulnerable (please refer back to the notes you made previously, in Box 2.1)

To date, in this chapter we have examined some definitions of vulnerability and established the link between vulnerability, health, and healthcare. What we need to do now is to further explore the different theoretical explanations of vulnerability, so that we can appreciate the complexity of this phenomenon and be better placed to understand why some individuals (including ourselves) may experience feeling vulnerable.

Different theoretical explanations for vulnerability

As we have acknowledged, an individual experience of vulnerability can occur for many different reasons and we need to understand these in order to:

1   Have a better understanding of why people can experience feeling vulnerable
2   Be effective in minimising individual experiences of feeling vulnerable
3   Better understand the ways in which vulnerability is seen by practitioners

There are different theoretical explanations of vulnerability (Box 2.6).

Each of these different explanations will now be considered in turn identifying the implications for professional practice.

Vulnerability as a mechanism to identify populations at risk of ill health

The predominant perspective of vulnerability in healthcare identifies vulnerable populations, as 'social groups who have an increased relative risk or susceptibility to adverse health outcomes … as evidenced by morbidity and premature mortality' (Flaskerud and Winslow 1998: 69). At the centre of this perspective is the notion of risk and harm; indeed, almost all uses of the term vulnerable in healthcare reflects epidemiological principles of population-based relative risk. As such this reflects the etic, normative perspective of vulnerability. Vulnerable groups therefore include people who are judged to be 'old' (Spiers 2000, Rydeman and Törnkvist 2006), 'poor' (Spiers 2000, Furumoto-Dawson *et al.*

> **Box 2.6** Theoretical explanations of vulnerability
>
> Mechanism to identify populations at risk of ill health:
> - Vulnerability is a way to identify individuals or groups at risk of ill health or potential death so that services can be developed to address their vulnerability.
>
> Mechanism to identify social groups in need of protection:
> - Vulnerability is a way to identify people who are at risk of being abused, so that we can put services in place to protect them.
>
> Consequence of social interaction:
> - Vulnerability is a dynamic process that occurs when two or more people interact and are influenced by societal values.
>
> Existential experience:
> - Feeling vulnerable is essentially a human experience, which is experienced by all human beings.
>
> Shifting experience:
> - Rather than a dichotomous experience (you are either vulnerable or you are not), vulnerability is a shifting experience, which means that individuals can have moments of feeling vulnerable depending upon the context they are in.
>
> Mutual vulnerability:
> - Within the context of a professional relationship, both staff and individual patients can experience feeling vulnerable, due to the nature of the work involved.
>
> Vehicle for personal growth:
> - Vulnerability is not always a negative experience; indeed, feeling vulnerable can be a positive experience as it drives us to learn new ways of coping or can open new opportunities.

2007), children (Hewitt-Taylor and Heaslip 2012, Clark 2007, Furumoto-Dawson *et al.* 2007), 'mentally ill' (Spiers 2000), and 'ethnic minorities' (Pitkin Derose *et al.* 2007). A key drive in this perspective is that vulnerability is seen as a problem to be solved which then drives statutory guidance and public health action.

So let us take the example of older people, who are often identified as a vulnerable group due to increased morbidity and mortality (Spiers 2000, Rydeman and Törnkvist 2006). We know that there is an association between aging and ones increased propensity to fall, and that when older people fall there is an increased likelihood of them sustaining an injury as well as a potential that they may die as a result of the fall (NICE 2004). This knowledge of their increased vulnerability to falling has led to a variety of practice initiatives geared at reducing the likelihood that people will fall. As such, there has been national guidance such as the National Service Framework for Older People (DoH 2000a) and Clinical practice guideline for the assessment and prevention of falls (DoH 2000a, NICE 2004) as well as the development of falls clinics in order to standardise and enhance the clinical care of older people who either fall or are at risk of falling. However, it must be remembered that not all older people fall. In addition, focusing upon vulnerability in this manner does not inform us of the lived experience of vulnerability in older age. Indeed, it can be argued that many older people may not define themselves as vulnerable and therefore what right do we as practitioners have to tell them they are.

Vulnerability as a mechanism to identify social groups in need of protection

Another way to explore vulnerability is the notion of a vulnerable adult identified within adult protection policy and safeguarding agenda. In this perspective, the term vulnerability is used to identify individuals and groups at risk of harm, as such providing the etic, normative judgement. The *No Secrets* document (DoH 2000b: 8–9) defines a vulnerable adult as 'Anyone aged 18 years + who is or may be in need of community care services by reason of mental or other disability, age or illness and who is or maybe unable to take care of him/herself'. As such groups of people identified as vulnerable under the *No Secrets* document included older people, people with learning disabilities, people with physical disabilities, traumatic brain injuries, or acquired brain damage, and people with mental health problems.

Box 2.7   Definition of a vulnerable adult is a person aged 18 or over who:

A person is vulnerable in the context of the setting in which they are situated or the service they receive as follows:

- Those in residential accommodation provided in connection with care or nursing or in receipt of domiciliary care services
- Those receiving healthcare
- Those in lawful custody or under the supervision of a probation officer
- Those receiving a welfare service of a prescribed description or direct payments from a social services authority
- Those receiving services, or taking part in activities, aimed at people with disabilities or special needs because of their age or state of health
- Those who need assistance in the conduct of their affairs.

These guidelines have also been supported by the Safeguarding Vulnerable Groups Act 2006 which was introduced in the House of Lords on 28 February 2006 and received Royal Assent on 8 November 2006. Section 59 of the Act and article 3 of the Order provides a definition of a vulnerable adult (Box 2.7) (Office of Public Sector Information 2007).

Box 2.8   Case study of Mary

Mary is an 83 year old woman and she has a 45 year old 'boyfriend' who is a cab driver. She lives in a large house and is very wealthy but has few friends and no close relatives. The boyfriend takes her out regularly in her Jaguar which he drives. However, her neighbour is concerned because Mary gives him a lot of money. Mary tells the neighbour to mind her own business; it is her money to do with as she sees fit. A nephew also lives locally but rarely visits. He is also unhappy about his aunt's relationship as he feels she is being swindled out of her money and demands something is done.

Again many of us would agree that this is a valid perspective and that society should aim to protect those who are vulnerable from harm. However, there are also potential problems associated with this perception of vulnerability linked to the notion of 'protection' and 'vulnerable', in that this perspective of vulnerability can be seen as restrictive, negative, and paternalistic. This can lead to a stigma being associated with the term vulnerability which becomes defined by terms such as weakness, failure, inequality, inferiority, and dependence (Batchelor 2006). Let us consider this further by exploring the case of Mary (Box 2.8).

In this example, we may perceive that Mary is a vulnerable adult, who is experiencing financial abuse by her boyfriend, and as such she needs to be protected. However, on what basis are we making this decision, Mary's age? Just because Mary is 83 we cannot assume that she is not competent to make her own decisions as an autonomous adult. Potentially, seeing Mary as a vulnerable adult to be protected could also negatively influence our working with her. Focusing upon our perceptions of her perceived weakness could lead us to become paternalistic in our approach (thinking we know what is best for her) which could result in us not facilitating her choice and control, thus disempowering her. The key point to note here is whilst we would not automatically discount abuse occurring, neither should we automatically assume Mary is being abused because of her age.

In addition, Penhale and Parker (2008) assert that it attaches a 'victim status' to the individual which appears to apportion blame to the individual rather than the person, agency, or society responsible for it. It is only when we align a less stigmatising conceptualisation of vulnerability will we be better equipped to interact with vulnerable populations in ways which encourage choice and openness to decisions that have a positive impact upon lifestyles and health outcomes (Purdy 2004) For example, in the case of Mary, it is about seeing her as an adult with the right to make autonomous decisions regarding her life even if we do not necessarily agree with her choices and about being open with her regarding the concerns that her nephew has raised. In 2007, the term 'protecting vulnerable adults' was superseded by 'safeguarding adults', in part to reflect that vulnerable adults are not different people – they are about us – and that all human beings can potentially be vulnerable. The perception of the term vulnerable as patronising and disempowering to the individual concerned was further highlighted in the consultation of the No Secrets guidance viewed in relation to abuse (DoH 2009).

Vulnerability as a consequence of interaction between different groups in society

Both of the theoretical perspectives presented to date (vulnerability as a mechanism to identify populations at risk of ill health and vulnerability as a mechanism to identify social groups at risk of abuse) largely focus upon vulnerability being something that is linked to the individual rather than recognising some of the wider societal forces. So another way to explore vulnerability is to examine it from a sociological perspective, which is in the relationships between people and the relationships between individuals and society. Some groups could be identified as vulnerable because they hold a lower position within society or are not valued by society; examples of such groups are people who are homeless, people with mental health conditions, and some ethnic minorities such as gypsies and travellers. These groups are typically impoverished, disenfranchised, or who are subject to discrimination, intolerance, and stigma (Peternalj-Taylor 2005). This perspective is supported by Vasas (2005) who recognised the link between marginalisation and vulnerability. Marginalisation conveys a sense of disadvantage and injustice. In nursing, it reflects individuals and/or groups who are peripheralised on the basis of their identities, associations, experiences, and environments (Vasas 2005).

Box 2.9   Social status of the gypsy/travelling community

- *Ideological* – Nomadic lifestyle pathologised and criminalised
- *Economic* – Increased financial vulnerability due to erosion of traditional working practices
- *Political* – Gypsies are a politically marginalised group, vilified not only by the media but also politically (Turner 2002)
- *Psychological* – Feeling of not belonging
- *Social* – Cemlyn (2000) identified that the travelling community could be perceived as vulnerable due to structural inequalities experienced (e.g. access to healthcare, education etc.)
- *Ethical* – Gypsies/travellers experience discrimination and are marginalised within society (Karner 2004), despite legal protection as a result of their ethnic minority status

Adapted from Redwood and Heaslip (2010)

A core determinant of health vulnerability at a population level is the social status of a group, as any material and psychosocial stresses imposed by social inequalities impact upon the individual across their whole life trajectory. For example, let us just consider the gypsy/travelling community (Box 2.9) who are one of the most socially excluded marginalised groups (Van Cleemput *et al.* 2007, McCaffery 2009).

A child born within this community may experience difficulties with regards to travelling, in that current UK law has criminalised a nomadic lifestyle restricting the extent to which gypsies and travellers are able to roam. Both Van Cleemput (2007) and Brown and Scullion (2009) note the difficulties experienced by gypsy/travellers in obtaining planning permission for private caravan sites, even though there is insufficient provision of both private and rented caravan sites. A clear example of this was Dale Farm, a former scrap yard site that was purchased by Irish travellers who then struggled to obtain planning permission to reside there. Before we can really understand the difficulties that surrounded Dale Farm, we need to look at the history surrounding gypsy/traveller sites. In 1968, the Caravan Sites Act placed a duty on councils to provide sites for gypsies and travellers; however, this act also created problems in that each city council had to provide sites which could accommodate a maximum of 15 families (Okely 2011). However, there were often many more gypsies and travellers requiring accommodation, the councils from the Act gained power to remove any more gypsies and travellers beyond their boundaries to semi-rural communities (Okely 2011). The country councils in return argued that they did not have responsibility for these families as they were not local, resulting in many gypsies and travellers having nowhere to settle. This was resolved in the 1994 Criminal Justice and Public Order Act which removed the responsibility of councils to provide sites and identified that gypsies and travellers should purchase their own land on which to live. Many gypsies and travellers therefore purchased land and applied for planning permission; however, 95% of planning permission is turned down for gypsy/traveller applications (Okely 2011). What was interesting was little of this history was publicised during the media coverage on Dale farm. During the process of Dale Farm evictions, I was undertaking data collection for my PhD, and many gypsies and travellers I was speaking to were very affected by Dale Farm – even though they did not live there. To them, it was another example of how the settled (non-gypsy) community do not accept them, and this further perpetuated a view that they do not belong within society, increasing their feelings of not being accepted.

Karner (2004) and Turner (2002) identify that gypsies/travellers often experience discrimination, both within schools as well as wider society. The bullying that some gypsy/traveller children experience in school can lead to those children not attending school, and this coupled with a transient lifestyle can make accessing education problematic, which has long-term implications both for employment and also for literacy levels. There is also a reduction in traditional working practices, as historically many gypsies and travellers would work on the land harvesting crops which is now largely undertaken by machinery resulting in an increased financial vulnerability of some members of the community.

Accessing healthcare is also difficult for some gypsies and travellers. A study by Peters *et al.* (2009) identified that only 69% were permanently registered with a GP, whilst research by Hodgins *et al.* (2006) identified that the community were dissatisfied with health services due to inadequate information and inequitable and poorly delivered services. It must be remembered that people of diverse cultures have different beliefs about the cause, diagnosis, and healthcare treatment, and these discrepancies in the belief system between the patient and nurse can lead to treatment failure and frustration equally on both parties (Martino Maze 2004). For example, within the gypsy/travelling community there is a large fatalistic belief in health which can make health promotion very difficult. Dion (2007) asserts that practitioners need to understand these deeply embedded beliefs and attitudes and need to address them in a way that makes a real difference to their health outcomes. If we consider the implications of all of these factors across the life trajectory, then the picture is not a positive one; there is evidence that the gypsy/travelling community experience poorer physical health than that of the general population (Goward *et al.* 2006). A study by Parry *et al.* (2007) identified that gypsies and travellers reported poorer health status over the preceding year than their age- and sex-matched counterparts and were significantly more likely to have a long-term illness, health problem, or disability. There is also evidence that the gypsy/travelling community experience poorer mental health than the general population (Goward *et al.* 2006, Parry *et al.* 2007).

Gypsies and travellers can experience feeling vulnerable due to these structural inequalities highlighted earlier as well as a tendency to pathologise them which reaffirms them as other, which results in increasing their vulnerability (Cemlyn 2000). In addition, gypsies and travellers experience discrimination and are marginalised within society (Karner 2004), resulting in them being one of the most socially excluded groups despite their legal protection as a result of their ethnic minority status (Van Cleemput *et al.* 2007). They are often vilified by the media, who present a certain picture of gypsies as individuals involved in criminal/illegal activity, leave mess, and devastation. This further perpetuates a 'them and us' mentality when referring to gypsies excluding them from society – this will be further explored in Chapter 8.

> **Box 2.10**   Continuum of vulnerability (Archer Copp 1986)
>
> - *Potentially vulnerable* – Including individuals of high risk (genetic disposition to specific diseases, low-birth-weight infant, teenage mother, chronic illness, and many more. It also includes individuals who may live in high-crime neighbourhoods and/or are homeless
> - *Circumstantially vulnerable* – Including individuals during time of war, famine, poverty, trauma, and expatriation
> - *Temporarily vulnerable* – Individuals experiencing trauma, incarceration, depression, divorce or other family disruption; kidnapped victims; welfare; hostages; sexual assault; and abuse
> - *Episodically vulnerable* – Noting recurrent diseases such as AIDS and sickle cell anaemia
> - *Permanently vulnerable* – Individuals with birth injuries, hemiplegics, and war wounds
> - *Inevitably vulnerable* – Including old age

Vulnerability as a shifting experience

Archer Copp (1986) provided another perspective of vulnerability (Box 2.10), arguing that rather than a dichotomous experience, vulnerability needs to be expressed as a continuum, upon which individuals will move depending upon their experience at that time. Rather than just a focus on the individual per se, this approach recognises that some individuals may be more susceptible to experiencing vulnerability due to a balance of both features inherent to the individual as well as some of the wider forces of society. This approach adds a different dimension to the study of vulnerability as it recognises the complex multifractional nature, using the analogy of an onion; vulnerability from this perspective can be seen as having multiple layers.

This approach reflects the shifting nature of vulnerability as well as identifying the potential of acquired vulnerability due to wider circumstances, in that clients can be temporarily vulnerable. This perspective I think is useful to us as practitioners, as it enables us to explore how an individual could be vulnerable due to a variety of factors, as well as demonstrating the complexity of vulnerability. However, I also feel that as practitioners we need to be cautious making assumptions regarding the vulnerability of others, remembering the individual experience of vulnerability. So whilst one individual living with AIDS, for example, may feel vulnerable another might not, recognising the importance of the emic perspective as well as the etic.

Vulnerability as an existential experience

A contrasting perspective identifies that all human beings are vulnerable (Erlen 2006), as part of their humanity, for human beings are never totally free from the risk of harm (Sellman 2005). Anthropological features identify that as a species human beings are poorly equipped physiologically and sociologically, which has enabled us, as a species, to grow and develop whilst also highlighting our vulnerability (Kottow 2004). Thus, vulnerability is a 'condition humana' which affects us all (Kottow 2003: 461). Within this perspective, it does recognise that some groups may be more than ordinarily vulnerable due to outside factors, whilst respecting the individualistic nature of vulnerability.

This approach has advantages as it avoids assuming that vulnerability is an inevitable consequence of gender, age, and socio-economic status. Vulnerability therefore exists as a lived experience of the individual's perception of self and their resources to withstand such challenges, identifying that vulnerability is based on the experience of exposure to harm through challenges to one's integrity (Spiers 2000).

Spiers' (2000) emic perspective (Table 2.1) fits with this existential perspective of vulnerability as vulnerability is defined by the individual perceptions of oneself and of the resources to withstand challenges; therefore, only the individual can define their vulnerability. Few nursing scholars have attempted to understand vulnerability as an experiential quality of life (Spiers 2000), even though qualitative research could illuminate the experience of vulnerability from the individual perspective (Rogers 1997).

Mutual vulnerability

> **Box 2.11**   Time for reflection
>
> Think about a time when caring for a patient induced a feeling of vulnerability within you. Try to identify what contributed to your feelings of vulnerability, and what you did (if anything) to reduce those feelings of vulnerability.

Building upon the perspective of vulnerability as a human experience is the notion of mutual vulnerability in that both staff and patients can simultaneously experience feeling vulnerable due to the nature of the caring role (Box 2.11).

There may be multiple reasons why practitioners may experience feeling vulnerable (Heaslip and Board 2012) and these may be due to:

- The close relationship that practitioners have with patients which includes an emotional investment in caring about them.
- Working with patients can actually remind us of our own morbidity and mortality, especially when we may look after people who are the same age as ourselves.
- The unpredictable nature of the patient and/or disease. For example, working in areas such as the emergency department, in mental health, acute medical wards, etc.
- We may feel vulnerable due to our own lack of understanding and/or knowledge regarding a situation or experience.
- The dynamics of the team in which you work which may have made you feel vulnerable.
- The environment in which you work (lone worker, emergency department, etc.).

Edward and Hercelinskyj (2007) recognise that nurses often witness traumatic or life changing situations which can be difficult to make sense of. From my own professional practice, whilst working as a staff nurse in an emergency department, I remember participating in the resuscitation of an 8-month-old baby who subsequently died. The resuscitation was at the start of a 12 hour shift and I distinctly remember being shell shocked initially, trying to acknowledge my feelings whilst also recognising my professional responsibilities in that at any second I could be called back to the resuscitation area for another person who required care. I remember my colleagues asking me if I was okay and not wishing at that time to discuss it with them, instead asking them not to ask me how I was. Later that evening, I went home and sobbed about the death of that child, not being able to make sense that despite our best efforts we were unable to save her.

Caring carries an emotional burden for the nurse (Edward and Hercelinskyj 2007); a study by Duffy *et al.* (2009) in a dementia care setting identified that 68.6% of the staff experienced moderate levels of burnout and were emotionally exhausted by their work. This emotional labour of nursing (Smith 1992, Gray 2009) can increase our own sense of vulnerability as we are opening ourselves up to 'harm' both physically and psychologically. However, this emotional commitment to people is vital in order to establish a true therapeutic relationship with patients (Heaslip and Board 2012). Through working with undergraduate students, I know that there is still a sense within nursing that nurses have to be seen to be distancing themselves from the patient, and need to 'toughen up' or 'harden up'. However, I think we have to question whether this should be true or whether exposing ourselves to feeling vulnerable by caring about people is actually a negative experience but a facet of providing good quality care. Indeed we have to question whether denying our own emotional engagement with patients through caring in order to reduce our own experience of feeling vulnerable may actually unintentionally contribute to theirs. There have recently been numerous reports such as Dignity in Practice (Tadd *et al.* 2011) and the Francis Report (2010) questioning whether caring in the National Health Service has been lost and I wonder if this mutual vulnerability may have contributed to nurses 'switching off their emotions'.

Positive dimensions of vulnerability

The views presented thus far regarding vulnerability identify it as a negative experience; however, Purdy (2004) and Batchelor (2006) both argue that vulnerability can have positive dimensions including the opening up of new possibilities. A study by Huta and Hawley (2010) identified that vulnerability is not merely the opposite of strength; indeed, in many cases strengths and vulnerabilities together had a unique relationship with well-being, making incremental contributions to life satisfaction, positive affect, self-esteem, and meaning. A study by Leroux *et al.* (2007) identified that in order for positive dimensions of vulnerability to occur it required two fundamental aspects of the relationship: firstly, that the practitioner had some investment, not only in the therapeutic agenda but also in caring about the client as an individual, and secondly, the feeling that each share some measure of vulnerability within the relationship.

Models of vulnerability

There are a variety of models of vulnerability that exist in order to assist practitioners to be able to assess the degree of a person's vulnerability. One such model is that by Proot *et al.* (2003) which was developed from a study exploring the needs and experiences of family members caring for a terminally ill person at home in the Netherlands. The findings identified that caregivers expressed a continuous balancing between the care burden and their capacity to cope which they expressed as balancing on a tight rope, thus reflecting vulnerability as a shifting perspective. They identified factors which reduced their experiences of feeling vulnerable including feeling hope for the future and a sense of being in control. In light of this, it is really important for us as practitioners to empower patients and carers when working with them, enabling them to have a sense of control over their environment and their care whenever possible. Conversely, loneliness and lack of support increased their feelings of vulnerability and as such it is really important that we recognise that social support acts as a buffer against vulnerability and therefore facilitates opportunities for patients and their families to access support.

Another model which can be used to understand vulnerability was Rogers (1997) which identified vulnerability is a balance between the interactions of two variables, those of personal resources and environmental supports which combined lead to vulnerability (Figure 2.2). Rogers identified that a subjective assessment could be made of an individual's personal and environmental resources which could help to assess their potential vulnerability.

Within this model, an individual level of vulnerability could be ascertained by examining the balance between a person's level of personal resources on one side and their environmental supports on the other side. In order to understand how we can use this model to identify an individual's potential levels of vulnerability, let us consider the case study of James (Box 2.12).

Personal components

- Age
- Gender
- Ethnicity/race
- Genetic predisposition
- Lifestyle
- Income
- Past health history
- Learned abilities
  e.g. coping skills
- Education
- Self-concept
- Attitudes/motivation

Environmental components

- Family/friends
  e.g. support harmony discord
- Community
  e.g. unemployment
- Society
  e.g. attitudes to health, disability, age,
- Immediate environment
  (e.g. pollution, noise, light)

Dynamic continuum – balance

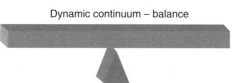

Figure 2.2   Adapted from Rogers (1997).

Box 2.12   Case study of James

James is a 47 year old man admitted to the local hospital with hematemesis (vomiting blood). James is well known within the department as he had had several previous admissions before of a similar nature. James lives in a bedsit and admits that he does not have many friends locally, and the friends that he does have also drink heavily. James can sometimes be verbally abusive to staff, especially when he is withdrawing from alcohol.

Examining the personal resources pertinent to James, it can be identified that

- *Age* – James is 47 and is able to communicate his needs to the care staff.
- *Gender* – Male. This potentially could be an issue as predominately the majority of nurses on the ward are female and James could potentially feel embarrassed having to rely on the nurses to provide personal care for him. Conversely, the fact that James is male and sometimes verbally aggressive could also increase the nurses' feelings of vulnerability as they may be frightened of him, resulting in them restricting their access to James (in an attempt to reduce their own vulnerability) whilst inadvertently increasing James' feeling of isolation and lack of control.
- *Ethnicity/Race* – James is white British and as he is admitted to a hospital in the UK; the staff speak the same language as James which could reduce his feelings of vulnerability as he can easily communicate his needs to them.
- *Lifestyle* – James chooses to drink to excess even though it is having a negative impact upon his health. James diet is poor; he admits he often misses meals as he cannot always afford to buy food.
- *Income* – Due to his drinking James has very little money; therefore, he does not really go out and at times struggles to pay his bills.
- *Past Health History* – James has had previous episodes of vomiting blood which have resulted in admission to hospital. So whilst James is aware of what may happen in terms of treatment, he knows that the staff are going to be cross with him as he has been told on numerous occasions that alcohol is 'his own worst enemy'.
- *Learned abilities* – James has had many failed attempts in the past to stop drinking, and he believes he cannot stop drinking.
- *Self-concept* – James defines himself as an alcoholic and does not see that he will ever stop drinking. Indeed, he will often say to the staff that his drinking will kill him.
- *Attitudes/Motivation* – James at times will get very upset and tearful about his life, especially as his drinking has affected his relationships with his ex-partner and children. He admits that drinking is his only comfort and as such his motivation to stop drinking is very low.

From examining these personal resources, whilst it has to be identified that James has some such as his age and ethnicity which facilitates communication with the staff, they are minimal in comparison to all of the other personal resources. Within Rogers (1997) diagram of vulnerability (Figure 2.3), it can be seen that his personal resources have been identified towards the few end of the few to many continuum (line a). From this point, a line is then drawn to the opposite apex of the triangle (point b).

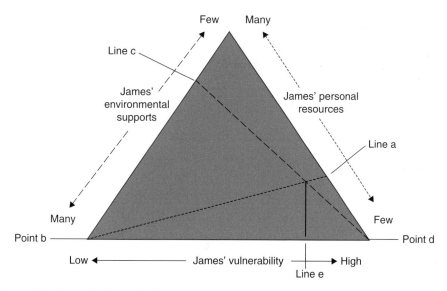

Figure 2.3   James' vulnerability (adapted from Rogers 1997).

Examining James' environmental supports

- *Family/friends* – James does not have any visitors during his admission nor did he on previous admissions. He currently does not have a relationship with his children, due to his drinking. The only friendships that James does have are his drinking buddies.
- *Community* – James is largely isolated within his community; he does not really go out much, apart from shopping.
- *Society* – In society, there is a negative perception about people dependent on alcohol. James believes that the staff caring for him (doctors, nurses, therapists, etc.) have little time for him; he knows he makes them cross because he does not stop drinking even though they tell him he must.
- *Immediate environment* – James is in hospital and as he feels unwell he is dependent upon the staff assisting him with his activities of daily living. James has little control over his environment; he is currently in a room with four other patients and they are aware of his drinking, as they overhear the conversation James has with the nursing and medical staff.

Within Rogers (1997) diagram of vulnerability (Figure 2.3), it can be seen that his environmental supports have also been located towards the few end of the few to many continuum (line c); this is due to a lack of family and friends, the perceptions that society has upon him, as well as his immediate environment. Again we would draw a line from this point to the opposite apex of the triangle (point d). Where these two lines intersect is the degree of vulnerability that the client has experienced; for James, we can see his level of vulnerability is high (line e).

A critique of this model, however, is that it does not offer any units of measurement to identify the level which the personal resources and environmental supports impact upon his experience of feeling vulnerable. Therefore, it only provides a subjective interpretation of James' vulnerability. I would argue that this model is best used as an aide memoire to remind practitioners of the different elements that together contribute to someone's subjective feelings of vulnerability so that they can explore each of these factors with the client (reflective on the emic approach see Table 2.1). However, I also acknowledge that this model can be used, utilising the practitioner's external judgement of James' personal resources and environmental supports (reflective of an etic approach, Table 2.1). Ultimately, the models enable us as practitioners to have a better understanding of some of the factors that contribute to an individual's experience of feeling vulnerable.

Conclusion

At the start of the chapter, we explored some definitions of vulnerability, examining these in light of our own personal experiences of feeling vulnerable. Identifying that vulnerability is a holistic concept that can affect us physically, emotionally, and socially. We then continued to explore the links between vulnerability, health, and healthcare, stressing that feeling vulnerable has health implications to individuals both physically and psychologically and is potentially damaging to one's health.

In light of the association between vulnerability, health, and healthcare, the importance of practitioners being aware of patients' potential feelings of being vulnerable was highlighted, and as such it can be argued that understanding vulnerability is central to good healthcare practice.

Professional definitions of vulnerability were then explored, enabling us to develop a better understanding of both the external perspective of vulnerability (etic) as well as the subjective lived experience (emic). This understanding of vulnerability was then explored from differing theoretical perspectives including:

- Mechanism to identify populations at risk of ill health
- Mechanism to identify social groups in need of protection
- Consequence of social interaction
- Existential experience
- Shifting experience
- Mutual Vulnerability
- Vehicle for personal growth

The links to professional practice were illuminated through case studies and reflective activities.

Links to other chapters

- Chapter 3 will explore how power can create an experience of vulnerability for patients, service users, and others.
- Chapter 4 explores further lived examples of vulnerability to examine the underlying processes of oppression which have subtly but powerfully contributed to the experience.

- Chapter 5 develops our understanding of how we make judgements about people as well as further examining how the label of 'Vulnerable' can impact on service users' lived experience.

References

Appleton, J. (1994) The concept of vulnerability in relation to child protection: Health visitors' perceptions. *Journal of Advanced Nursing*, 20, 1132–1140.

Archer Copp, L. (1986) The nurse as advocate for vulnerable persons. *Journal of Advanced Nursing*, 11, 255–263.

Batchelor, D. (2006) Vulnerable voices: An examination of the concept of vulnerability in relation to student voice. *Educational Philosophy and Theory*, 38 (6), 787–800.

Brown, P. and Scullion, L. (2009) 'Doing research' with gypsy-travellers in England: Reflections on experience and practice. *Community Development Journal*, 17 March, 1–17. (45, 2, 169-185)

Cemlyn, S. (2000) Assimilation, control, mediation or advocacy? Social work dilemmas in providing anti-oppressive services for traveller children and families. *Child and Family Social Work*, 5, 327–341.

Clark, C. (2007) Understanding vulnerability: From categories to experiences of young Congolese people in Uganda. *Children & Society*, 21, 284–296.

Department of Health (DoH) (2000a) *National Service Framework for Older People*. Stationary Office. London.

DoH (2000b) *No Secrets*. HMSO, London.

DoH (2008) *Confidence in Caring*. DoH, London.

DoH (2009) *Safeguarding Adults: A Consultation on the Review of the 'No Secrets' Guidance*. DoH, London.

Dion, X. (2007) What is means to 'be healthy' for Gypsy Traveller women; seeking causative factors of health and ill-health. MSc Dissertation. Bournemouth University, Bournemouth.

Duffy, B., Oyebode, J. and Allen, J. (2009) Burnout among care staff for older adults with dementia. *Dementia*, 8, 515–540.

Edward, K. and Hercelinskyj, G. (2007) Burnout in the caring nurse: Learning resilient behaviours. *British Journal of Nursing*, 16 (4), 240–242.

Erlen, J. (2006) Who speaks for the vulnerable? *Orthopaedic Nursing*, 25 (2), 133–136.

Flaskerud, J. and Winslow, B. (1998) Conceptualizing vulnerable populations: Health-related research. *Nursing Research*, 47, 69–77.

Francis, R. (2010) *Independent Inquiry into Care Provided by Mid Staffordshire NHS Foundation Trust January 2005–March 2009*. Stationary Office, London.

Furumoto-Dawson, A., Gehlert, S., Sohmer, D., Olopade, O. and Sacks, T. (2007) Early-life conditions and mechanisms of population health vulnerabilities. *Health Affairs*, 29 (5), 1238–1248.

Goward, P., Repper, J., Appleton, L. and Hagan, T. (2006) Crossing boundaries. Identifying and meeting the mental health needs of gypsies and travellers. *Journal of Mental Health*, 15 (3), 315–327.

Gray, B. (2009) The emotional labour of nursing – Defining and managing emotions in nursing work. *Nurse Education Today*, 29, 168–175.

Heaslip, V. and Board, M. (2012) Does nurses' vulnerability affect their ability to care? *British Journal of Nursing*, 21 (15), 912–916.

Hewitt-Taylor, J. and Heaslip, V. (2012) Protecting children or creating vulnerability? *Community Practitioner*, 85 (12), 31–33.

Hodgins, M., Millar, M. and Barry, M. (2006) '… it's all the same no matter how much fruit or vegetables or fresh air we get': Traveller women's perceptions of illness causation and health inequalities. *Social Science and Medicine*, 62, 1978–1990.

Huta, V. and Hawley, L. (2010) Psychological strengths and cognitive vulnerabilities: Are they two ends of the same continuum or do they have independent relationships with well-being and ill-being? *Journal of Happiness Studies*, 11, 71–93.

Karner, C. (2004) Theorising power and resistance among travellers. *Social Semiotics*, 14 (3), 249–271.

Kottow, M. (2003) The vulnerable and the susceptible. *Bioethics*, 17 (5–6), 460–471.

Kottow, M. (2004) Vulnerability: What kind of principle is it? *Medicine, Health Care and Philosophy*, 7, 281–287.

Leroux, P., Sperlinger, D. and Worrell, M. (2007) Experiencing vulnerability in psychotherapy. *Existential Analysis*, 18 (2), 315–328.

Little, M., Paul, K., Jordens, C. and Sayers, E.J. (2000) Vulnerability in the narratives of patients and their carers: Studies of colorectal cancer. *Health*, 4 (4), 495–510.

Martino Maze, C. (2004) Registered Nurses' personal rights vs. professional responsibility in caring for members of undeserved and disenfranchised populations. *Journal of Clinical Nursing*, 14, 546–554.

McCaffery, M. (1968) *Nursing Practice Theories Related to Cognition, Bodily Pain, and Man-Environment Interactions*. University of California at LA Students Store, California.

McCaffery, J. (2009). Gypsies and travellers: Literacy, discourse and communicative practices. *Compare*, 39 (5), 643–657.

National Institute for Clinical Excellence (NICE) (2004) *Falls; the Assessment and Prevention of Falls in Older People*. NICE, London.

Nursing and Midwifery Council (NMC) (2002) *Practitioner – Client Relationships and the Prevention of Abuse*. Nursing and Midwifery Council, London.

Okely, J. (2011) The Dale Farm eviction. *Anthropology Today*, 27 (6), 24–27.

Office of Public Sector Information (2007). *Safeguarding Vulnerable Groups Act*. Available from http://www.opsi.gov.uk/acts/acts2006/en/06en47-c.htm [accessed on 29 March 2012].

Parliamentary and Health Service Ombudsman (2011) *Care and Compassion? Parliamentary and Health Service Ombudsman*. Stationery Office, London.

Parry, G., Van Cleemput, P., Paters, J., Walters, S., Thomas, K. and Cooper, C. (2007) Health status of gypsies and travellers in England. *Journal of Epidemiology and Community Health*, 61, 198–204.

Pearsall, J. (2002) *Concise Oxford English Dictionary*. 10th ed., Oxford University Press, Oxford.

Penhale, B. and Parker, J. (2008) *Working with Vulnerable Adults*. Routledge, Abingdon.

Peternalj-Taylor, C. (2005) Conceptualizing nursing research with offenders: Another look at vulnerability. *International Journal of Law and Psychiatry*, 28, 348–359.

Peters, J., Parry, G., Van Cleemput, P., Moore, J., Cooper, C. and Walters, S. (2009) Health and use of health services: A comparison between gypsies and travellers and other ethnic groups. *Ethnicity & Health*, 14 (4), 359–377.

Pitkin Derose, K., Escarce, J. and Lurie, N. (2007) Immigrants and health care: Sources of vulnerability. *Health Affairs*, 26 (5), 1258–1268.

Proot, I., Abu-Saad, H., Crebolder, H., Goldsteen, M., Luker, K. and Widdershoven, G. (2003) Vulnerability of family caregivers in terminal palliative care at home; balancing between burden and capacity. *Scandinavian Journal of Caring Science*, 17, 113–121.

Purdy, I. (2004) Vulnerable: A concept analysis. *Nursing Forum*, 39 (4), 25–33.

Redwood, S. and Heaslip, V. (2010) Equality and diversity in practice development. In: *Implementing Excellence in your Healthcare Organization* (McSherry, R. and Warr, J. eds), pp. 170–185. Open University Press, Berkshire.

Rogers, A. (1997) Vulnerability, health and healthcare. *Journal of Advanced Nursing*, 26, 65–72.

Rydeman, I. and Törnkvist, L. (2006) The patients' vulnerability, dependence and exposed situation in the discharge process: Experiences of district nurses, geriatric nurses and social workers. *Journal of Clinical Nursing*, 15, 1299–1307.

Sellman, D. (2005) Towards an undertsading of nursing as a response to human vulnerability. *Nursing Philosophy*, 6, 2–10.

Shepard, M. and Mahon, M. (2002) Vulnerable families: Research findings and methodological challenges. *Journal of Family Nursing*, 8 (4), 309–314.

Smith, P. (1992) *The Emotional Labour of Nursing*. Macmillan, London.

Spiers, J. (2000) New perspectives on vulnerability using emic and etic approaches. *Journal of Advanced Nursing*, 31 (3), 715–721.

Sykes, J. (1982) *The Concise Oxford Dictionary*. The Clarendon Press, Oxford.

Tadd, W., Hillman, A., Calnan, S., Calnan, M., Bayer, A. and Read, S. (2011) Dignity in practice: An exploration of the care of older adults in acute NHS Trusts. NIHR Service Delivery and Organisation Programme.

Turner, R. (2002) Gypsies and British parliamentary language; An analysis. *Romani Studies, 5*, 12 (1), 1–34.

Van Cleemput, P. (2007) Health impact of gypsy sites policy in the UK. *Social Policy and Society*, 7 (1), 103–117.

Van Cleemput, P., Parry, G., Thomas, K., Peters, K. and Cooper, C. (2007) Health related beliefs and experiences of gypsies and travellers: A qualitative study. *Journal of Epidemiology and Community Health*, 61, 205–219.

Vasas, E. (2005) Examining the margins: A concept analysis of marginalisation. *Advances in Nursing Science*, 28 (3), 194–202.

Chapter 3

Power, discrimination, and oppression

Julie Ryden and Chris Willetts

Introduction

This chapter will explore the relationship between vulnerability and two other terms often used in relation to vulnerability: discrimination and oppression. The inter-connectedness of these three concepts is explored in the early part of this chapter. We have looked closely at definitions of each term to illustrate the relationship between them and to help in understanding the nature and experience of vulnerability in healthcare situations. After this we will look at the concept of power as it is a key aspect of these three terms. The chapter explores different theories and perspectives on power, considering what it is, how it can affect people, and, most importantly, in relation to vulnerability, who has power and who does not have power.

Defining oppression and discrimination

Within the literature there is a problem in differentiating between the terms 'oppression' and 'discrimination'. The two terms are used in different ways and authors offer different interpretations, so it can be hard to distinguish between them. Whilst the debate about the differences in meaning is important, it should not be allowed to get in the way of the hard reality of vulnerability that is faced by individuals every day within healthcare. The two terms will be distinguished here, for the sake of clarity; however, the reader should be aware that different interpretations exist elsewhere. If possible, the reader should look beyond the semantic differences and focus more on the underlying issues which affect the vulnerability of people.

Thompson (2011: 90) identifies discrimination as:

> … the process (or set of processes) by which people are allocated to particular social categories with an unequal distribution of rights, resources, opportunities and power. It is a process through which certain groups and individuals are disadvantaged and oppressed.

This is supported by other authors who suggest discrimination as 'differential treatment' (Banton 1994, cited in Northway 1997: 739) or 'unfair and unjust treatment' (Northway 1997: 739). So discrimination is about the way people are treated or, more particularly,

Understanding Vulnerability: A Nursing and Healthcare Approach, First Edition. Edited by Vanessa Heaslip and Julie Ryden.

the way 'difference' is treated, and for Thompson, discrimination is the fundamental process which leads to and causes oppression.

Dominelli views discrimination as a 'much smaller part of oppression' Dominelli (2008a: 119). So whilst Thompson suggests that discrimination is a separate entity which *leads to* and *causes* oppression, Dominelli sees it as *a part* of the bigger picture of oppression; discrimination is a sub-element of the overall concept of oppression. For Dominelli (2008a), the concept of discrimination fails to consider the 'complex web of attitudes and behaviours' embedded in oppression (119) and ignores the humiliation and attack on a person's sense of self that comes with oppression. This text will follow Dominelli's perspective that whilst the term 'discrimination' is a distinct concept, referring to unequal and differential treatment, it is a part of the wider concept of oppression, which will now be examined further. Let us commence by looking at discrimination and oppression within the context of healthcare, please take some time to complete the activity in Box 3.1.

Thompson offers a comprehensive definition of oppression:

> Inhuman or degrading treatment of individuals or groups; hardship and injustice brought about by the dominance of one group over another; the negative and demeaning exercise of power. It often involves disregarding the rights of an individual or group and is thus a denial of citizenship. (Thompson 2006: 40)

Whilst comprehensive, this might at first sight appear too much to take in and even difficult to apply to healthcare situations. Let us just explore each element of this definition with some real life scenarios in the health service (see Box 3.2, Box 3.3, and Box 3.4).

It should be clear from the aforementioned examples that each element of Thompson's definition of oppression can be linked to vulnerability and that oppression can 'harm' or 'wound' patients/clients; it presents a threat and a danger to clients and thus fits with the definitions of vulnerability explored in Chapter 2.

Now take some time to reconsider the service users/patients you identified in Box 3.1 and explore them in light of Thompson's categories of oppression, go to Box 3.5 to reflect further on the people you have cared for.

Oppression is a word which can often be associated with dictatorships or oppressive regimes in other countries (Northway 1997). However, we would suggest that oppression

---

Box 3.1 Time for reflection

Oppression is the devaluing of people – who they are and What they have to offer to others.

(Dominelli 2008a: 116)

- Have you ever seen any patients/service users who are devalued?
- Does the healthcare team take the time to value each patient/client for whom they are?
- Does the healthcare team value each patient/client for what they have to offer to others?
- Are patients/service users always seen as 'people' who are worthy in their own right?

After answering these questions, are there any patients/service users that you have cared for, who might be seen as oppressed according to Dominelli's definition? Make a list of the patients/ service users you are thinking of.

Box 3.2 Inhuman or degrading treatment of individuals or groups

- In March 2005, seven care home workers were jailed for bullying, kicking, slapping, hair pulling, and humiliating mentally and physically disabled service users – none had the capacity to speak or complain (BBC 2005a).
- Soraya was bedbound as a result of a stroke. She was a large woman with a high body mass index. The ward she was on did not have a suitable hoist and the staff had not found the time to order one yet. Soraya was told that she should 'wet the bed' when she needed to urinate as the staff were unable to lift her onto a commode or a bedpan.
- The Francis Report on the Independent Inquiry into the Mid-Staffordshire NHS Trust (2010) identified the following occurrences amongst many others:
  - incontinent patients left in degrading conditions;
  - patients left inadequately dressed in full view of passers-by;
  - patients moved and handled in unsympathetic and unskilled ways, causing pain and distress;
  - failures to refer to patients by name or by their preferred name;
  - rudeness or hostility.

Box 3.3 Hardship and injustice brought about by the dominance of one group over another

- Cicely was in hospital for rehabilitation following a stroke. During the handover of staff, the nurse in charge said that Cicely was a 'typical Jewess' who was very lazy and did not make any effort. Later Cicely wanted to go to the toilet, and usual practice was to place her wheelchair about 5 metres away from the toilet, so that she could maintain and improve her walking ability. On this particular day (as a result of the handover report), the healthcare assistants placed Cicely's wheelchair over 10 metres away. Cicely was then told she must walk the extra distance. Cicely was unable to even attempt this and felt upset and humiliated at her inability.
- Gareth is a recovering substance user who was admitted to a general hospital for treatment of a medical condition. Gareth also smokes over 20 cigarettes a day. When he was assessed, the doctor announced that he would be unable to smoke within the hospital due to the smoking ban and was not able to leave the ward because of his condition. She did not offer Gareth any substitute medication. Gareth became very anxious in the following hours, and staff warned each other to 'be wary' of him. One of the student nurses later started chatting to him in the bay and discovered that he was struggling without cigarettes. The student nurse asked the staff nurse if he could be prescribed Nicorette patches and was told that they were far too busy at that time and it would need to wait. The student nurse persisted and later managed to ask the doctor to prescribe the patches. This was now some 12 hours after Gareth's last cigarette – it had been a distressing and difficult period of time for Gareth.
- Emma died on 25 July 2004. She had been diagnosed with cancer and her mother was told she had a 50% chance of survival with active treatment. However, doctors decided that Emma would not cooperate with treatment because of her learning disability. She was not treated and died aged 26 (Mencap 2007).

---

can be seen to be operating within healthcare settings and is a key cause of vulnerability. Indeed, Harvey (1999) introduces the concept of 'civilised oppression' to capture the more subtle, less obvious forms of oppression. This involves many apparently small actions, which exclude, denigrate, and subordinate the individual:

Box 3.4 The negative and demeaning exercise of power

- Nurse Caroline Lowe refused to bring a jug of water to an ill and distressed patient. Then when he rang his wife to tell her what had happened, she said 'what lies are you telling now' or words to that effect, and later threatened to remove his mobile phone (Fagge 2010). The nurse was later struck off the register of Nurses and Midwives.
- In June 2011, a BBC Panorama programme revealed how residents at a Castlebeck assessment unit for adults with profound learning disabilities were slapped and kicked, pinned to the floor, and drenched with cold water (Brindle 2011). One client was forced into the shower fully clothed and then placed outside until she shivered from the cold (Curtis and Mulholland 2011).
- An analysis of calls to the Elder Abuse Response helpline found that 34% of abusers of older people are paid care workers (Action on Elder Abuse 2004).

Box 3.5 Time for reflection

Consider the service users/patients you identified in Box 3.1.
Now see if any of their experiences fall within Thompson's categories of oppression:

- *Inhuman or degrading treatment of individuals or groups*
- *Hardship and injustice brought about by the dominance of one group over another*
- *The negative and demeaning exercise of power*

Are there any other service users/patients that you would now add to this list?
Keep this list available for when you read Chapter 4 – which will further explore the experiences of these service users.

---

apparently trivial acts that often pass under the social radar screen [and] can wreck the lives of those systematically at the receiving end (Harvey 2010: 15).

These acts are less brutal and less conspicuous but are no less damaging to someone's emotional, social, and physical well-being. Chapter 4 identifies the processes of oppression and includes many actions which may be deemed 'small' and yet powerful in their ability to undermine, devalue, exclude, or oppress. These acts may often be 'well intentioned' (Young 1990) or unintentionally oppressive; oppression is not always committed by evil abusers. All of us are capable of oppressing others, without meaning to and without realising the extent of the damage or harm we may be causing. Therefore, reflection is a key skill for any practitioner who wishes to reduce vulnerability, with a commitment to be honest and see the full impact of our 'small' actions, even when this may trouble us or offend our sense of our own innate goodness.

The PCS model of oppression

Thompson (2011) has produced a useful model to capture or demonstrate the wide and complex nature of oppression. The model acts as a framework for analysing oppression, and since we assert that oppression leads to, or causes, vulnerability, it may also be useful

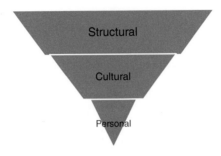

Figure 3.1   Adaptation of PCS model of oppression (data based on Thompson 2011).

in analysing vulnerability. Put simply, the model represents oppression as occurring at three different levels or layers, the *personal* level (P), the *cultural* level (C), and the *structural* level (S) – see Figure 3.1. This is very similar to Dominelli's account of three dimensions of oppression – personal, cultural, and institutional (2008a, 2008b), although Dominelli distinguishes her own model as different from Thompson's, in seeing both the cultural and institutional dimensions as structural issues. However, use will be made of her account within the description of Thompson's model.

P – personal level of oppression

This level refers to the individual level of oppression and includes the thoughts, beliefs, feelings, attitudes, and actions of individuals towards another. This level can be seen in the face-to-face personal experiences of oppressed individuals in everyday life and professional settings. It can include the expression of prejudices towards individuals or professional practice that is influenced by a personal prejudice. For instance, a nurse previously told one of us that whenever she went in to care for a man with HIV/AIDS, she made sure a window was open, so that she could breathe in 'fresh uncontaminated air'. This is a personal prejudice, based upon a personal belief, which would have affected the experience of the man she cared for. How must he have felt whenever she went to the window for fresh air? How must her prejudice have affected how close she got to him, and how did this feel for him?

However, this example illustrates well why Thompson places the *personal* level within the other circles. This is because this nurse could not have chosen this prejudice and this belief on her own without the influence of the media at the time. When the human immunodeficiency virus and acquired immunodeficiency syndrome (HIV/AIDS) first appeared, there was a level of panic and misinformation spread by the media (BBC 2005b). The prevailing culture at the time was influenced by this panic, and many myths and prejudices about HIV/AIDS began at this time. So whilst the aforementioned nurse chose to act in a prejudicial and frighteningly oppressive manner with the patient/client at an individual level, her behaviour could be said to have been influenced by wider cultural factors. Hence, Thompson suggests that the *personal* level is 'embedded' within the *cultural* level (2011: 26), so that the actions, beliefs, attitudes, and feelings of individuals are strongly affected by the cultural context in which the individual exists and works.

Chapter 4 includes further examples of discriminatory processes which may be experienced at the personal level, like dehumanisation, infantilisation, and stigmatisation.

C – cultural level of oppression

The *cultural* level refers to a broad level of influence that affects each of us, mostly in ways that we are entirely unaware of. Culture has been referred to as:

> … an inherited lens, through which the individual perceives and understands the world … and learns how to live within it. Growing up within any society is a form of enculturation, whereby the individual slowly acquires the cultural lens of that society (Helman 1994, cited in Burch 2001: 135).

Here, Helman is suggesting that culture is like a set of spectacles given to us by the society we belong to. This set of spectacles shapes how we see the world and the people we meet, the situations we encounter, the roles we take, and the choices we make, so that we see these in the way that society wants us to. It also means that we learn how to behave within that society; we know what is 'acceptable' behaviour and what is not. It is only possible to see within the confines of the spectacles, which restricts what is seen and revealed. Some aspects of the world around are brought into sharp focus, whilst others are not seen. So culture is a code of behaviour, a guide for how to 'be' in the world – and this code or guide can supply us with oppressive styles of behaviour, but without us necessarily realising. This is because we trust and believe that the spectacles show us reality, not realising that they only show us *one* of many possible versions of reality (see Chapter 6 for further discussion on this issue).

Peacock views culture as:

> … the taken-for-granted but powerfully influential understandings and codes that are learned and shared by members of a group…(Peacock 1986, cited in Dobson 1991: xv)

Here Peacock points to the subtle, hidden, and 'taken-for-granted' nature of culture, but also its power to shape our behaviour. Therefore, culture provides us with a way to behave, which may be oppressive, but which we may be unaware of. Peacock reflects the more contemporary view of culture, which is that culture exists in any group of people no matter what the size of the group. Culture does not just exist within a 'society', it also occurs in smaller groupings, for example, professional groups such as 'nursing' or even smaller ward, unit, or community teams (see Chapter 5 for further exploration of this issue). You can explore this in more depth in Box 3.6).

The *cultural* level of oppression for both Thompson (2011) and Dominelli (2008a, 2008b) refers to the cultural norms, values, beliefs, and traditions which oppress individuals and which are seen as acceptable by members of the group to which the individual is exposed. This group may be society as a whole, or it may be a healthcare environment, a social group, or any work environment. Within this chapter, we are concerned with how the norms, values, beliefs, and traditions of both wider society culture *and* the healthcare setting culture can devalue, degrade, disempower, or undermine patients/service users and thus cause or increase their vulnerability.

Box 3.6   Activity

Think back to a practice setting that you have joined, such as on going on placement or taking up a new post.

How did you feel when you joined? Did you feel you belonged immediately, or did you have to try and 'fit in'? What aspects did you need to consider in trying to 'fit in'?

- Were there rituals or routines that everyone else knew but you did not?
- Was there certain language you needed to learn, or language you needed to avoid?
- Were there certain beliefs or values that were shared by team members?
- Were there 'in-jokes' that you needed to learn about and understand?
- Were some members of staff more valued than others?
- Did you have to learn who had the 'real power'?
- Were some patients/ service users more valued than others?
- Did patients/ service users also have to 'fit in' to the team expectations and 'rules'?
- Which patients/service users did not 'fit in', and why was this?

All of these aspects are part of the 'culture' of the team, and when you join a new team, you often have to 'learn' their culture in order to feel that you belong and to feel accepted. Culture is also most noticeable to new members of a team, rather than to the existing members, because it is 'taken for granted'. So the team may not be aware of the learning you had to go through in order to 'fit in'.

Having undertaken this activity, can you see any ways or instances when a practice setting's culture might be seen as oppressive to service users or patients?

Keep your notes from this activity as the issues will be revisited in Chapter 5.

Cultural norms, values, beliefs, and traditions can be seen all around us; however, to recognise them requires that we try to become 'strangers' in what is a very familiar world. Unless we look with the 'eyes of a stranger', just like when you were new to healthcare, then it is hard to see the taken-for-granted assumptions, beliefs, rituals, rules, and practices. Without that willingness to step back and 'disengage' yourself from the cultures you belong to, it will be very difficult to identify the cultural level of oppression. This is why active and empathic listening to patients/service users can be a very useful insight, seeing the world of healthcare from their perspective can help you to see the cultural level of oppression.

To 'see' the cultural level of oppression, it is worth examining:

- Culture and media representation and portrayals of individuals or groups. For example, the media portrayal of HIV/AIDS, mental illness, single mothers.
- Language and labels used about individuals or groups. For example, the term 'bed blockers' is now common within healthcare environments, consider what this term infers about the person referred to. It suggests that they are wasting valuable health service time, they are not in the right place, and time they moved on.
- Stereotypes about that group (see Chapter 4 for further discussion and illustrations).
- Social roles that people are allowed or forced to play. For example, whether people are encouraged into the workplace or restricted from work, e.g. people with mental health issues, people with disabilities, homeless people, older people.
- Values – whether the group are socially valued or not. For example, the dominant cultural values (in Western society) are geared towards the able-bodied majority. The

emphasis is on physical perfection and academic achievement as high status characteristics. This immediately devalues people with learning disabilities, physical disabilities, people of larger body size, people with facial differences, e.g. skin graft, skin
blemishes.

- Humour and jokes made about the group. For example, in the BBC comedy programme
'Little Britain', there is a character who is unable to remain continent. This is deemed
humorous, and the humour derives from her incontinence. This could make members of
the audience who have continence difficulties embarrassed to reveal their condition, as
they may risk laughter or ridicule.
- Invisibility of certain types of people or issues in media or everyday life. For example,
how many television or magazine adverts include disabled people or a 'gay family'?
This invisibility can reinforce the ignorance which fuels prejudice.

S – structural level of oppression

This is an examination of the way in which the organisation of society reinforces
discrimination and oppression. This *structural* level, according to Thompson's model, is
concerned with the ways in which social divisions are created and maintained (e.g. class,
race, gender), the ways in which power is used to create and maintain inequalities, and the
ways in which wealth and other resources are distributed amongst groups. Additionally,
we would like to include Dominelli's (2008a, 2008b) conception of 'institutional
oppression' within this level, which refers to:

> … policies and practices that carry social authority by being enshrined in legislation, and in
> policies that endorse specific kinds of goods and services as entitlements for particular types
> of people (Dominelli 2008a: 117).

This clearly overlaps with Thompson's explanation of the structural level, but in particular
this specifies the role of policy in creating and maintaining oppression.

Some readers may at this point be thinking 'what has this structural level got to do with
me as a healthcare practitioner working with patients/service users, this is more the role
of managers'.

We would urge you to think again – your role here is considerable. Let us look at an
example of the *structural* level of oppression within healthcare (please see Box 3.7).

Other examples of structural level factors which can affect the vulnerability of patients/
clients might include the Nursing and Midwifery Council (NMC) requirements for the
depth and range of experience students have with different branches of nursing, the range
and type of dietary options offered, mixed sex wards, and the dignity afforded by the
gowns purchased in each hospital. The *structural* level is clearly a factor in the vulnerability of many service users/patients, and without considering this level and your role within
it would be to ignore the full complexity of vulnerability.

The argument of Thompson and Dominelli is that all three levels or dimensions are
crucial in understanding oppression – to neglect one is to take an incomplete view. Equally
all three levels are overlapping and interconnected, they lead to and from each other. For
example, the NMC (2008) code of conduct is an example of a structural mechanism to

---

Box 3.7   Returning to Soraya's story

Soraya was bedbound as a result of a stroke. She was a large woman with a high body mass index. The ward she was on did not have a suitable hoist and the staff had not found the time to order one yet. Soraya was told that she should 'wet the bed' when she needed to urinate as the staff were unable to lift her onto a commode or a bedpan.

   Firstly the provision of 'bariatric equipment' is the responsibility of the hospital management and is an example of a *structural* level factor. Who decides how much of the budget will be spent on such equipment? Do they provide sufficient equipment for any service user to have immediate access? Do they offer only enough money to allow for shared access to such resources?

   Secondly the urgency with which the staff on the ward did or in this case *did not* order the equipment is an issue of power and as such is a *structural* level issue. The nurse in charge had the authority and power to ensure the equipment was available but did not prioritise this as urgent.

   In this case, there was insufficient equipment available, as a result of both hospital management spending and also the decisions of the nurse in charge. This resulted in Soraya facing an inhuman and degrading experience as a result of *structural* oppression. Equally, the wider nursing team also had a responsibility to make senior nurses and management aware that the structural resources were insufficient to provide care with dignity and compassion. Thus, all nurses played a key role in Soraya's vulnerability.

Box 3.8   Time for reflection

From the list of service users you collected together in Box 3.1, choose one and try to identify examples of:

- Personal oppression
- Cultural oppression
- Structural oppression

---

reduce the vulnerability of service users, and yet on its own it clearly does not achieve this – see Chapter 5 for discussion on recent examples where this has come to light. This suggests that whilst the NMC code of conduct is one valuable *structural* mechanism to protect against vulnerability, it also requires efforts at the *cultural* and *personal* level to ensure that people are protected from vulnerability.

   Let us consider the personal, cultural, and structural oppression further in Box 3.8.

   You may have found it difficult at times to decide whether a situation is personal, cultural, or structural, and at times the factors can straddle two or more levels. This is not always as important as the fact of being forced to look wider than just personal and individual explanations for oppression and hence vulnerability. The strength of the PCS analysis is that it shows the inadequacy of any explanations that stop short by looking at personal level explanations alone, ignoring wider cultural and structural factors. Reducing vulnerability requires a multi-level approach, taking account of the significance of each level.

   So far this chapter has explored the concepts of discrimination and oppression and linked these to vulnerability. A key theme within this book is that oppression and discrimination cause, or create a susceptibility to, harm or danger. They are processes which can wound clients both physically and psychologically, and these processes occur within healthcare settings in Britain. We now want to focus on the role that *power* plays in vulnerability.

The role of power

The concepts of vulnerability, discrimination, and oppression can be seen as relationships of *power* between an individual and the threats or harms that they may face. For example, from looking at the definitions in Chapter 1, vulnerability implies feeling threatened or out of control. This can be interpreted as a state of being or feeling 'powerless', subject to the power of an external threat, or a feeling of being powerless against an internally evaluated threat.

What follows (Box 3.9) is an example drawn from the very critical report of the treatment of older people in the health service (Parliamentary and Health Service Ombudsman 2011). In it, there were numerous examples where older people or their partners/family members felt powerless against the neglect or uncaring treatment offered by some heath service staff.

The case of Mrs N shows that she and her family were powerless. On one level, it is uncertain whether the cancer was preventable or detectable earlier. What was certainly preventable, according to the Ombudsmen, was the lack of awareness of the extent of the pain she was experiencing, and what was required was a quick and appropriate response of the medical and nursing staff to that pain and the need for the prompt prescription and administration of adequate pain relief. Without a definitive diagnosis, the family was also powerless to get full attendance allowance.

Box 3.9   Mrs N's story (from Parliamentary and Health Service Ombudsman 2011)

In October 2007, Mrs. N was provisionally diagnosed with lung cancer by her GP. She went to her local general hospital. According to the first consultant she saw, the tests were inconclusive and she was sent to another hospital for further protracted tests.

'While waiting for the results of the hospital tests, Mrs N began to suffer from severe pain. Her daughter told us that because her mother had not been given a diagnosis she was not given adequate pain relief. The lack of a diagnosis also prevented Mrs N claiming full attendance allowance – something that would have helped the family to care for her. The Christmas period was a particularly distressing time for everyone, as Mrs N's family witnessed her suffering without being able to help. Another daughter, who spent a large part of each day caring for Mrs N, became ill herself as a result of the distress.

A few days later Mrs N – who described herself as 'disorientated and in extreme pain' at the time – was admitted to hospital to control her increasing pain. A pain management plan was drawn up specifying that Mrs N should receive medication on an "as required" basis, but it was five days before she received adequate pain relief. Mrs N said that she was in 'unbearable pain'. On one occasion, Mrs N had asked for pain relief, only to be told that she had already taken it. However, when the Macmillan nurse checked the drugs chart, that was not the case. As her daughter observed "our mother continued to suffer for too long"' (from Parliamentary and Health Service Ombudsman 2011: 37–38).

What made this even more concerning was when Mrs N was not believed when she was complaining of severe pain until the Macmillan nurse actually checked the drugs chart. Clearly, as her daughter summed up, her mother and her family were powerless to help and she 'continued to suffer for too long'. Mrs N and her family were left *power*-less and vulnerable; therefore, we will now move on to an analysis and discussion of power.

About power – what is it?

The concept of power is a large and significant topic within social and political sciences, and this chapter could never offer a definitive or exhaustive review of the concept. The ideas and concepts drawn from the wider social sciences about power can be useful to understand it in relation to vulnerability in healthcare, so we recommend you use the references in this chapter to read further about power.

Power is a hotly contested concept: there are many disagreements and disputes about the nature of power, about what it is, how it affects people, and where it comes from (Wenman 2005, cited in MacKenzie 2005). The concept is most associated with politics and political science (Mackenzie 2005, Heywood 2007) and many of the definitions of power highlight the political nature of the concept.

In a classic analysis of 1936, Lasswell says that politics is essentially about *who gets what, when, and how*. For Bilton *et al.* (2002), the study of power is similar – the study of power is concerned with *who has it, to what purpose it is used, is it equally distributed*, or when it is not, *how and why is it distributed in the way that it is*. This is an overtly political view of power in that it asks us to consider who has power over us, as it assumes that power is not equally distributed but is concentrated in the hands of a few, such as in the hands of different powerful groups. It also asks us to consider *who* may have less power or *who* may be relatively or very power-*less*. It also asks us to question to what purpose power is used for and what goals those with power are pursuing. Definitions of power can be found in Box 3.10.

However, as Thompson (2007) notes, power could also be seen as a psychological concept. For example, someone who is more assertive and confident may be more able to achieve their ends or goals, which could be seen as a form of psychological power.

Looking at different definitions of power, whether one takes a political or psychological perspective, many definitions emphasise power as an ability to achieve your aim or goal,

---

Box 3.10 Power defined

- The ability of individuals or the members of a group, to achieve aims to further the interests they hold … (Giddens 2009: 1128).
- The probability that one actor in a social relationship will be in the position to carry out their will despite resistance … (Weber 1968, cited in MacKenzie 2005: 372).
- The ability to achieve a desired outcome (Heywood 2007: 7).

or the ability to exercise power over something or someone. Worsley (1964: 16–17) suggests:

> we can be said to act politically when we exercise constraint on others to behave as we want them to, and the exercise of constraint in any relationship is political.

Thus, it could be argued that even the psychological power to achieve ones aims is a form of personal political power. The extent to which nurses and healthcare staff influence or constrain the actions and behaviours of service users within the caring situation is political; therefore, all power is political.

Two types of power?

Both Heywood (2007) and Thompson (2007) suggest that there are different types of power. One type of power is 'the ability to achieve a desired outcome' (Heywood 2007: 7). This could be the ability to keep oneself alive, to be healthy, to work, to find a partner, or even to buy a cup of coffee if thirsty. This type of power is often referred as the 'power to' (Heywood 2007, Thompson 2007). The second type of power sees power as a *relationship*, where we possess the ability to influence or control the behaviour or actions of others, not (necessarily) of their own choosing (Heywood 2007). This second type of power is often referred to as 'power over' (Heywood 2007). Thompson calls this domination over others (2007).

Both of these types of power ('power to' and 'power over') have relevance to the study of vulnerability and oppression. It concerns how we as practitioners enable or restrict service users in their 'power to' achieve desired outcomes. We as nurses or healthcare staff could exercise our 'power to', to help patients and service users to stay alive, to have full rewarding life opportunities, and to have pain relief or help when they want or wish it or the power to help them become or remain independent. We as nurses and healthcare staff may on the other hand deny or restrict our use of our 'power to' help or support patients or service users. Therefore, the use, non-use, or inappropriate use of our 'power to' help patients/service users to 'achieve a desired outcome' is part of understanding vulnerability in the context of nursing and healthcare.

On the other hand, the second type of power described by Heywood and Thompson, the 'power over', also has great relevance to the study of vulnerability. For example, to what extent do nurses and healthcare staff have 'power over' their patients and service users by making decisions about when they can have pain relief, when they can have a drink or something to eat, or when they can have a bath or shower or even the 'power over' what they know about their own health problem and treatment. Now take a few moments to reflect on your own personal power – go to Box 3.11.

Power exists in many aspects of the relationship between healthcare professionals and their patients and service users (Barry and Yuill 2008, Cooke and Philpin 2008). Thompson (2007, 2011) suggests that power can operate at different levels along the lines of his PCS model. That is to say that power can operate on the personal level, the cultural level, and/or at the structural level. However, it is not always easy to see or detect: it is easier to see power when it is 'directed against you' and not so easy to see when 'you possess it' (Nzira and Williams 2009: 25). Thus, reflection is a key tool to expose the power we hold.

Box 3.11 Time for reflection

Spend some time thinking about and make some notes on how YOU may have 'power' in your work with service users/patients?

- Thinking of the first type of power, power to, what power(s) do you have to help service users and patients to achieve their desired outcomes?
- Thinking of the second type of power, power over, what power(s) do you have over service users and patients?

Reflection points:

- Is this power ('power to' and 'power over') always 'beneficial' for service users/patients or is it used in their best interests?
- What factors might make it difficult to exercise beneficial 'power to' or 'power over' when working with service users of patients?
- In what ways could 'power to' or 'power over' be misused or even abused in working with patients and service users.
- Consider possible reasons for such misuse or even abuse of 'power to' or 'power over' in working with patients and service users.
- Reflect on what you can do as a healthcare professional or a healthcare team if you believe that 'power to' or 'power over' is being misused or even abused in working with patients and service users.

Possible responses to many of these reflection points are contained in this chapter or elsewhere in this book.

Now that we have tried to define power, let us look at some of the uses and abuses of power, considering who uses it and for which reasons.

The effect of power

Power can have a positive effect, something to be valued and welcomed, or could be negative, as a potentially destructive force that can be used to exploit, oppress, or abuse (Thompson 2007). Any of us could think of examples of where a nurse, a doctor, a teacher, or any other professional has helped us achieve our desired outcomes through their positive and beneficial use of their 'power to' help us or the positive and beneficial use of their 'power over' us. However, as much of this chapter illustrates, there may be situations and times where 'power to' and 'power over' is used against us in a negative, destructive way that could leave us being, or feeling, vulnerable and oppressed.

Weber, one of the founding figures in sociology, identified these two aspects of power, one positive and potentially helpful and the other negative, abusive, and potentially destructive. For Weber, *authority* is a form of power accepted as legitimate by those upon whom it is exercised (Weber undated cited Giddens 2009: 989–990). Authority should and can be beneficial for the recipient, such as when a doctor or nurse uses their expertise, skill, and care in providing good quality treatment or healthcare for their patients or service users. On the other hand, coercion is the use of a power not accepted as legitimate by those upon whom it is exercised (Weber undated cited Giddens 2009: 989–990) (see Box 3.12).

These examples would all fit Weber's notion of 'coercion' as they restrict or restrain someone's rights, freedoms, and options, ethically go against the NMC Code (2008), are legally questionable, and could be seen as abusive and destructive. They would also be

> **Box 3.12 Examples of coercion?**
>
> Weber's concept of coercion could be used to describe any of the following:
>
> - Denying or taking away food or drink on the pretext that it is not the 'right time for a drink' or 'you cannot have a dessert unless you finish your dinner';
> - Making someone unnecessarily wait to go to the toilet or use a commode if they need assistance;
> - Mistreating or verbally/physically abusing someone, using sarcastic language, or 'telling someone off';
> - The excessive and inappropriate use of physical control and restraint, 'cot sides' on beds or using furniture and locks on doors to restrict someone's movement;
> - Being treated in a way which makes us feel unnecessarily upset, degraded, vulnerable, or even oppressed;
> - Being forced or manipulated into doing something, or agreeing to do something against their will or preference because of threats or intimidation.

unwelcome and unasked for (even if the recipient does not complain at the time). It is important to note that although we may believe we have the best of intentions in our use of 'power to' or 'power over', we cannot and should not assume that our actions or interventions are always welcomed by the recipient (Thompson 2003, 2011; Nzira and Williams 2009). What we see as the beneficial use of our authority/power, could be construed as unwelcome abuse and coercion by the recipient.

Thompson (2007, 2011) and Nzira and Williams (2009) suggest that we should constantly reflect when exercising our 'power to' or 'power over' in working with others or providing care. For example, if someone were to accept the use of our power without question or challenge, is it because they genuinely agree with us and give us their free and informed consent, have we manipulated them into agreeing with us, or have they been abused or coerced at some point in the past, making them more submissive and compliant into accepting their powerlessness.

Equally, if someone were to question or challenge our authority or decision, even if we believe we have the best of intentions, we should try to explore the reasons why someone may choose to resist our power or decision and acknowledge their fundamental right to question and challenge our authority. It is also important to note that there may be other personal, cultural, or structural reasons why a patient or service user or even a colleague may be unable or unwilling to challenge what we believe is a beneficial and acceptable use of our authority, even if they do not like what we suggest (see Chapters 8 and 9).

So, if offering to help a service user or patient or offering them some intervention, we should constantly reflect on what we are doing and how we are coming across to them in our interaction. By doing this we might avoid using undue influence or pressure, giving them as free an opportunity as possible to consent or not consent to the choice we offer, and value their right to accept or reject our help or suggestion on that occasion.

The abuse of power

Another possible consequence of power is that unaccountable and concentrated amounts of power can lead to corruption and abuse. There is a famous saying about power attributed to the nineteenth century British politician, Lord Acton (undated cited in Heywood 2007: 7), who said 'Power tends to corrupt, absolute power corrupts absolutely'. According to Lord Acton, all power, its possession, and use can lead to abuse of that power and the abuse of others. The more power one has, the more abuse of power is possible.

> Abuse is the harming of an individual (physically, psychologically or emotionally) by a person in a position of power, trust or authority over that individual. (Centre for Policy for Ageing 1996, cited in Lawson 2001: 289)

No Secrets (DoH 2000), in its multi-agency guidance to prevent the abuse of adults, defined a broad range of categories of potential abuse:

1 Physical abuse
2 Sexual abuse
3 Psychological abuse
4 Financial or material abuse
5 Neglect or acts of omission
6 Discriminatory abuse

As seen in Chapter 2, the government has also identified key groups of 'vulnerable people' who are particularly at risk of abuse, thus adopting an etic approach to vulnerability. Clough (1988 cited in Lawson 2001: 289) adds further depth by arguing that the presence of certain factors can make an individual such as a patient or service user vulnerable to the abuse of power when:

1 They are vulnerable and dependent on services provided
2 They have to live with the consequences if they complain
3 They despair that nothing will be done, thinking no one will listen
4 They do not know their rights
5 They fear threats from staff
6 They have ambivalent feelings towards their 'abusers', almost excusing the abuse by trying to justify it on the staff being 'busy' or 'overworked', or 'short staffed'
7 They think they will be blamed for complaining
8 The patients'/service users' personal confidence and self-esteem are low and they feel devalued or even 'worthless'

Naylor lists similar factors that may make someone vulnerable to abuse which may include (Naylor 2006: 113–115, Naylor 2010: 115):

- Over compliance and dependence on a service or practitioner
- Fear of retaliation for complaining
- No support networks outside of a service
- Social isolation
- Unable to communicate a complaint
- Practitioner/organisation factors: over work, low pay, low status of work, and other psychological factors in the abuser

---

Box 3.13   Time for reflection

Look at the risk factors identified previously that might make some vulnerable to abuse as described by Clough (1988 cited in Lawson 2001: 289) and Naylor (2006) and (2010).

* Which factors might apply to the people you work with?
* Are the people you work with vulnerable to abuse?
* Make a note of why and what it is that makes them vulnerable to abuse.
* If only a few or none of these factors apply, are there other factors that would make them vulnerable, which should be added to the lists?

According to Williams *et al.* (2003, cited in Monk 2010), even people not in residential/hospital care, but dependent on family or other informal carers, may be reluctant to complain about abuse for the same reasons. Their dependence on the carer and fear of consequences may leave them feeling powerless and thus vulnerable to the abuse of power.

Before we continue, let us just consider what has been said to date within the context of practice (see Box 3.13).

Power and power relations in the care setting are central to understanding all abuse situations (Penhale and Parker 2008). In most, if not all, cases of the misuse and abuse of power, abuse and harm can result in serious or even extreme harm. Just in recent history, some of the biggest multiple killers in UK criminal history were healthcare professionals. Beverly Allitt, a nurse, killed five children in her care in 1993; Anne Grigg-Booth was charged with killing three patients in 2005 but died from an overdose before her trial; Colin Norris, a nurse, murdered four elderly patients in Leeds in 2008; and nurse Benjamin Green was convicted of killing two patients and deliberately harming sixteen others in 2006 (all cases cited in Laurance 2011). Indeed, the most prolific serial killer in UK criminal history was Harold Shipman who was convicted in 2000 of killing 15 patients, but according to the official Shipman Inquiry Final Report (2005), he is strongly suspected of killing at least 250 vulnerable people.

Prevention of abuse

In order to prevent abuse arising from the accumulation and exercise of unaccountable power, many professions work within sophisticated systems of accountability and legal safeguards. Therefore, there are 'checks' on the power that nurses and healthcare professionals have and use. For example, nurses, like other healthcare professions, must work within the legal constraints of common and civil law in order to prevent any abuse of the undoubted power that they have. They should also adhere to key ethical principles (as described by Beauchamp and Childress 2008) such as the duty to beneficially help others and not harm them, to uphold the principle of informed consent, and to respect the rights and autonomy of others to make decisions about their own care. These principles are also now legally enshrined in legislation such as the Human Rights Act 1998, the Mental Capacity Act 2005 and the Deprivation of Liberty Safeguards amendment, the Mental Health Act 1983 and 2007, and the Equality Act 2010.

The NMC has a legal duty to set standards regarding the education of nurses, about standards of nursing care itself, and to regulate and hold nurses to account to check and prevent any abuse of their power. Using Thompson's PCS Model, this is an example of structural level measures to prevent abuse but also reflects a cultural level expectation of the values within which nursing care should take place.

It is clear that structural processes alone cannot prevent all instances of abuse, as evidenced by the earlier examples of abusive healthcare practitioners, thus emphasising the role of cultural and personal strategies. At the personal level, Nzira and Williams (2009: 26) suggest professionals should:

- Use their power for the benefit of others and not to oppress others
- Develop the self-awareness and reflective practice needed to do this
- Understand and accept that we can become defensive when we feel our power or authority is being challenged by others; it is essential to not be threatened by this
- Recognise that the abuse or inappropriate use of power can harm others
- Recognise that power can be also good: power is the engine that drives both oppression or can drive anti-oppression

Thompson (2007, 2011) says that we have choice and control over our use of power. He argues that as a professional, we have choice about whether and how to use our power, to help or to harm; we have the ability to increase our own power or to 'give away' or lessen our power; and we also have choices about the purposes we use our power for, the intention behind it.

Ideally, our 'power to' should be used for the benefit of service users, in their best interests, and most importantly where ever possible, directed and dictated by the patient or service user in order to be *person centred* rather than professional or service centred. Power *over* service users and patients should be minimised to be replaced by *power with*, based on partnership and equality with patients and service users. This partnership basis for therapeutic and helping relationships is advocated by many sources such as Peplau (1998), Rungapadiachy (1999), Heron (2001), Cambridge and Carnaby (2005), and Strega (2007), to name just a few.

However, Thompson does acknowledge that there may be limits or constraints on any of us exercising choice and acting independently. For example, Thompson (2011) and Lukes (2005) are just two authors who suggest that our goals, aspirations, and even ability to exercise or resist power may be affected by structural or cultural processes and influences. According to both, some people because of their age, gender, or social class may never have had the socialisation, encouragement, opportunity, or skills to develop the confidence to challenge or resist medical or nursing decisions. Instead, many may just defer to medical power without question. This is an example of the power contained within beliefs, ideologies, or 'discourses' (see Chapter 6 for further discussion of discourses).

Up to now, we have seen that power can be exercised through the actions or behaviours of 'powerful' people, but power can also be seen to exist in ideas, such as in and through the powerful idea of the medical model. Power, in particular, the amount of our relative *power* or *powerlessness*, may be linked to societal structure and our membership of a

> **Box 3.14   Perspectives on power**
>
> 1   Traditional 'pluralist' perspective of power: This perspective suggests that power is derived from social role or that power is a disposition or attribute that one can possess and can be increased or decreased like the ownership of a commodity.
> 2   Marxist/structuralist perspective: The power we possess is dictated by our position in the social system or hierarchy, linked to our social class, gender, age, race or ethnicity, or any other aspect of our social identity. In this view, some groups are said to be more powerful than other social groupings, such as in the concept of a ruling class or elite.
> 3   The 'dispersed power' perspective: According to this perspective, power is immediate and everywhere, so that our lives are shaped by the people around us such as partners, children, neighbours, managers and work colleagues, and others so that for many feminists, the 'personal is the political' (Hanisch 1969, Wright Mills 1999). This perspective also encompasses the view that power is everywhere in the form of discourses and ideas, so that the words and language we use, and the way we think and talk about 'things', in narrow and limited ways can influence us and our social structure in ways that we may not always be aware of.

particular social identity such as our social or occupational class, our age group, and our gender. Therefore, it will be useful to now explore where power comes from, why and how some people have *it*, and others seem to have less.

Theories of power

Many authors suggest that there are different perspectives about the source and origin of power (Dearlove and Saunders 2000; Bilton *et al.* 2002; MacKenzie 2005; Goodwin 2007; Heywood 2007; Thompson 2007, 2011). These can all be encompassed within three broad perspectives (Box 3.14) on the nature of power which will each be considered in turn in the rest of the chapter.

Perspective one: Traditional 'pluralist' theories

Many theories of where power may come from suggest that power is like a commodity that anyone can accumulate and possess; hence, it is often referred to as a pluralist perspective in that any of us can possess power if we know where it comes from and know how to exert or use it (Dahl 1989). In order to understand this further, please undertake the Time for reflection activity (Box 3.15)

One well-known analysis of power suggests that it depends on whether we possess particular qualities or attributes that derive from particular *sources* of power (French and Raven 1959). Although dating from 1959, this source could now appear old, but it is still widely cited and seen as influential: (French and Raven 1959 are cited in Podsakoff and Schriescheim 1985, Hinkin and Schriesheim 1989, Yukl and Falbe 1990, and Aguinis *et al.* 1998).

French and Raven suggest that people can derive their power through particular sources (or *bases*) of power as outlined in 'Sources of power' (French and Raven 1959).

Box 3.15   Time for reflection

1   Make a list of people you think are powerful.
2   Look back at the people on your list. (*You might have included particular people like The Queen, the current UK Prime Minister, USA President, the Pope or the Dalai Lama, or famous celebrities such as Cheryl Cole or David Beckham. You may have included abstract people based on their roles such as police officer, a judge, traffic warden, or doctor. You may have included powerful or influential people from your own social circle or immediate experience such as partner, parent, or your own children.*)
3   Where do these people get their power from, what exactly gives them their power?
4   Does their power come from having or using any particular qualities, skills, or resources that they possess, or does it come from their occupational or social roles/positions, or does it come from something else?

The following discussion of theories of where power comes from may help you answer this further: it may well be worthwhile returning to this activity once you have read the rest of this chapter to see if you have a better idea of where power comes from.

Sources of power

1   *Reward power*:

This power comes from the ability of an individual to reward others who can then give them power or influence over others. These rewards can take the form of money, promotion, praise, and recognition. So, political leaders and managers have the power that comes from being able to reward with money, promotions, well-paid jobs and appointments, and honours such as OBE's and MBE's, knighthoods, and even peerages. Teachers, nurses, and doctors can reward their students and patients by offering qualifications or better treatment. Police officers and traffic wardens may have reward power if they decide to 'let you off' from a parking or speeding ticket if you are friendly and courteous to them. Partners and children may reward you by providing you with emotional *rewards* if you do as they want. Chapter 6 discusses the concept of the 'unpopular patient' which illustrates the use of reward power by nurses.

However, Devito (2008) argues this form of power is limited as it is dependent on how desperate you are to receive that particular reward. Therefore, people are not and should not be thought of as performing dogs: chocolate will not serve as a reward for someone who either does not like chocolate or is otherwise sated with chocolate, money may diminish as a potential reward if someone does not value it highly or desperately need it, and praise and recognition will only enhance someone's reward power if it is seen as coming from someone valued and respected.

2   *Coercive power*:

This power derives from the ability of certain people to punish you or even 'force' you to do something, even against your will. The most obvious form of this power is that certain people can physically force you to do certain things or achieve it through threats and intimidation, or limit and restrain your free movement. This may match Weber's concept of coercion described earlier in this chapter. This may be illegal coercion, but some coercion can be legal, when exercised by people by virtue of their legally allowed role or occupation. This could include people such as police officers, a prison officer, or a mental health professional if a patient is detained under the Mental Health Act. Again, Chapter 6 discusses the concept of the 'unpopular patient' which also illustrates the use of coercive power by nurses.

3   *Legitimate power:*

French and Raven (1959) describe this power as given to people through legally permitted or sanctioned means, so that some people have a legal right or authority to exert certain types of power over or with someone else. So in terms of coercion, which might ordinarily be thought of as abusive, some people in certain contexts are legally permitted to use force or restraint within boundaries set by relevant legislation. As described earlier in terms of coercive power, police officers, prison officers, psychiatrists, and approved mental health professionals have legally permissible powers to detain someone, but they are accountable for this power.

Other people have this legally permitted or 'allowed' power: the Queen and Prime Minister as well as other political figures may be seen to have legitimate power and influence as their role and position is enshrined in the British Constitution, or they have been elected to office through due democratic process. Other people have legitimate power because of their professional role and their qualification. For example, it is illegal to stab someone with a sharp object, but it is legally permissible to do so in the *right context*. This could be a surgeon or doctor who is *legally permitted* to cut someone in the context of a surgical procedure or for a doctor or nurse to inject a patient or service user if that medication was legally prescribed and the patient or service user consents.

However, legitimate power, when exercised, is highly dependent on the context. People hold legitimate power because they hold certain professional or occupational roles and have the necessary training and accreditation to carry out the action or procedure in the right legally permitted context. So a doctor and nurse should not, and cannot, legally inject someone out of the legitimate context.

However, even though this sort of legitimate power is legally permissible, the way that a procedure or action is carried out is significant. For example, giving someone an injection, even *if* legitimately prescribed and to be carried out by an accredited person, could still be abusive, unethical, and coercive. Giving an injection in a rushed, unskilled, or uncaring way could be construed as unethical and coercive, even if technically speaking it met the legitimate criteria for action.

4   *Referent power:*

French and Raven (1959) recognise that some people who have power have it because they are influential on the views and actions of others, people *refer* to the view of people who are seen to be moral or social leaders. These people may have no ability to directly reward others, they may not have direct legitimate authority over others, and cannot or do not use force or coercive power, and yet can still be influential on others.

So religious leaders such as the Pope or Archbishop of Canterbury, Dalai Lama, Chief Rabbi, or Imam may have referent power because they may act as role models and their views influence the thoughts and actions of many others. Political and moral philosophers can also be influential and be said to have referent power on the thoughts and actions of others such as Confucius, Aristotle, or Karl Marx.

Today, famous celebrities may hold referent power such as David Beckham or Cheryl Cole, so that people may buy products they endorse in advertising and marketing or imitate their look and lifestyle wherever possible. This can have consequences in terms of making some people feel vulnerable as there is plenty of evidence that the rise in 'celebrity worship' and the aspiration to imitate them can undermine our self-esteem and self-confidence (Higgins 1987, Deetz 1992, Alvesson and Willmott 2003).

Doctors and nurses may still hold some referent power in that patients and service users might be persuaded by their advice or recommendation on whether to agree to healthcare procedures as they may be seen to be health role models. The view of nurses as 'angels' is still powerful today (Hart 2004).

However, again whether this power and influence is a good thing depends on the quality of advice and the intention when making recommendations to patients and service users and how directive we should ever be with people who look to us for support. The NMC in its code (NMC 2008) insists that nurses should base their nursing practice on best available evidence and urges caution on what advice nurses should give to patients and service users: they are clear about the unacceptability of nurses using their qualification to endorse or market commercial products and services.

5   *Expert power*:

French and Raven (1959) describe a fifth type of power they describe as expert power. This is where someone is powerful because they are perceived as having real or assumed expertise. Therefore, people with qualifications or people who are believed to be expert and knowledgeable in their field may have an influence and power over the actions of others.

Just to show how the types of power described by French and Raven can overlap, a doctor may have referent power and legitimate power, but this may be reinforced and amplified if they are believed to be expert in their field. This expertise may be real or may be assumed in that sometimes people may use long complex words, jargon, and technical terminology which can both confuse people, but leave the impression, deserved or otherwise, that this person knows what they are talking about.

However, like many other types of power, expert power can be a force for good as we would all like to be operated upon by an expert surgeon or supported by nurses with expertise, and yet one of the factors that enabled Harold Shipman to kill so many people, with the cooperation of his victims, was that they did not suspect him and they trusted in his expertise as a general practitioner (GP) (The Shipman Inquiry 2005).

Since French and Raven's original analysis of power, others have tried to add further bases of power. Raven (1974) has suggested that the possession of knowledge and factual information can give the owner of that information power, which he called *informational power*. It reflects the old truism 'knowledge is power'. This can be a manipulative and ethically questionable form of power if the person withholds information from others, in order to increase their own power at the expense of disempowering others and keeping them in ignorance.

However, *informational power* could be turned into a positive form of power if one uses the skill of finding and having information in order to disseminate it and enlighten and inform others. Therefore, as Thompson (2011) suggests, the ability to identify and search for relevant information and evidence on which to base care, to act on this sound evidence base, and to share that with others could be a more positive use of *informational power*, as a key anti-oppressive strategy.

Thompson (2007) also argues that power may be 'dispositional' or comes through a person's 'attributes' or through the qualities that they may possess or have acquired. He adds further characteristics or attributes that can enhance the power and influence that an individual may have. The first one is quite controversial in that he argues that some individuals may have power because of their charisma or sexual attractiveness, Thompson (2007: 5). Certainly some other authors such as Conger and Kanungo (1987) and Goodwin (2007) agree that 'charismatic power' can be a source of power and influence. There are questions about whether charisma (if possible to define and identify it) and sexual attractiveness can and should be used to gain power and influence over others, and the use of such attributes to gain influence or even power over patients and service users must be seen as ethically questionable.

Thompson also suggests that some people may have power and influence through the particular skills that they have, particularly in communication and interpersonal skills. 'Emotionally intelligent' people may have power because they have good communication and interpersonal skills (Thompson 2007, also Yukl and Falbe 1990 and Devito 2008). Thompson goes onto say that presenting certain attitudes can amplify or reinforce the influence one has, such as being confident and having self-belief (Thompson 2007).

These psychological or personal forms of power can be learnt or developed over time: the caveat remains in that they should not be misused to gain power or domination *over* others.

This pluralist conception of power as a set of qualities or attributes has been criticised because it ignores the more cultural and structural determinants of power. The pluralist view of power is a relatively socially neutral concept of power as it assumes that anyone, given the right skills and qualities or if occupying appropriate occupational or professional roles, can be as powerful and influential as anyone else.

It ignores the possibility that wider structural factors may determine power, such as whether the power one has may be related to position in the overall social hierarchy. To ignore structural factors could be to ignore the effect of our social class, gender, racial and ethnic, and any other aspect of our social identity or social position, which might really determine how powerful we really are and our potential to increase or reduce vulnerability in others.

Perspective two: Marxist and 'system' theories of power

According to Poulantzas (1976), power is determined by one's position in the wider social system, so that when we are 'born' we are merely slotted into the existing power relations of a capitalist system (i.e. our inherited social class, gender) that we can do little to change without wider societal change. Therefore, our position in the social hierarchy dictates our fortune, life chances, and the power we will have. This social position is largely inherited and passed on from one generation to the next, even if small and rare examples of modest social mobility occur (Poulantzas 1976). According to Miliband (1969, 1982), Wilkinson and Pickett (2009), and Saunders (2010), in a country like the UK with an inherited monarchy and aristocracy, inherited wealth, income inequality, and rigid social class system, any significant upwards mobility is still very unlikely and rare.

Since the time of Karl Marx and Frederick Engels in the mid-1800s (1845–1846, 1863–1883a, 1863–1883b and 1863–1883c), many authors (often referred to as neo-Marxists or structuralists) have argued that power, inequality, and oppression are structurally determined (Gramsci 1968, 1971; Bacharach and Baratz 1970; Althusser 1971; Poulantzas 1976; and Lukes 2005, to name a few). They would ask us to look for evidence that the structural and social class inequalities exist and affect life chances. For example, in terms of health, there is increasing and continued evidence that your social class position affects your health chances and life expectancy (see these reports on health inequalities in the UK spanning the last thirty years: the Black Report, DoH 1980, the Acheson Report 1998, the Marmot Review 2010, and DoH 2010). The gap between the richest and poorest in the UK is increasing and in 2010 was the largest it has been in over 30 years, since before the 1970s (Joseph Rowntree Foundation 2009, 2010). Child poverty is at higher levels today than in the 1960s (Child Poverty Action Group 2011).

This is not a definitive list of evidence of structural inequalities but is indicative that power, influence, and opportunity are linked to position in the social hierarchy. It suggests too that vulnerability and powerlessness could be structural. Indeed, other authors suggest that power and powerlessness are linked to other aspects such as one's position in the social hierarchy. Sylvia Walby (1990) suggested that gender inequalities and oppression are structural and she called this systemic gender oppression 'patriarchy'.

> A society is patriarchal to the degree that it promotes male privilege by being male dominated, male identified, and male centred. It is also organized around an obsession with control and involves as one of its key aspects the oppression of women (Johnson 2005: 5).

According to Walby (1990), patriarchy is structural and institutional so that oppressive and discriminatory gender roles and the subordination of women are perpetually reinforced. Institutions such as marriage and the family, the continued physical and sexual violence towards women, the lack of affordable childcare and restrictions on promotion opportunities at work, cultural expectations of women reinforced through media and pornography that women should be submissive and ornamental are all institutionally and systematically socially sanctioned. Many feminist writers have continued to publish evidence which suggests that the patriarchal subordination of women continues in this new millennium: Hunnicutt (2009), Monagan (2010), Sultana (2010), and Norman (2010), to name just four.

The oppression associated with other social dimensions is equally claimed to be socially structured and reinforced: the concept of structural disablism has been identified by Oliver (1990), Swain *et al.* (1993, 2004), and Barnes and Mercer (2006). The concept of institutional racism was made famous by the Macpherson Inquiry into the murder of Stephen Lawrence and the subsequent 'mishandled' police inquiry. It was defined as:

> The collective failure of an organisation to provide appropriate and professional service to people because of their colour, culture, or ethnic origin. It can be seen or detected in processes,

attitudes and behaviour which amount to discrimination through unwitting prejudice, ignorance, thoughtlessness and racial stereotyping which disadvantage minority ethnic people. (Macpherson Report 1999: Clause 6.34)

The term had originally been coined by Carmichael and Hamilton (1968) and Mason (1982) to mean the subordination of a racial group or groups and maintaining control over those groups, often covertly by the active and pervasive operation of anti-black attitudes.

Other forms of structural and institutional oppression are also said to exist, such as ageism, healthism, and heterosexism (Thompson 2007, 2011; Nzira and Williams 2009). There is no space in this particular chapter to further explore these possible structural and institutional forms of oppression, but if interested you may want to look for your own evidence that they exist and that they have a structural and institutional dimension.

When adopting a Marxist or feminist view of power, structural level factors will be significant in understanding that power. However, Thompson (2007) urges us to be cautious and to avoid taking an oversimplistic view of structuralist power. Whether an individual has power or not is not just a matter of their position in the social hierarchy. For example, women may now increasingly get promotion at work, which may involve having a leadership role with a male workforce, and with the Equality Act (2010), job opportunities and equal pay with men now has a legal basis.

By that same Equality Act, discrimination on the grounds of race and ethnic identity, age, and sexual orientation are now illegal, so the structural mechanisms to address inequalities and structural oppression exist. However, despite the amount of anti-discrimination and pro-equality legislation that exists in the UK today, legislation has failed to eradicate gender, age, or race oppression or to promote real equal opportunities for everyone (Dalrymple and Burke 2006, Thompson 2011).

For neo-Marxists and others who adopt this structural analysis of power and social inequalities, this suggests that power is equally exercised at the ideological, cultural, and philosophical level, and is not a product of social structures alone. For many of these theorists, a ruling *ideology* is used to reinforce and justify the existing social hierarchy (Adorno *et al.* 1950; Marcuse 1964; Gramsci 1968, 1971; Althusser 1971; Postman 1985; and Clegg 1989). For these authors, if the social system is grossly unequal, unfair, and even oppressive, a ruling ideology might serve to *justify* the existence and even *desirability* of that system.

Putnam (1973) defines an ideology as a life-guiding system of beliefs, values, and goals which shape views about what is to be done to organise society as well as how best it should be done. For theorists like Gramsci and Althusser, the ruling elite would find the use of force to impose their domination both expensive and inefficient. Witness the success of the revolutions in Eastern Europe and Russia from 1989 to 1990 and in northern Africa in 2011 even in the face of violent crackdowns by armed state forces. They argue that the ruling elites, whether political, economic, or religious, would use *ideology* to persuade people to be governed and dominated, rather than the use of direct military force. Gramsci (1968) suggested that this domination takes the form of the manipulation and shaping of a society's value system by the ruling class to justify its position, a concept he termed as *hegemony* (1971). In order to understand this further, let us examine some examples of 'dominant' values of beliefs in the Time for reflection activity (Box 3.16).

Box 3.16   Time for reflection

- People are responsible for their own situations: they can be blamed for getting themselves into situations, such as becoming ill or addicted or poor, and they should then be held responsible for getting themselves out of those situations.
- 'Deserving' and 'undeserving' people: some people are seen as being the victims of circumstances and are deemed worthy and deserving of help and support, whereas others are deemed as undeserving and unworthy because they have got themselves into their situation.
- 'Abuse' is often construed in narrow ways: abuse is often legally defined as physical or sexual assault or abuse; in policy and legislation, child or adult poverty is not construed as a form of 'abuse'.
- 'Free market is best': there is a widely held belief that the introduction of a competitive market into healthcare and education 'drives up standards' and gives consumers greater choice. This belief persists even through instances which might suggest that the introduction of the free market and the spread of profit-driven service providers in health and social care has not necessarily driven up standards in services for vulnerable people needing social care ['Southern Cross set to shut down and stop running homes' (BBC 2011a, 2011b)] or in services for people with learning disabilities (CQC investigation of Castlebeck services, 2011a, 2011b).

Try to identify any 'opposing values' that are hidden or obscured by these beliefs – even if you do not agree with them.

- Who gains from the aforementioned values, whose interests do they serve?
- Can you identify any dominant values within healthcare which maintain power for some groups over others?

It can be suggested that the aforementioned values might uphold the interests of the ruling elite in that they can blame individuals for their troubles and deny any state responsibility for having to take action, so that those higher up in the social hierarchy will not need to pay more tax.

Dominelli (2002: 8) argues that:

> … the ruling group … draw on mechanisms of normalisation that promote dominant values and priorities to impose a range of social control systems aimed at curtailing the activities of subordinate groups within the grounds that the dominant group designates as legitimate.

This suggests that the aforementioned beliefs and values serve the purpose of 'controlling' the behaviour of individuals and limiting the resources required to support a population – thus in the process potentially increasing or reducing the vulnerability of certain groups or individuals. This represents Gramsci's concept of hegemony where ideas and ideologies become accepted as dominant, so that the ruling interests can generate a consensus reinforcing their dominance and maintaining existing power relationships and social structure (Thompson 2007). It is argued from this perspective that control and domination, if it exists, is exercised by any ruling group through the creation and manipulation of a ruling belief system and ideology which explains and justifies their domination and creates a mental or ideological acceptance of that domination in the subordinate class or grouping.

Lukes and the three faces of power

Lukes (2005), in his radical concept of power, argues that power has three faces or comes in three different forms. He argues that the most persuasive aspect of it has this more psychological and ideological quality. To paraphrase Lukes (2005: 12), he said that power could be when 'person *A* exercises power over person *B* (*or has the capacity or potential to exert power*), when *A* affects *B* in a manner that may be contrary to *B*'s interests (even if *B* is unaware of this)'.

For Lukes, the challenge was to understand how person A can exert power over person B, even against their will, given that force or coercion may be illegal, inefficient, or ineffective. He was concerned that power may be more subtle and be operating on more than one level. Therefore, according to him, power could contain elements of coercion, but more often operates through forms of 'persuasion' and 'manipulation'.

Lukes argued that power has three dimensions, or, as he calls them, 'faces'.

The first face of power is that of decision making

This is the more traditional pluralist view of power, in that power may lie with the person who makes decisions. This could be with a government minister, the person who chairs a meeting, or the doctor or nurse who decides on treatment. This is a very obvious form of power which can often be seen or measured. In this face of power, the powerful person uses their qualities or attributes to achieve their goal as described in the pluralist perspective earlier.

The second face is that of non-decision making

This form of power was principally identified by Bacharach and Baratz (1962, 1963, 1970). Following their analysis, Lukes (2005) recognises that power is more than just the ability to make decisions: it can also involve the power to deny decisions. This form of power can include the setting of the agenda so that certain other or alternative options are never mentioned or discussed, so the person can decide which options, choices, and decisions are permissible. Equally, by using this form of power, powerful individuals can ensure that options that they dislike are not even discussed, so in effect they are influencing or constraining decisions. An example of this form of power is when a government minister or the chair of a meeting decides the agenda of a meeting or the options to be consulted upon, but ignores or leaves out suggestions that they find unpalatable or unacceptable. Alternatively, they may put items at the end of the meeting agenda so that little time left is for discussion on that issue, or is left late when people need to leave.

In relation to healthcare, a practitioner may put a range of options to someone in order to make an informed decision, for example, about care options, where they may leave out or omit options that they do not agree with when discussing those care choices with the patient or service user. Or they may spend less time discussing some options than others, so the client has less information available to make their choices. People can also exercise this *non-decision making power*, by delaying certain decisions that they may disagree with by setting up a working group, all proposing that a discussion paper or report be written so as to delay, hopefully forever, the decision that they find unpalatable. Therefore, by omitting options and choices by manipulating the agenda or through delaying certain decisions, some people can exert this *non-decision making power*.

The third face of power involves the ability to shape the desires, wants, and needs of others

Shifting the desires, wants, and needs of others so that they accord with your own and which may be contrary to the individual's or social groups' interests. Lukes describes this as when

> person A exercises power over B, not just by getting them to do what they may or may not want to do, but by influencing, shaping or determining their very wants.... to secure their compliance by controlling their thoughts and desires (Lukes 2005: 27).

In this form of power, thought control or the shaping of wants and desires can take many forms, many of them mundane and everyday. It can be through control of information by ruling groups, through the mass media, public relations (*spin*) and marketing, as well as through the socialisation process where we acquire our social values (Lukes 2005: 27). In this view of power, Lukes argues that political and social leaders do not *follow* and *respond* to public opinion but, through clever manipulation of public opinion and management of the news media, create and lead public opinion.

Another example of this is in the use of marketing and advertising to shape consumer tastes for a particular brand and to promote brand loyalty. Nationalism or political party loyalty in elections could be an example of brand loyalty as a result of day-to-day marketing and advertising on the political scale. The use of negative propaganda in order to 'demonise' opposing groups, individuals, or their view points and to sell the virtues of the desired course of action or groups could be examples of positive propaganda (Heywood 2007).

Again, governments may try to create the view that certain courses of action are in the 'public interest' or for the 'common good', such as the current round of public sector spending cuts or in spending large amounts of the national wealth to subsidise failing banks (Osborne 2010).

Perspective three: The 'dispersed power' perspective

This perspective suggests that power lies in the everyday and is dispersed widely and not monopolised or controlled by any one ruling grouping. In this perspective, the most important consideration about power is that it is immediate and everywhere but does not necessarily have a 'purpose'.

Power – the 'personal is the political'

On the most fundamental and basic of levels, our lives are shaped by the people around us such as partners, children, neighbours, managers and work colleagues, and others so that for many feminists and writers about gender and sexual politics, the 'personal is the political' and that 'politics is in everyday life' (Millett 1968, Hanisch 1969, Wright Mills 1999). In this view, power over us is not necessarily exercised by people in legitimate power roles of government, or necessarily through the structural system, but is ever present in the everyday relationships and dealings we have with the people around us.

The French philosopher Michel Foucault described the ever present nature of power in every relationship when he said 'every human relation is to some degree a power relation. We move in a world of perpetual strategic relations' (Foucault 1988: 168). He argued that we have a personal responsibility as to how and to what goals we exercise that power, but we also have a choice in whether we accept or resist the power of others.

Devito (2008) in his analysis of human interactions equally suggests that *power* permeates all aspects of our relationships and interactions. He also argues that we have a level of choice in our interactions with others, we can choose to increase our power *over* or *with* other people, or we can choose to withhold or limit the use of our power *with* or *over* others. Therefore, from this perspective, our partner may be a more powerful influence over our thoughts, behaviours, and day-to-day actions than any prime minister or president. Further, if someone is pleasant and friendly towards us, or if they are unfriendly and hostile, that may have more impact on us and our lived experience than any government law or policy, or a membership of any particular social class or grouping. Many radical theorists and radical feminists of the 1960s and 1970s coined the expression *the personal is the political* (Millett 1968, Hanisch 1969 and Wright Mills 1999) to illustrate this everyday nature of power.

Therefore, it is again asking us to be mindful of our own behaviour and the way we interact with others to avoid the negative and dominating use of any power we might have and to avoid underestimating the impact we can have on others. In the same way, we can hope that others will treat us in the same courteous and respectful way so that they do not seek to dominate us. This is one of the key anti-oppressive strategies explored later in the chapter, so that if power is everyday and in all our actions, there is something we can do to prevent or at least limit the vulnerability that someone else might feel at our hands.

Discourse and power

This third perspective also encompasses the view that power is everywhere in the form of the discourses and ideas, even in the words and language we use. These discourses represent the way we think and talk about 'things'; they affect how we see and interpret the world, people, and situations around us. Their influence is often subtle in ways that we may not always be aware of, and they may narrow or limit our vision of the world, people, or situations to a particular perspective. Power comes in the ways we are influenced to see the world and also in the way that our vision may be restricted to a particular version of events. Power is exercised through the way a discourse can guide and shape our thinking, utterances, and even our social structures. The key difference between 'discourse' and 'hegemony' is that in the second perspective, ideology and 'thought control' are used to purposely maintain existing power structures and the hold of ruling elites: in the dispersed power perspective, although power is exercised through discourse, language, and ideology, it is not specifically used consciously or purposely to uphold any single ruling interest.

Discourses are a significant component in any consideration of power; however, a fuller explanation and discussion can be found in Chapter 6.

Foucault and the concept of disciplinary power

Michel Foucault wrote much about the mechanisms of power in day-to-day interactions. He called this day-to-day power, *disciplinary power*. He argued that this disciplinary power is necessary to 'train' the individual and make us governable. In his book, *Discipline and Punish* (1979), he tried to analyse how power is exercised to make the running of complex societies possible.

Foucault argues that in modern societies, practices and technology have evolved that can give the impression that we are being constantly monitored, observed, and measured. This idea that we are being 'watched' or are under constant surveillance is sufficient to make us more conscious of what we are up to, so that we may self-monitor, self-regulate, and self-censor our own behaviour. This sense of being surveilled reinforces our 'inner cop' so we do not necessarily need external coercion; the coercion comes from within.

To reinforce the two-way effect of this process, just as we sense that we might be under surveillance, other people may be regulating their own actions because they believe that we have them under surveillance. Foucault says this sense of watchfulness and the sense of being observed is ever present, even if it is not really taking place. This *sense* or *perception* that we may be observed and judged is sufficient to secure our governability (Foucault 1979). He called this process 'governmentality' a play on words to suggest that power is psychologically exerted over ourselves by ourselves (Foucault 1983).

Foucault (1979) used the term 'gaze' to describe this surveillance and identified a number of possible processes and practices where the *gaze* of others can create a sense of being observed. He argued that these processes of 'gaze' permeate many aspects of our social world where we are frequently conscious that we may be observed and surveilled; the frequent sense that we are observed and surveilled may make us more accepting of that surveillance (Foucault 1979). Additionally, he claimed that the more visible and obvious the sense of being observed is, the greater the hold of disciplinary power.

Foucault says that there are three interconnected processes involved in this 'gaze', which facilitate this 'observational' power and control over each other (Box 3.17).

Box 3.17 Foucault's three processes of disciplinary gaze (Foucault 1979 and 1983)

1 *Hierarchical observation through gaze and surveillance –*
   - Through perpetual surveillance, information is collected about each of us, often by 'authorities', and through this we become accustomed to our place in the social order, we cooperate, and we even volunteer information about ourselves.
   - This gaze happens through educational assessments, medical investigations, censuses, job applications, and so on, even nursing assessments. These processes give us the sense that information has been collected on us.

2 *The examination* –
  ○ As well as simple observation, we are also expected to subject ourselves to regular examination whether it is educational, medical, or some other form of appraisal.
  ○ The ritual and regular collection of information about people is a symbolic act of their disempowerment.
  ○ The examined are expected to obediently submit themselves to the examination.
  ○ Humiliation may sometimes be part of this examination process.
3 *Normative judgements are then made about people*:
  ○ As a result of surveillance, observation, and examination, normative judgements are made by powerful people about the subject of their observation and examination.
  ○ Such judgements may be about someone's behaviour, willingness to cooperate, and reputation.
  ○ There may be 'penalties' for unacceptable behaviour or treatment for 'abnormal' behaviour.

These three processes of 'disciplinary gaze' facilitate what Foucault calls 'governmentality', where we all become governable and submissive to power (Foucault 1979, 1983).

Example of disciplinary gaze in medical and nursing context

Medical surveillance

Twigg (2000, cited in Forbat *et al*. 2009: 308) suggests that the 'the medical encounter is the supreme example of surveillance' . Forbat *et al*. (2009) carried out a study to test the effect of the use of handheld monitors by cancer patients to monitor their symptoms, as these devices regularly fed information back to the care team. The researchers theorised that patients might find this level of surveillance intrusive and intimidating in that information about their biological functioning was constantly being collected.

However, in this study, many of the patients interviewed found the constant surveillance and collection of this intimate biological data was comforting and reassuring, that rather than passive and docile patients, they felt empowered when data collected led to changes and modification to their treatment. This reinforces Foucault's notion that surveillance and gaze should be seen as neither inherently bad nor good.

> There is a need to question the straightforward assumption that being a patient with cancer and being under surveillance are uncritically negative … It is clear that the system is not a problem for people using it, and that the technologies of power are welcomed as aids in promoting patient empowerment, (Forbat *et al*. 2009: 313).

However, it also confirms some of Foucault's view about medical gaze in that patients came to be reduced down to sets of medical symptoms and shows the potential power of the bio-medical discourse in that they came to accept and welcome this surveillance of their medical symptoms as important in their sense of well-being.

According to Foucault, power does not reside in or with people or structures but is a result of the relationships between people. For him, power is dispersed and fluid. Power does not reside in governments but in people's willingness to go along with 'government direction', not through force or coercion, but whether they agree or believe in that course of action. Therefore, for Foucault, discourses (the beliefs, values, and ideologies of people) shape and create social structures and social practices (social behaviour). There is a two-way interaction; discourse shapes social structures yet social structures can create the discourse too (Foucault 1988). This effect can be manifested through the three processes of disciplinary power offering a much richer but more complex view of how power may operate.

Having considered the three possible theoretical perspectives on power, it is possible to use Thompson's PCS model to show the different levels at which these perspectives operate. The pluralist, dispositional theories of power suggest that it lies in the personal qualities, attributes, or roles that people have, reflecting a more *personal* level of analysis. The second perspective of power suggested by the Marxist and radical social structuralist theorists reflects a more structural view of power as reflected in Thompson's *structural* level. The final perspective on power, the 'dispersed view', which emphasises the role and power of everyday relations and discourse in shaping individuals and their social world, corresponds to a more *cultural* level analysis.

This emphasises that power is never simply understood by considering any one of these three levels: a more complete analysis is only possible through considering the interaction of all three of these possible levels of power. Equally we should aim to avoid oversimplistic analysis. People do not fit easily into *powerful* or *powerless* groupings; they sometimes have membership of both at the same time. Someone may be powerful at work, but as a woman may experience oppression outside of work. Equally someone may belong to a powerful and successful occupational group, but when admitted to a healthcare setting may become powerless and vulnerable. Also, people experience power and empowerment in different ways: what is empowering for one person might be experienced as disempowering by another (Fook 2002: 47).

Thompson (2007) argues that another analytical oversimplification of power is the assumption that power is always a bad thing. For some theorists such as Foucault, power is neither inherently good nor bad, it just *is*. Although it may have the capacity to hurt or harm others, it can also be creative and productive (Thompson 2007). Therefore, Thompson summarises that there may be four types of power:

1   *Power to*: the power to hurt or harm someone
2   *Power over*: to exert power and domination over someone and make them feel oppressed and vulnerable
3   *Power with*: the sharing of power to achieve real partnership with service users and others
4   *Power within*: the inner strength and resources to cope with life experiences and may require the practitioner to help build such qualities as self-esteem, self-efficacy, and resilience in others (Thompson 2007: 17)

The latter two forms of power can be the basis for more empowering approaches that can help reduce vulnerability and will be explored later in Chapters 5 and 9.

Conclusion

This chapter has explored the concepts of discrimination and oppression demonstrat ing their key role in the experience of vulnerability. Power has been presented as a core theme underlying each of these three concepts, as they all imply a level of helplessness or powerlessness in the face of some harm or threat. The concept of power has been defined and examined, pointing to its complexity and diversity. The manner in which power permeates through many levels of our social existence is illustrated by the different perspectives examined. It would be no exaggeration to suggest that 'power is everywhere'; it resides in our everyday lives, no matter how much we may prefer not to see it. It is a significant factor in the everyday experience of vulnerability, and as practitioners, we need to be prepared to recognise the multiplicity of ways in which it infiltrates our working practices if we are to reduce the potential for vulnerability.

Links to other chapters

- The 'Processes of oppression' whereby people can be oppressed and made to feel vulnerable are explored in Chapter 4. Many of these processes are further illustrations of the power to harm or hurt.
- The role of professional cultures and the way they may contribute to the vulnerability felt by patients/service users as well as care staff is contained in Chapter 5.
- Chapter 6 explores power of discourse and language to construct the experience of vulnerability and oppression.
- Practical suggestions of how to minimise or address the factors that can lead to oppression and vulnerability are covered in Chapter 9.

References

Acheson, D. (1998) *Independent Inquiry into Inequalities in Health*. Stationary Office, London.

Action on Elder Abuse (2004) *Hidden Voices: Older People's Experience of Abuse*. Action on Elder Abuse, London.

Adorno, T.W., Frenkel-Brunswik, E., Levinson, D. and Sanford, R. (1950) The authoritarian personality. Studies in Prejudice Series. American Jewish Committee Archives. Available from http://www.ajcarchives.org/main.php?GroupingId=6490 [accessed on 29 October 2012].

Aguinis, H., Simonsen, M. and Pierce, C. (1998) Effects of nonverbal behavior on perceptions of power bases. *Journal of Social Psychology*, 138 (4), 455–469.

Althusser, L. (1971) *Lenin and Philosophy, and Other Essays*. New Left, London.

Alvesson, M. and Willmott, H. (eds) (2003) *Studying Management Critically*. Sage, London.

Bacharach, P. and Baratz, M. (1962) Two faces of power. *The American Political Science Review*, 56 (4), 947–952.

Bacharach, P. and Baratz, M. (1963) Decision and non decisions: An analytical framework. *The American Political Science Review*, 57 (3), 947–952.

Bacharach, P. and Baratz, M. (1970) *Power and Poverty*. Oxford University Press, Oxford.

Barnes, C. and Mercer, G. (2006) *Independent Futures: Creating User-Led Disability Services in a Disabling Society*. Policy Press, Bristol.

Barry, A. and Yuill, C. (2008) *Understanding the Sociology of Health: An Introduction*. 2nd ed., Sage, Los Angeles.

BBC (2005a) Carers Jailed in Home Abuse Probe. Available from http://news.bbc.co.uk/1/hi/england/humber/4367587.stm [accessed on 7 July 2011].

BBC (2005b) *The 1980s AIDS Campaign*. Available from http://news.bbc.co.uk/1/hi/programmes/panorama/4348096.stm [accessed on 11 July 2011].

BBC (2011a) *Southern Cross Set to Shut Down and Stop Running Homes*. Available from http://www.bbc.co.uk/news/health-14106430 [accessed on 11 July 2011].

BBC (2011b) *Southern Cross: Your Stories*. Available from http://www.bbc.co.uk/news/business-14115183 [accessed on 11 July 2011].

Beauchamp, T. and Childress, J. (2008) *Principles of Bio-Medical Ethics*. 6th ed., Oxford University Press, Oxford.

Bilton, T., Bonnett, K., Jones, P., Lawson, T., Skinner, D., Stanworth, M., Webster, A. (2002) *Introductory Sociology*. 4th ed., Palgrave Macmillan, Basingstoke.

Brindle, D. (2011) Abuse at Leading Care Home Leads to Police Inspections of Private Hospitals. *The Guardian*, 1 June 2011. Available from http://www.guardian.co.uk/society/2011/may/31/abuse-at-leading-care-home [accessed on 21 July 2011].

Burch, S. (2001) Cultural and anthropological studies. In: *Health Studies – An Introduction* (Naidoo J. and Wills J eds), 1st ed., pp. 185–220. Palgrave Macmillan, Basingstoke.

Cambridge, P. and Carnaby, S. (eds) (2005) *Person Centred Planning and Care Management with People with Learning Disabilities*. Jessica Kingsley, London.

Care Quality Commission (CQC) (2011a) *CQC Calls on Castlebeck to Make Root and Branch Improvements*. Available from http://www.cqc.org.uk/newsandevents/newsstories.cfm?widCall1=customWidgets.content_view_1&cit_id=37478 [accessed on 27 July 2011].

CQC (2011b) Castlebeck Reports. Available from http://www.cqc.org.uk/newsandevents/castlebeck/reports.cfm [accessed on 27 July 2011].

Carmichael, S. and Hamilton, C. (1968) *Black Power: The Political Liberation in America*. Cape, Boston.

Child Poverty Action Group (2011) *Poverty in the UK*. Available from http://www.cpag.org.uk/povertyfacts/index.htm [accessed on 29 July 2011].

Clegg, S. (1989) *Frameworks of Power*. Sage, London.

Conger, J. and Kanungo, R. (1987) Towards a behavioural theory of charismatic leadership in organisational settings. *Academy of Management Review*, 12, 637–647.

Cooke, H. and Philpin, S. (2008) *Sociology in Nursing and Healthcare*. Churchill Livingstone/Elsevier, Edinburgh.

Curtis, P. and Mulholland, H. (2011) Panorama Care Home Abuse Investigation Prompts Government Review. *The Guardian*. Available from www.guardian.co.uk [accessed on 1 June 2011].

Dahl, R. (1989) *Democracy and its' Critics*. University of Yale Press, New Haven, CT.

Dalrymple, J. and Burke, B. (2006) *Anti Oppressive Practice: Social Care and the Law*. 2nd ed., Open University Press, Maidenhead.

Dearlove, J. and Saunders, P. (2000) *Introduction to British Politics*. 3rd ed., Polity Press, Cambridge.

Deetz, S. (1992) *Democracy in the Age of Corporate Colonisation: Developments in Communication and the Politics of Everyday Life*. State University of New York Press, Albany.

Department of Health and Social Security (1980) *The Black Report – Report of the Working Group on Inequalities in Health*. Station Office, London.

Department of Health (DoH) (2000) *No Secrets*. HMSO, London.

DoH (2010) Health Inequalities Archived Page. Available from http://www.dh.gov.uk/en/Publichealth/Healthinequalities/index.htm [accessed on 27 July 2011]

Devito, J. (2008) *The Interpersonal Communication Book*. 12th ed., Pearson, Harlow.

Dobson, S.M. (1991) *Transcultural Nursing*. Scutari Press, London.

Dominelli, L. (2002) *Anti Oppressive Social Work Theory and Practice*. Palgrave Macmillan, Basingstoke.

Dominelli, L. (2008a) Anti-oppressive practice as contested practice. In: *Value Base of Social Work and Social Care: An Active Learning Handbook* (Barnard, A., Horner, N. and Wild, J. eds), pp.115–127. Open University Press, Maidenhead.

Dominelli, L. (2008b) *Anti-Racist Social Work: A Challenge for White Practitioners and Educators*. Palgrave Macmillan, Basingstoke.

Fagge, N. (2010) Nurse Refused Dying Man Glass of Water. *Daily Mail*, 16 September 2010. Available from http://www.dailymail.co.uk/news/article-1312345/ Nurse-refused-dying-man-glass-water-took-mobile-phone.html?ito=feeds-newsxml [accessed on 08 July 2011].

Fook, J. (2002) *Social Work: Critical Theory: Critical Theory and Practice*. Sage, London.

Forbat, L., Maguire R., McCann L., Illingworth, N. and Kearney, N. (2009) The use of technology in cancer care: Applying Foucault's ideas to explore the changing dynamics of power in health care. *Journal of Advanced Nursing*, 65 (2), 306–315.

Foucault, M. (1979) *Discipline and Punish* (Trans. A Sheridan) Penguin, Harmondsworth.

Foucault, M. (1983) *The Government of Self and Others: Lectures at the Collège de France 1982–1983*. Palgrave Macmillan, Basingstoke.

Foucault, M. (1988) *Politics, Philosophy, Culture: Interviews and Other Writings, 1977–1984*. Routledge, London.

Francis, R. (2010) *Independent Inquiry into Care Provided by Mid Staffordshire NHS Foundation Trust January 2005–March 2009*. Stationary Office. London.

French, J. and Raven, B. (1959) The bases of social power, In: *Studies in Social Power* (Cartwright, D. ed.), University of Michigan Institute for Social Research, Ann Arbor, Michigan.

Giddens, A. (2009) *Sociology*. 6th ed., Polity Press, Cambridge.

Goodwin, B. (2007) *Using Political Ideas*. 5th ed., John Wiley and Sons, Chichester.

Gramsci, A. (1968) *Prison Notebooks*. Lawrence and Wishart, London.

Gramsci, A. (1971) *Selections from the Prison Notebooks* (Hoare, Q. and Nowell-Smith, G. eds), Lawrence and Wishart, London.

Hanisch, C. (1969) The Personal is Political in the Redstockings Collection. *Feminist Revolution* (204–205). Available from http://www.carolhanisch.org/CHwritings/PIP.html [accessed on 28 July 2011].

Hart, C. (2004) *Nurses and Politics: The Impact of Power and Practice*. Palgrave Macmillan, Basingstoke.

Harvey, J. (1999) *Civilised Oppression*. Rowman and Littlefield Publishers Inc., Maryland.

Harvey, J. (2010) Victims, resistance and civilized oppression. *Journal of Social Philosophy*, 41 (1), 13–27.

Heron, J. (2001) *Helping the Client: A Creative Practical Guide*. 5th ed., Sage, London.

Heywood, A. (2007) *Politics*. 3rd ed., Palgrave Macmillan, Basingstoke.

Higgins, E. (1987) Self discrepancy: A theory relating self and affect. *Psychological Review*, 94, 319–340.

Hinkin, T. and Schriesheim, C. (1989) Development and application of new scales to measure the French and Raven (1959) bases of social power. *Journal of Applied Psychology*, 74 (4), 561–567.

Hunnicutt, G. (2009) Varieties of patriarchy and violence against women: Resurrecting 'patriarchy' as a theoretical tool. *Violence Against Women*, 15 (5), 553–573.

Johnson, A. (2005) *Gender Knot: Unravelling Our Patriarchal Legacy*. Temple University Press, Philadelphia.

Joseph Rowntree Foundation (MacInnes, T., Kenway, P. and Parekh, A.) (2009) Monitoring Poverty and Social Exclusion 2009. Joseph Rowntree Foundation/New Policy Institute, York. Available from http://www.jrf.org.uk/publications/monitoring-poverty-2009 [accessed on 29 July 2011].

Joseph Rowntree Foundation (Parekh, A., MacInnes, T. and Kenway, P.) (2010) Monitoring Poverty and Social Exclusion 2010. York. Joseph Rowntree Foundation/New Policy Institute. Available from http://www.jrf.org.uk/publications/monitoring-poverty-2010 [accessed on 29 July 2011].

Lasswell, H. (1936) *Politics: Who Gets What, When and How ?* McGraw Hill, New York.

Laurance, J. (2011) The dangerous power of healing. *Independent on Sunday* online. Available from http://www.independent.co.uk/life-style/health-and-families/features/jeremy-laurance-the-dangerous-power-of-healing-hands-2325861.html [accessed on 30 July 2011].

Lawson, J. (2001) The role of citizen advocacy in adult abuse work. In: *Good Practice with Vulnerable Adults* (Pritchard J. ed.), pp. 288–305. Jessica Kingsley, London.

Lukes, S. (2005) *Power: A Radical View*. 2nd ed., Palgrave Macmillan, Basingstoke.

MacKenzie, I. (ed.) (2005) *Political Concepts: A Reader and Guide*. Edinburgh University Press, Edinburgh.

Macpherson Report (1999) *The Inquiry into the Murder of Stephen Lawrence*. TSO. Available from http://www.archive.official-documents.co.uk/document/cm42/4262/sli-06.htm#6.6 [accessed on 26 November 2009].

Marcuse, H. (1964) *One Dimensional Man: Studies in the Ideology of Advanced Industrial Society*. Routledge Classics, London.

Marmot Review (2010) *Fair Society, Healthy Lives, 'The Marmot Review' 2010*. Available from http://www.marmotreview.org/ [accessed on 28 July 2011].

Marx, K. and Engels, F. (1863–1883a) *Capital: A Critique of Political Economy Volume I*. Available from http://www.marxists.org/archive/marx/works/1867-c1/ [accessed on 1 March 2013].

Marx, K. and Engels, F. (1863–1883b) *Capital: A Critique of Political Economy Volume 2*. Available from http://www.marxists.org/archive/marx/works/download/Marx_Capital_Vol_2.pdf [accessed on 1 March 2013].

Marx, K. and Engels, F. (1863–1883c) *Capital: A Critique of Political Economy Volume 3*. Available from http://www.marxists.org/archive/marx/works/download/Marx_Capital_Vol_3.pdf [accessed on 1 March 2013].

Marx, K. and Engels, F. (1845–1846 [1999]) *The German Ideology*. Prometheus Books Publ., New York.

Mason, D. (1982) After Scarman: A note on the concept of institutional racism. *Journal of Ethnic and Migration Studies*, 10 (1), 38–45.

Mencap (2007) *Death by Indifference*. Available from http://www.mencap.org.uk/document. asp?id=284 [accessed on 08 July 2011].

Miliband, R. (1969) *The State in Capitalist Society: The Analysis of the Western System of Power*. Weidenfeld and Nicolson', London.

Miliband, R. (1982) *Capitalist Democracy in Britain*. Oxford University Press, Oxford.

Millett, K. (1968) Sexual Politics. Available from http://www.marxists.org/subject/women/authors/millett-kate/sexual-politics.htm [accessed on 28 July 2011].

Monagan, S. (2010) Patriarchy: Perpetuating the practice of female genital mutilation. *Journal of Alternative Perspectives in the Social Sciences*, 2 (1), 160–181.

Monk, J. (2010) To what extent is self-direct support actually self directed by people with learning disabilities. In: *Vulnerable Adults and Community Care*. 2nd ed (Brown, K. ed.), pp. 60–77. Learning Matters, Exeter.

Naylor, L. (2006) Adult protection for community care/vulnerable adults. In: *Vulnerable Adults and Community Care*. 2nd ed (Brown, K. ed.), pp. 111–128. Learning Matters, Exeter.

Naylor, L. (2010) Safeguarding adults for community care. In: *Vulnerable Adults and Community Care* (Brown, K. ed.), Learning Matters, Exeter.

Norman, L. (2010) Feeling second best: Elite women coaches' experiences. *Sociology of Sport Journal*, 27 (1), 89–104.

Northway, R. (1997) Disability and oppression: Some implications for nurses and nursing. *Journal of Advanced Nursing*, 26, 736–743.

Nursing and Midwifery Council (NMC) (2008) *The Code: Standards of Conduct, Performance and Ethics for Nurses and Midwives*. NMC, London.

Nzira, V. and Williams, P. (2009) *Anti Oppressive Practice in Health and Social Care*. Sage, London.

Oliver, M. (1990) *The Politics of Disablement*. Macmillan, Basingstoke.

Osborne, G. (2010) *Spending Review Statement to Parliament*, H.M Treasury 20 October 2010. Available from http://www.hm-treasury.gov.uk/spend_sr2010_speech.htm [accessed on 1 August 2011].

Parliamentary and Health Service Ombudsman (2011) *Care and Compassion? Report of the Health Service Ombudsman on Ten Investigations into NHS Care of Older People*. The Stationery Office, London.

Penhale, B. and Parker, J. (2008) *Working with Vulnerable Adults*. Routledge, Abingdon.

Peplau, H. (1998) *Interpersonal Relations in Nursing*. Macmillan, Basingstoke.

Podsakoff, P. and Schriescheim, C. (1985) Field studies of French and Raven's bases of power: Critique, reanalysis, and suggestions for future research. *Psychological Bulletin*, 97 (3), 387–411.

Postman, N. (1985) *Amusing Ourselves to Death: Public Discourse in the Age of Show Business*. Penguin, London. Available from Community Audio http://www.archive.org/details/Amusing_Ourselves_to_Death [accessed on 30 July 2011].

Poulantzas, N. (1976) *Political Power and Social Classes*. New Left Books, London.

Putnam, R. (1973) *The Beliefs of Politicians*. Yale University Press, New Haven.

Raven, B. (1974) The comparative analysis of power and power preference. In: *Perspectives in Social Power* (Tedechi, T. ed.), pp. 172–198. Aldine, Chicago.

Rungapadiachy, D. (1999) *Interpersonal Communications and Psychology for Health Care Professionals*. Butterworth Heinneman, Oxford.

Saunders, P. (2010) *Social Mobility Myths*. Civitas, London.

Shipman Inquiry (2005). Available from http://www.shipman-inquiry.org.uk/fr_page.asp?id=187 [accessed 30 July 2011].

Strega, S. (2007) Anti-oppressive practice in child welfare. In: *Doing Anti Oppressive Practice: Building Transformative Politicised Social Work* (Baines, D. ed.), pp. 67–83. Fernwood, Halifax.

Sultana, A. (2010) Patriarchy and women's gender ideology: A socio-cultural perspective. *Journal of Social Sciences*, 6 (1), 123–126.

Swain, J., Finkelstein, V., French, S. and Oliver, M. (eds) (1993) *Disabling Barriers, Enabling Environments*. Sage, London.

Swain, J., French, S., Barnes, C. and Thomas, C. (eds) (2004) *Disabling Barriers, Enabling Environments*. 2nd ed., Sage, London.

Thompson, N. (2003) *Promoting Equality: Challenging Discrimination and Oppression*. 2nd ed., Macmillan, Basingstoke.

Thompson, N. (2006) *Anti Discriminatory Practice*. 4th ed., Palgrave Macmillan, Basingstoke.

Thompson, N. (2007) *Power and Empowerment*. Russell House, Lyme Regis.

Thompson, N. (2011) *Promoting Equality: Working with Diversity and Difference*. 3rd ed., Palgrave Macmillan, Basingstoke.

Walby, S. (1990) *Theorizing Patriarchy*. Blackwell, Oxford.

Wilkinson, R. and Pickett, K. (2009) *The Spirit Level: Why More Equal Societies Almost Always Do Better*. Penguin, Harmondsworth.

Worsley, P. (1964) The distribution of power in industrial societies. *Sociological Review Monograph*, 8 (1), 15–34.

Wright Mills, C. (1999) *The Sociological Imagination*. Oxford University Press, Oxford.

Young, I. (1990) *Justice and the Politics of Difference*. Princeton University Press, Princeton.

Yukl, G. and Falbe, C. (1990) Influence tactics and objectives in upward, downward and lateral relations. *Journal of Applied Psychology*, 75, 132–140.

Chapter 4

Processes of oppression

Julie Ryden

Introduction

Having explored power as a phenomenon, we will now explore some ways in which power can be exerted, illegitimately, to create vulnerability. In many instances, the user of power is unaware of the power they are exerting; indeed, it is a feature of the processes discussed that they can become 'taken for granted' ways of interacting with clients, 'unthinking practices' which are shared by the staff group. Therefore, readers are urged to be open to reflecting upon their own practice as they read the following section. All of us have at some time used these processes or been present when the processes are used by others, and yet not realised the harm and vulnerability that may be caused.

Thompson (2011) has identified a number of processes which create discrimination thus leading to oppression, and for a fuller description of these processes, the reader is recommended to read Thompson's chapter on 'Discrimination and oppression' (2011). In this section, the processes will be outlined and linked to clear examples of their presence within contemporary healthcare. The processes represent various ways in which dominant groups or individuals can use their power to treat certain powerless groups or individuals differently and thus create vulnerability.

Overview of the processes

Thompson (2011) discusses eight processes (Box 4.1); however, he does recognise that this list is not exhaustive. Stigmatisation has been added for explanation here as it is particularly relevant within healthcare. A further process of 'othering' will be explained within Chapters 6 and 8.

As Thompson (2011) notes, these processes do not necessarily occur on their own, they may overlap or combine with others; thus, at times, it may be difficult to see one process in isolation. However, they will be addressed as separate entities here for the sake of a clearer explanation, whilst recognising the limits of such an approach.

Understanding Vulnerability: A Nursing and Healthcare Approach, First Edition. Edited by Vanessa Heaslip and Julie Ryden.
© 2013 John Wiley & Sons, Ltd. Published 2013 by John Wiley & Sons, Ltd.

Box 4.1 The processes of discrimination

Stereotyping
Marginalisation
Invisibilisation
Infantilisation
Welfarism
Medicalisation
Dehumanisation
Trivialisation
Stigmatisation

Stereotyping

Psychologists suggest that humans need to process a huge amount of social information each day, through meeting others, interacting with others, or watching and listening to media sources. As a result we can face an 'information processing burden' (Blaine 2007: 21) or overload, just getting through each day, and therefore we use 'categories' to label and distinguish between different individuals or groups (Allport 1988, Smith and Mackie 2007, Kessler and Mummendey 2008, Sanderson 2010). These categories such as man, woman, black, Asian, white, old, young, teenager, and baby enhance our efficiency in processing the vast amount of social information we face in our day-to-day interactions. However, we need more than a label to inform our interactions, so we attach stereotypes to the labels or social categories.

Blaine (2007) uses a filing system analogy to understand the process of categorisation and its connection to stereotyping. Instead of having our information about people on different bits of paper and in different books thrown around the floor, we place all the information into a filing system, with clear labels to differentiate between each file. This enables us to avoid sifting through ALL the information presented to us by social situations by only focusing on general categories. 'Stereotyping' then goes a step further than the file label and offers a *summary* of what we will find in the file; it gives more information than just the social category but saves us the effort of going through all the information presented in the file. The stereotype summarises key information about the social category; it is a bite-sized, 'all you need to know' shortcut to people and situations.

Thus, a stereotype provides us with a 'cognitive short cut' (Hargie 2011: 202), which enables us to react or manage our experiences without making the effort to find out about the other person. It provides us with a summary of pre-information on 'personality traits, behaviours, and motives' (Blaine 2007: 27). So for some people the category of 'woman' may come with an accompanying stereotype or summary of 'emotional, irrational, sentimental, soft hearted, and nurturing'. Equally, the category of 'lesbian' may come with the accompanying stereotype of 'masculine, dislikes make-up and feminine styling, and sexual predator'. As you can see the stereotypes may be true for some individuals but can be very inaccurate and untrue for many others in the category. However, the stereotype gives

---

Box 4.2 Time for reflection

1 Consider the following social categories:
   a Single parent
   b Person over 70 years old
   c Gang member
   d Substance user
   e Traveller/gypsy
   f Homeless person
   g Person with learning difficulties
   h Person with HIV
   i Gay man
   j Transsexual person
   k Person with multiple body piercings
2 Make a note of the *immediate* 'stereotype' that is conjured by the aforementioned social categories. Your first reaction is important here. What are the publicly held images of these categories? What behaviours, abilities, preferences, or desires would the stereotype lead you to expect when you meet someone in this category?
3 Choose two of these and find some writing, a magazine article, poetry, TV clip, song, or a film which portrays how a member of this social category might feel. Try to find material where someone from this social category tells you about their life or their feelings. Try to see the world as they would see it.
4 Now compare the results of points (2) and (3). Does the stereotype match the persons themselves?

---

us the illusion of knowing the person without having to spend the time getting to know them and suggests that all individuals in this category will fit the same summary.

This is a feature of stereotypes; they encourage a view where members of a group (social category) are seen as 'homogenous, with identical traits and behaviour patterns' (Hargie 2011: 202). This means that all those who share the same category are deemed to be the same and to have the same desires, abilities, and styles of behaviour. As a result, our interactions with such individuals are less objective; the uniqueness of the person in front of us is ignored, not appreciated, or dismissed. This can lead to irrational or emotional reactions to the person rather than reasoned and rational interactions (Hargie 2011). The stereotype fills us in on the information we need to make inferences about and understand the behaviour of those we meet, in a more immediate and quick way. However, the stereotype only prepares us for meeting the stereotype, not the unique individual who is in front of us. In order to consider this further, please undertake the activity in Box 4.2.

It would be highly unusual for the individual to completely match the stereotype. Stereotypes are often based upon small grains of truth for some people and sometimes lead people to 'become' the stereotype they are given (Blaine 2007, Sanderson 2010); however, in general, they are inaccurate characterisations of the full diversity of individuals. Stereotypes tend to be rigid, inflexible, and difficult to adjust or discard, even when further information and research challenges the stereotype (Thompson 2011). Additionally, they may on occasions occur automatically, outside of our awareness and with unintentional use (Blaine 2007). Thus, stereotypes can have serious consequences for the vulnerability of patients receiving healthcare.

Now let us return to the stereotypes you listed for the social categories in Box 4.2 and explore these further in Box 4.3.

Box 4.3   Time for reflection

1 Consider how these stereotypes might affect the care of patients.
2 Consider how a nurse who holds any of those stereotypes might treat a patient in that category.
3 Have you ever seen a patient treated differently as a result of a stereotype?

Box 4.4   Case study of Emma

Emma had a severe learning disability, which meant that she sometimes exhibited challeng-ing behaviour and had difficulty in communicating how she felt. Emma died on 25 July 2004. She had been diagnosed with cancer and her mother was told she had a 50% chance of survival with active treatment. However, doctors decided that Emma would not cooperate with treatment because of her learning disability. She was not treated and died aged 26. While she was in hospital, Emma was distressed and in pain. Emma was not provided with any pain relief for over two weeks; her mother sought legal enforcement for the hospital to provide pain relief. Eventually, Emma went to a hospice where her pain was well controlled until she died (Mencap 2007).

Now let us consider the real life experience of Emma (Box 4.4).

Is it possible that Emma's experience and the judgements made about her ability to 'cooperate with treatment' were based upon a stereotype of people with learning disabili-ties? One survey which asked members of the public to describe 'a typical person with a learning disability' found that their responses revealed a frequently negative portrayal focusing on 'characteristics such as having poor social skills, lack of confidence, shout-ing, being aggressive or slurred speech' (Turning Point, cited in Williams 2010). Possibly this public stereotype influenced the expectations of Emma's potential reaction rather than any full assessment of her actual reactions. Perhaps this stereotype dominated think-ing so much that Emma's distress was seen as being due to her learning disability rather than her pain. Potentially, Emma's distress and early death were increased by a dominant and negative stereotype attached to the category of 'learning disability'.

Consider finally, in this section, the following poem whose origins are uncertain (Box 4.5) but was thought to have been found in the bedside locker of a patient who had died after spending time in a care unit. Consider how many 'crabbit' old women or men are created in care environments by the stereotype of older people as 'frail, weak, unat-tractive and useless' (Williams and Giles 1998: 136). The exhortation of 'see me' not the stereotype is evidence of the harm that can be done by stereotyping.

Stigmatisation

A process which has close links to stereotyping is 'stigmatisation'; this refers to the pro-cess of allocating or creating a *stigma* for individual characteristics or behaviours. Erving Goffman initiated exploration of the concept of *stigma* in 1963, and this has produced continued research and debate within many disciplines ever since (Link and Phelan 2001).

Box 4.5 'Crabbit Old Woman' – Anonymous

What do you see, what do you see?
Are you thinking, when you look at me-
A crabbit old woman, not very wise,
Uncertain of habit, with far-away eyes,
Who dribbles her food and makes no reply
When you say in a loud voice,
I do wish you'd try.
Who seems not to notice the things that you do
And forever is losing a stocking or shoe.
Who, unresisting or not; lets you do as you will
With bathing and feeding the long day is fill.
Is that what you're thinking,
Is that what you see?
Then open your eyes,
nurse, you're looking at me...
...I'm an old woman now and nature is cruel-
Tis her jest to make old age look like a fool.
The body is crumbled, grace and vigor depart,
There is now a stone where I once had a heart,
But inside this old carcass, a young girl still dwells,
And now and again my battered heart swells,
I remember the joy, I remember the pain,
And I'm loving and living life over again.
I think of the years all too few- gone too fast.
And accept the stark fact that nothing can last-
So open your eyes, nurse, open and see,
Not a crabbit old woman, look closer-
See Me.

Goffman's original definition of the core concept of *stigma* referred to 'an undesired differentness' (Goffman 1968: 15) or a person who is 'less desirable...reduced in our minds from a whole and usual person to a tainted, discounted one' (Goffman 1968: 12). Stigma encourages us to focus upon '...an attribute that is deeply discrediting...' (Goffman 1968: 13). The important point to note here is the negative taint that is associated with the characteristic or behaviour, the 'differentness' of the characteristic or behaviour is to be seen in a negative, devalued, and inferior manner. It is crucial to note that the 'negative taint' is a view which is *created* by people, groups, or processes rather than referring to any real or objective truth or fact. This process of *creating* and applying a negative taint is the process of stigmatisation.

Stigmatising attitudes are evident within society; for example, Crisp *et al.* (2000) conducted a survey of public attitudes to people with mental illness. People with schizophrenia, alcoholism, and drug addiction were frequently viewed as dangerous to others and unpredictable. People with alcoholism and drug addiction were frequently rated as being to blame for their disorders and capable of helping themselves. Green *et al.* (2003) reported a general feeling from mental health service users that the illness 'marks you out as strange, and affects the way people relate to you' (228). Clearly they feel the effects of a negative taint created and applied by society.

Rogge *et al.* (2004) report that obese people are stigmatised, portrayed as 'unnatural, abnormal and unhealthy' (305), and experience similar judgement and condemnation as people with sexually transmitted diseases or lung cancer. Puhl and Heuer (2010) identified that Western cultures portray obese people as 'lazy, weak-willed, unsuccessful, unintelligent, lack self-discipline, [and] have poor willpower' (1019).

There are many other reports of groups of people who have been stigmatised by society or the environment they live in. For example, people living with AIDS (Scott 2009), people with chronic pain (Cohen *et al.* 2011), people who smoke (Bell *et al.* 2010), injecting drug users (Simmonds and Coomber 2009), people with epilepsy (Fernandes *et al.* 2011), people who are lesbian or gay (Balsam and Mohr 2007), and many others.

Given that these stigmatising views are held within wider society, it is highly likely that healthcare practitioners will also be vulnerable to holding such views. Ross and Goldner (2009: 562) cite research where people with mental health issues were deemed as wasteful of scarce health resources by general medical nurses. They were seen as 'not really sick', they had 'brought it on themselves', they were 'less deserving', and were 'blocking a bed'(Bailey 1994, Mavundla 2000, Happell 2005, Lethoba *et al.* 2006, SSCSAST 2006, Thornicroft 2007 and Picard 2008, all cited in Ross and Goldner 2009: 562). Creel and Tillman (2011) similarly reported on the stigmatisation of overweight patients by nurses. They found that nurses perceived overweight patients as 'unhealthy, "not smart", sedentary, and unclean…illnesses were attributed to their weight' even when there was no link between the illness and weight (Creel and Tillman 2011: 1346). The patients in their study perceived that care was 'reluctantly or grudgingly provided' (2011: 1346). These are all examples of a negative taint being applied, clearly these individuals have an 'undesirable differentness' (Goffman 1968: 15) in the eyes of the nurses. Please read Stefan's case study (Box 4.6).

Stefan's 'differentness' was the fact that he no longer had a medical need, he had been diagnosed and treated and now he needed to be 'somewhere else'. He was thus different from the other patients on the ward. His difference was devalued by the nurses; he was seen as not being worthy of the bed, that others were more worthy and more deserving of the nurses attention. Stefan had been reduced in the minds of some staff to a 'bed blocker'; his needs were not discounted, but perhaps given lower priority as a result of this view. This could be seen as the process of stigmatisation of Stefan who did not fit with staff expectations of 'worthy patient', someone who is worthwhile for them to spend their time and efforts on. Before we move on, let us take a moment in Time for reflection (Box 4.7) to consider this further within the context of practice.

Box 4.6   Case study of Stefan

Stefan had completed his treatment in hospital but it had been decided that it would be unsafe for him to return to his home alone, and therefore he was waiting for further assessment on possible residential care. In handover, the nurses would refer to him as a 'social', and this was accompanied by 'sighs', raising of the eyes upwards as if to suggest that it was a nuisance to have him on the ward when he did not need the care offered. One nurse stated that it was a shame when there were other people who were more deserving of the bed. Some of the staff left Stefan to the end of the morning to help him with his hygiene needs, as they felt his nursing needs were not as important as other patients.

Box 4.7   Time for reflection

Think back over your experiences in healthcare as a practitioner. Can you identify any patients or clients who were deemed by yourself or other staff as:

1   Worthy patients, i.e. worthy of staff time and attention
2   Unworthy patients, i.e. unworthy of staff time and attention

For each person you identify, try to think what was it that marked them out as 'worthy' or 'unworthy'? Which factors caused this judgement?

Link and Phelan (2001: 367) have identified five key elements in the process of stigmatisation:

1   People distinguish and label human differences.
2   Dominant cultural beliefs link labelled persons to undesirable characteristics – to negative stereotypes.
3   Labelled persons are placed in distinct categories so as to accomplish some degree of separation of 'us' from 'them'.
4   Labelled persons experience status loss and discrimination that lead to unequal outcomes.
5   Stigmatisation is entirely contingent on access to social, economic, and political power that allows the identification of differentness, the construction of stereotypes, the separation of labelled persons into distinct categories, and the full execution of disapproval, rejection, exclusion, and discrimination.

To apply this process to Stefan:

1   The nurses identified him as different from other patients on the ward because he no longer needed acute medical attention. He was therefore given the label of a 'social'.
2   The nurses as the dominant group in the environment then attached certain undesirable characteristics to Stefan – he was a nuisance, he was wasting valuable healthcare resources, and he was blocking a bed needed by someone more worthy of their attention. He was stopping them doing their job of caring for the acutely sick.
3   In Stefan's situation, he was placed in a separate category of 'unworthy patient' as opposed to the other patients who were deemed as 'worthy patients'. Additionally, it was clear that Stefan was positioned as 'them', since clearly the staff and their families (us) would never dream of being in the same position as Stefan.
4   Stefan then found that on occasions he was left until the end of the morning for help, and sometimes the help was rushed and he felt that his hygiene needs were not fully met. Thus, he experienced unequal care compared to other patients on occasions.
5   The whole process was allowed to happen because key people i.e. healthcare staff had 'power over' Stefan's daily routine, and the label had been allowed to be stated publicly in handover thus conveying that this belief was acceptable within this cultural group. The group had used their collective social power to approve of this stigma.

Box 4.8   Activity

- Choose one of the patients identified as 'unworthy' in your list (see Box 4.7).
- Try to apply Link and Phelan's five step process of stigmatisation.
- In particular, what were the consequences for the client (point 4)?

The next activity enables you to explore Lin and Phelan's five step process further (Box 4.8).

People who have, may have, or are rumoured to have a stigmatised characteristic are likely to be seen as inferior and not having equal status or rights (Serafini *et al.* 2011). Cohen *et al.* (2011) support this suggesting loss of status, discrimination and loss of voice; they become 'the unheard' (1639). Equally Green *et al.* (2003) point to lowered self-esteem, self-hatred, and shame. Clearly, stigmatisation has a major impact on the vulnerability of stigmatised individuals.

Marginalisation

This is a process whereby individuals or groups are excluded, isolated, pushed out to the margins, ignored, or not taken seriously (Hall *et al.* 1994, Thompson 2011). Hall *et al.* (1994) define the term as:

> ...the process through which persons are peripheralized on the basis of their identities, associations, experiences, and environments (25).

It is this concept of being placed on the *periphery* which sums the process up, being put or pushed to the borders or edges of a place, group, or society. In the process of being peripheralised, individuals are silenced or 'rendered voiceless' (Meleis and Im 1999: 96). They are devalued in this process, deemed as unimportant, or made to feel unimportant. The concept of being or feeling a 'second class citizen' is relevant here (Concannon 2009).

The process overlaps with a similar process of *social exclusion* (Vasas 2005) where individuals are denied access to, or participation in, societal or community life through various:

> ...exclusionary processes that are driven by unequal power relationships operating across four dimensions, economic, political, social and cultural, and at different levels, individual, households, country and global regions. (Popay 2010: 296)

Thus, marginalisation refers to a socio-political process that occurs at the personal (P), cultural (C), and structural (S) levels. Clearly, 'power' is a key element of this process, with power being used to push or place people on the margins. Let us have a look at some examples of how this may occur.

1   Geographical moving or placement of people or groups, for example, the previously familiar practice of positioning residential homes or hospitals for people with learning

---

Box 4.9 Case study of Bella

Bella was placed in a side room when she was discovered to have methicillin-resistant *Staphylococcus aureus* (MRSA). Bella hated being in the side room, and she found the isolation difficult to bear as she was a sociable person; however, she understood the reasons. Once she became clear of MRSA, a student nurse asked the nurse in charge if she could now be moved back to a bay. The nurse replied 'No – it's easier to keep her in the side room' and added as an afterthought 'Anyway who'd want to be looking at that'. Bella had a high body mass index and was labelled as 'clinically obese'.

---

disabilities or mental illness outside of urban locations, out in rural areas (Livingstone 1990, Killaspy 2006): Equally, this could apply to the movement of unpopular patients or noisy patients to side rooms or the furthest part of the ward. Certainly, placement of a patient is crucial in the experience of the individual themselves and other patients; however, when the movement of patients occurs more for the benefit of nurses, then marginalisation might be occurring (see Case study of Bella in Box 4.9).

It is essential that placement of patients in side rooms is carefully considered to ensure that the process is a reasoned and non-marginalising one. Initially, Bella's location in a side room was based upon clear and valid health reasons for herself and other patients; however, once she became clear of MRSA, the decision to keep her there might be seen as based upon invalid and marginalising reasons.

2 Social attitudes which exclude people through devaluing or dismissing the individual or group, thus reducing the ability to feel included and valued (Thompson 2011). Previous examples of stigmatisation would be relevant here in creating attitudes which devalue the individual and where such attitudes lead to their exclusion. Van Den Tillaart *et al.* (2009) researched the experiences of women with a mental health diagnosis and found that in common with other studies of this group, the women reported that their stories were discounted or not taken seriously in general healthcare settings. Their own self-knowledge was ignored by healthcare practitioners as if they did not know what they were talking about. Their voices were silenced.

Similarly, the Report of the Independent Inquiry into access to healthcare for people with learning disabilities (Michael 2008) found clear evidence of a dismissal of the contribution of parents and carers of adults and children with learning disabilities when accessing general healthcare facilities. Their opinions and assessments were ignored by the healthcare professionals, despite their expertise in understanding the individual and managing their care. Again their views were silenced by the attitudes of healthcare practitioners. It is argued that the attitudes lead to a dismissal and peripheralisation of the individuals.

3 Lack of effort or attention to ensure inclusion for all individuals in social, political, and economic activities or processes (Thompson 2011): Whilst this can refer to wider processes such as access to voting, employment opportunities, and community involvement, there are also more individual examples (see case study of Afaf in Box 4.10).

For Afaf, it was the lack of effort of care home staff and activity coordinators to learn her communication style or to enable other residents to develop a relationship with her, which marginalised her and ensured she remained on the periphery. She was

---

Box 4.10 Case study of Afaf

Afaf is a woman of 53 who has learning disabilities. She lives in a residential home for people with dementia – she is the only person with learning disabilities in the home. The care home staff tend to leave Afaf out of the social activities within the home. They think that Afaf would not be able to join in on an equal basis because of her difficulties in communicating. Afaf can communicate well if you spend time with her learning her style of communication. The staff and activity coordinators do not feel they have the time to do this. Additionally, when Afaf eats her meals she tends to make some mess, for this reason staff put her on a table on her own away from the other residents.

---

excluded from the activities which might have enhanced her social life and general inclusion within the home. By not being involved, the other residents did not get to know her, nor she them; this resulted in her being isolated, something that was compounded by the physical separation when she ate meals.

4   Wilson and Neville (2008) through secondary research on studies with older women with dementia and Maori women identified that care which is 'problem based' rather than individualised or 'patient centred' leads to marginalisation. Such problem based care is focused on the needs of the nurses rather than the patient, whereby care is centred on the disease, illness, or presenting problem and the workload required of the nurse. Thus, the assessment and care provided is likely to ignore the unique needs and social contexts of the patient. In this way, the unique needs of the patient are peripheralised, whilst care is centred on the nurse's perspective and role.

5   Language is another means by which marginalisation can occur (Thompson 2011). This can include not making translators available for someone who does not speak English, using medical jargon or abbreviations when speaking with patients, or using a language style that is not understood by the recipient, for example, using text speak or multi-syllabled words when the recipient would not use such language themselves. All of these examples of language marginalisation have the impact of denying the recipient full access to the information available to them. They are thus barred from full participation in decision making or social interaction and are peripheralised.

Marginalisation is a powerful process that overlaps with several others identified in the chapter; however, it is the distinctive element of being excluded, silenced, or peripheralised which captures the essence of it.

Invisibilisation

This process refers to the way in which individuals and groups are 'rendered invisible' (Thompson 2011), as if they do not exist. Thompson uses this term exclusively to refer to the way in which language and imagery paint certain individuals and groups in strong and dominant positions, while the contribution and existence of others is hidden. For example, the use in nursing textbooks of the term 'he' to refer to doctors and 'she' to refer to nurses. This technique which is widely used instantly hides the contribution of male nurses and female doctors. Whilst there may be reasons of convenience for its use, it clearly hides and

---

Box 4.11   Examples of invisibilisation

Sinead is a resident in a care home. The carers come in each day to offer her a wash and help with personal hygiene. The two carers arrive to wash Sinead; they help her out of bed onto a chair ready for the wash. During the wash, the two carers stand on each side of Sinead and have a discussion about their own lives. Sinead is between them and is being washed, but at no point is Sinead included or encouraged to contribute to the discussion. The carers are washing Sinead's body, whilst their attention and obvious interest is caught up in the conversation between them.

Ahmed is on a cardiac ward awaiting an angiogram. Each day the nurses/carers come along to make his bed. Ahmed is asked to sit out on the chair beside the bed, whilst the health carers make the bed. They engage in a discussion about their own lives and what they did the night before. At no point is Ahmed invited to join the conversation nor is there any eye contact with him to suggest he might be involved. The health carers complete the bed and walk on to the next bed, with a cursory nod to indicate Ahmed can sit back on his bed.

---

invisibilises the significant contributions of key groups. Readers are referred to Thompson for further examples of language and imagery as a means to invisibilise. Here we would also like to explore the way in which actions, beliefs, and discourses can also invisibilise.

The examples in Box 4.11 suggest that nurses can invisibilise clients on an everyday basis. These scenarios offer evidence of invisibilisation through actions rather than words. The carers are going through the actions of care, but their interest and attention is not with the patient, it is with their own conversations. It is as though the patients are not present, they are merely part of the scenery, not even bit players – they are invisible. There are strong overlaps with dehumanisation here, but there is equally a strong sense of the patients being 'blanked out' and invisibilised. Almerud *et al.* (2007) identified a similar form of invisibilisation for patients within an intensive care environment. Participants in their study reported feeling invisible despite constant monitoring and observation. Clients felt that staff focused more on the apparatus and technology than the person in the bed, and thus felt invisible as a person:

> The roar of technology silences the subtle attempts of the critically ill or injured person to give voice to their needs. (Almerud *et al.* 2007: 157)

Hence, the actions of the healthcare staff reflected a privileging of the technology and a greater attention to this than the person, who thus became invisible and silenced.

Another means by which invisibilisation may occur is through the influence of dominant cultural assumptions and discourses (see Chapter 6 for further explanation of discourses). 'Discourses' shape how we see the world, and we can only 'know' the world through the discourses we have been given through our lives:

> Discourses are inherited and acquired 'guides' for viewing the worlds, events, situations and objects we encounter. (Allen and Hardin 2001: 166)

In short, discourses refer to the ways in which we are encouraged to view the world around us and also include the ways we are influenced *not to see* certain aspects of the world. For example, there is a dominant discourse of older people which includes the perception that they are asexual, that sexual activity and interest ceases at a younger age (Price 2005). This discourse, which is fed to us by media images, peer and family influence, or everyday conversations, can lead nurses and carers *not to see* the sexual needs of older people – thus a key aspect of human life is invisibilised for older people.

This invisibilisation is even greater for lesbian, gay, and bisexual older people, who Blando identifies as 'the most invisible of an already invisible minority' (Blando 2001: 87). This invisibilisation occurs because of an ageist discourse of older people as asexual, but also because of the assumed heterosexuality of all older adults (Pugh 2005). Thus, the uniqueness of older lesbian, gay, and bisexual clients may be ignored because key aspects of their identity and health needs are invisible. The invisibility comes not because as individuals we want or choose to ignore such people and their needs; it comes because the way we learn about the world feeds us a belief that all people are heterosexual unless they tell us otherwise. Therefore, society feeds us an assumption and belief within the discourses we learn, which encourages us to assume that all people we meet and care for are heterosexual and this invisibilises lesbian, gay, and bisexual people. The added discourse which sees all older people as asexual therefore further invisibilises or doubles the invisibilisation of older lesbian, gay, and bisexual people.

Further examples of discourses which invisibilise are offered in relation to gender and heart disease (Emslie *et al*. 2001) and older men (Fleming 1999). Emslie *et al*. (2001) show how cultural and medical discourses influence the perception of coronary heart disease as a *male* condition, amongst the lay public. Thus, the cultural and medical discourses invisibilise women as being at risk of coronary heart disease and potentially prevent women who are at risk from the condition from taking preventative action. Fleming (1999) on the other hand has pointed to the invisibilisation of men over the age of 65 within dominant perceptions of ageing. He suggests that contemporary discourses on ageing have been 'feminised' to the extent that the experiences of older men are hidden behind the dominant image of ageing being about the experiences of older women. Equally, he argues that the dominant discourses on masculinity have focused on younger men and that the presence of older men is given little attention, thus again invisibilising the experiences of a large and growing number of men.

In Box 4.12, you are provided with the opportunity to think about times in your life that you may have felt 'blanked out' or invisibilised.

Box 4.12   Time for reflection

Think back on your own experiences through life. Are there any times or instances where you have felt 'blanked out' or invisibilised?
  Think back to being a child, a teenager, being a young adult, being a student, your first job, and later jobs. Think about when you watch TV or read magazines. Think about particular events such as weddings, christenings, going to the theatre or nightclubs, particular people, meetings you attend, standing at the bar, etc.
If you have experienced this:

• How this was done, what methods were used?
• How did it feel?
• How did you react?

Make a note of your feelings and reactions, and then consider how it might feel for patients to be invisibilised.

Infantilisation

This refers to 'the act of treating older people as children' (Kayser-Jones 1990: 39). Kitwood defines it as:

> treating a person very patronizingly (or matronizingly!) as an insensitive parent might treat a child (Kitwood 1997: 46)

Thus, adults are treated in an 'age inappropriate' manner, which Salari (2005) argues is a form of 'psychological mistreatment'. Indeed Kayser-Jones (1990) also describes such behaviour as a form of abuse. However, Kitwood (1997) does make clear that such actions are often undertaken with 'kindness and good intent' (1997: 46) (see Case study of Monika in Box 4.13).

This is an example of an infantilising interaction. Salari (2005) identifies four different types of infantilisation: speech infantilisation, behaviour infantilisation, activity infantilisation, and environmental infantilisation.

Speech infantilisation includes 'baby talk' (high pitched, patronising, and exaggerated tone), simple content, and inappropriate verbal intimacy, such as 'lovey', 'sweetheart', 'darling', 'sweetie', or 'my love' (Whitbourne *et al.* 1995, O'Connor and Rigby 1996). It can also include assuming the right to address someone by their first name without having gained consent or abbreviating names, again without checking e.g. Maggie instead of Margaret, Fred instead of Frederick. Additionally, the practice of using collective pronouns such as 'shall *we* take this off?' or 'let's stand you up' are styles of address that are more commonly used with children rather than adults (Ryan *et al.* 1995). Additionally, in the example of Monika mentioned earlier, the carer talks to her as if she is 'being a good girl' and offers strong praise to reinforce her good behaviour. These are examples of how a parent might reward good behaviour with a child. Salari documents such speech infantilisation with older people; however, research also points to this behaviour with disabled people (Gouvier *et al.* 1994, Liesener and Mills 1999).

Behaviour infantilisation is closely linked to speech infantilisation in that it refers to the manner of using speech or the way in which people are communicated with. An example of this is public disclosure of private information, such as announcing or commenting upon bowel or toileting requirements in a public arena. It can also include use of 'reprimands' or 'punishments' as an incentive for behaviour as would be done with children.

Box 4.13   Case study of Monika

Monika has been admitted to hospital for investigations. She is 93 years old. The healthcare assistant came to help her in getting out of bed:

'OK sweetheart I'd like you to get out of bed into this chair. So let's see if we can sit on the edge of the bed first.

Oh well done, that's very good. We'll just pop these slippers on first.

Now I wonder if you can stand for me, do you think you could do that for me?

Oh that's marvellous, you are being good for me' [*All spoken in a higher pitched tone of voice.*]

For example, 'if you get up now I'll get you a cup of tea', or 'you'd better be good today…we only like good people here'. Lack of choice or autonomy can also be a feature of behaviour infantilisation, so that commands, directions, or statements are offered without any sense of choice being available, for example, 'I'll open the curtains now', or 'it's time for you to get up now'.

Activity infantilisation refers to the involvement of clients in child-orientated activities, such as games, songs, stories, television programmes, or toys. An additional element of this is the lack of choice in participation, where clients are made to feel they *must* join in or that they are a spoilsport or killjoy if they prefer to avoid such activities. Child-orientated or meaningless topics for discussion, or asking inappropriately easy/trivial questions, can also indicate a level of infantilisation. There may be occasions when a client's health condition requires the use of easy or simple questions; however, infantilisation occurs when such questions are used *irrespective* of the client's condition. Assuming that clients would not wish to discuss politics, or to engage in a political argument, and instead discussing favourite foods can indicate a lack of expectation of cognitive ability as with a child.

Environment infantilisation refers to child-orientated decor or equipment, lack of space to converse or rest privately, or being enforced to join in communal groups. For example, with the chairs in a resident's lounge being placed around the edges of the room, the presence of soft toys, and enforced participation in group exercise activities.

Medicalisation

Thompson suggests this term to mean ascribing the status of 'ill' to someone (2011). The definition will be expanded here to incorporate ideas developed by Illich (1975, 1990), Foucault (1975, 1979), and Szasz (1973). Certainly, the act of certifying someone as 'ill' is a key element of medicalisation, whereby the individual becomes the focus of medical investigation, treatment, and management. It also conveys the power of certain prescribed experts i.e. doctors as the sole agents in Western medicine who are able to diagnose and prescribe care. However, the term can also be seen as referring to the harm that is caused by allowing medicine to be seen as the sole and dominant reference point for 'health'. Here scientific enquiry is used to 'know' the body, there is a strong reliance on medical expertise, for managing health and ill-health, together with a corresponding reduction in self-management of health or ill-health (Illich 1975). Further to this, Foucault (1975) suggested that medical power has placed the body as an object, subject to a medical 'gaze' (see Chapter 3 for further explanation of this concept). The body becomes a 'docile body' which can be 'subjected, used, transformed and improved' (Foucault 1979: 136) through medical knowledge. Indeed, Szasz is a fierce critic of the damage caused by medicalisation or 'psychiatrisation' (Szasz 1973: 507) in the field of mental health, using warlike metaphors to describe the impact of psychiatry such as 'conquest of human existence', 'invasion of man's journey', and 'psychiatric take-over' (1973: 506).

> Indeed, it is no exaggeration to say that life itself is now viewed as an illness that begins with conception and ends with death, requiring, at every step along the way, the skillful assistance of physicians and especially, mental health professionals. (Szasz 1973: 506)

Thus, medicine/psychiatry has become the dominant means for 'explaining' the body/ mind and is seen as *the* authority on the body/mind. To reject the dominant medical explanations and prescriptions is to be deviant, to be irrational, and thus to be encouraged away from self-determination and self-care.

So what does this mean for vulnerability? How does medicalisation lead to vulnerability? Many sources have shown how the power of medicalisation can and has contributed to the vulnerability of individuals and groups:

- Disabled people have been fierce critics of medicalisation and the consequent result that disability has been seen as a medical 'problem' to be controlled and manipulated (Scullion 2010). Thus, making disability a problem for the individual rather than a problem caused by society. So instead of looking for environmental and societal changes as a means to reduce the disability of living in a world dominated by an able-bodied perspective, medicalisation has sought treatments, therapies, and procedures to reduce the individual's disability. Medicalisation has reduced the person with a disability 'to a dysfunctional body in need of care' (Hayes and Hannold 2007: 360). Medicalisation has led to the position where:

  > medicine and the health professions have come to exert a position of control/domination over the lives of people with disabilities through the development of a knowledge/power spiral which has made people with disabilities the object and target of professional discourse and practice. (Hayes and Hannold 2007: 354)

- Many feminist writers have criticised the process whereby 'normal' and 'natural' processes in women's lives such as menstruation, menopause, and childbirth have been labelled as pathological and in need of medical intervention (Harding 1997: 144). Childbirth and reproductive processes have been seen to be taken within the hold of medicine, so that Caesarean section is becoming the birth method of choice, with a consequent dehumanisation of the birth process and a focus on the physical rather than social and psychological elements of the process (Gould 2002).
- Illich (1990) and Clark (2002) have pointed to the medicalisation of death and the process of dying. This has led to the devaluing and possible trivialisation of family and traditional rituals surrounding death and dying, with a loss of the integration of death and suffering into everyday life experiences. Illich points to the end of the 'natural death' through medical intervention and control of the process of dying (Illich 1990: 210). Death has been removed from the realm of the individual and family, to the medical sphere, with expert medical control of the process seen as being required. This can tend to increase the sense of powerlessness and dependency of individuals and their families. It can also lead to a desire to 'control' and 'manage' physical symptoms, thus neglecting psychosocial and spiritual needs as intrinsic to the process (Clark 2002).
- Hall (2003) has used her own experiences of living with cancer to bring to the surface the cruelty of medicalisation for people with cancer, in terms of the medical control and manipulation which they face. The way in which healthcare professionals impose their own view of health and treatment methods, and the imperative to 'wage war' on cancer:

In order to shield myself from a surprise attack, I must attach myself with a permanent umbilical cord to my putative saviors in the health care system, and do exactly what they insist, even when it is clear that they have not much to offer. For the rest of my life, no matter how long life goes on, I am supposed to be monitoring it, thinking about it, and giving it my precious time, energy, and life. (Hall 2003: 54)

The world that medicalisation threw Hall into was one of constant fear and vigilance, one of disempowerment, where her own decisions were viewed with derision or disbelief, and one of being vulnerable to the whims of medical practitioners and their 'useless treatments' (Hall 2003). This theme is developed by Cowling *et al.* (2006) to consider the wider implications of medicalisation beyond Hall's experience and beyond cancer and is worthy of reflection for all healthcare practitioners. Have a look at the examples of medicalisation in Box 4.14.

Hall (2003), Thompson (2011), and Cowling *et al.* (2006) all point to the insidious nature of medicalisation, to the extent that healthcare practitioners are so immersed in the medical way of viewing the world that there is no ability to see outside of it. It becomes the dominant norm, with no alternative. Anyone who does not 'conform' to medical opinion or prescriptions is seen as deviant, odd, a burden, ungrateful, and not rational. In this way, Joyce was dismissed for expressing her own autonomy as an adult, it was inconceivable to the healthcare staff that anyone would want to avoid the distress of continued leg ulcers given the solutions that surgery and science was offering her. Her own autonomy and reasoning was not explored nor considered important – that is the power of medicalisation to diminish an individual. Sanjay's 'irrationality' in choosing a risky life with the possibility of 'premature death' was explained as disordered thinking brought on by his medical

---

Box 4.14 Time for reflection

To what degree does medicalisation influence the judgements you make about clients and the decisions they make? Here are two real-life case scenarios (details altered for confidentiality). Reflect on these and consider:

* *Have you seen such behaviour amongst nurses?*
* *Have you yourself felt this way and made similar judgements about clients?*
* *In what ways are these examples of medicalisation?*

Joyce is an 84-year-old woman who had previously been a model. Her body and how she looked to the outside world was important to her. Joyce was admitted to hospital with chronic leg ulcers. The medical team advised Joyce that she needed an amputation to prevent continued distress and future health problems. Joyce decided that she did not want an amputation, that she would rather live with her leg ulcers. After this Joyce felt that the nurses did not spend as much time with her, and she noticed that they seemed rather rushed when they carried out her leg ulcer dressings. In handover, the nurses commented on the time and expense wasted on carrying out the leg ulcer dressings.

Sanjay had lived at home with multiple sclerosis (MS) for 16 years. His condition had been slowly deteriorating, but he still managed to live at home. Sanjay had begun to develop choking fits when eating. The nurses advised Sanjay that he should consider moving to a care home, where he could receive more supervision. Sanjay was adamant that he did not want to leave his home; he believed that he was coping, and if he should choke then he would accept the consequences. The nurses found this hard to understand and made comments amongst themselves that it was Sanjay's MS that was affecting his decisions.

condition, as there could be no other explanation. Medicalisation supplied the blinkers which obscured wider vision and consideration of Sanjay as an autonomous being.

These scenarios show the power of medicalisation in creating prejudicial judgements as well as the potential harm to clients who challenge the dominant norm of medicalisation. Vulnerability is thus increased through medicalisation, and the unwitting and unthinking way in which healthcare practitioners 'enforce' this viewpoint should be a focus for reflection for each healthcare practitioner.

Welfarism

This term refers to the tendency to assume that certain individuals or groups 'need' or 'require' welfare services just because they belong to a particular group or share certain characteristics, such as older age, disability, and caring role (Thompson 2011). The assumption suggests that such individuals 'automatically' require support from health and social services e.g. benefits, day centres, respite, and referral to support services. The case of Sanjay is an example – where the automatic assumption was that he now 'needed' 24-hour care in a care home. However, Sanjay did not wish to fit into this 'box', his choice was to remain at home, to take the risk, and to choose his own care environment. It is this 'autonomous choice' that welfarism neglects. It offers benevolent assumptions of 'what is best' and 'what is needed', without consulting the individual or jointly negotiating an individual route. This can be seen as patronising, demeaning, and disempowering (Thompson 2011).

Older people in particular are often the target of such welfarism. Walker and Walker (1998) comment on the ageist assumptions underlying the services available for older people, which assume a 'service career' movement from domiciliary care through day care to residential care. Such a continuum of service provision assumes that older people will 'inevitably' decline in their abilities and become dependent. Yet this is not the case for the vast majority of older people. Comas-Herrera *et al.* (2001) identify that in 2000, 5.2% of people over the age of 65 were in institutional care settings, whilst 4.5% were in receipt of home help or home care services. Therefore, 9.7% of the over 65 population were requiring additional support, which suggests that 90.3% of this population were not requiring additional support. Taking account of the greater potential dependency of people in the over 75 or 80 group, and also the invisible care provided by family members – it is still suggested here that to assume dependency and additional support is 'required' for older people is, as Walker and Walker (1998) state, an ageist assumption and an example of welfarism.

Dehumanisation

Thompson (2011: 97) offers a simple definition of the term '…treating people as things', which is supported by Haslam's 'The denial of full humanness to others…' (2006: 252). Suggesting that individuals are treated as objects, where people are no longer seen as '… persons with feelings, hopes and concerns, but as sub-human objects' (Bandura 2002: 109). Thompson (2011) identifies a number of ways in which language use can infer and create the sense of an object, for example, the use of terms such as '*the* elderly' or 'spinals' (referring to people who have spinal injuries – anecdotally heard by the author). Equally, phrases such as 'the hysterectomy in bed 4' or 'the bariatric patient' or 'the diabetic in room 6' all convey a partial and limited picture of the person. The full personhood of the individual loses out to one defining characteristic (e.g. diabetes, hysterectomy, age, spinal injury), which is all that the healthcare practitioners need to know about that person. A person with diabetes is so much more than their illness, and yet the use of the term 'the diabetic' suggests that only this one health condition is important about them. So instead of being a person with 'feelings, hopes, and concerns', they become a 'condition' or a 'thing', and this would suggest dehumanisation.

Bar-Tal (2000, cited in Haslam 2006: 254) defines dehumanisation as:

> labelling a group as inhuman … by referring to negatively valued superhuman creatures such as demons, monsters and satans.

It could be suggested that the language and attitudes used to convey mental illness could fall into this description. The terms 'psycho', 'loony', and 'nutter' used for people with mental health issues (Rose *et al.* 2007) could be seen as inferring the frightening imagery of monsters or demons. Indeed, a study of television programme content found that 44% of storylines over a three month period presented people with mental illness as 'harmful and dangerous' (Philo *et al.* 2010). Such imagery enhances the depiction of people with mental illness as inhuman. Nurses have also been found to hold such images of people with mental illness (Ross and Goldner 2009), so it could be suggested that clients with mental health issues may equally be dehumanised within healthcare settings.

Dehumanisation is not just evident in language and labelling but is also illustrated in actions and beliefs. To consider this further, it is worth beginning with Kelman's (1973) identification of two aspects of dehumanisation. Kelman suggested that dehumanisation occurs when we deprive others of both 'identity' and 'community' (1973). The concept of identity refers to a perception of the person as:

> … an individual, independent and distinguishable from others, capable of making choices, and entitled to live his own life on the basis of his own goals and values (Kelman 1973: 48)

Whilst the concept of 'community' refers to a perception of the person as:

> … part of an interconnected network of individuals who care for each other, who recognize each other's individuality, and who respect each other's rights. (Kelman 1973: 48)

From Kelman's first dimension, denying a person 'identity', it is possible to see links to infantilisation and medicalisation, where the client is offered limited or no choice in their care or in their daily routines, for example. Indeed, Szasz suggests that the process of psychiatric classification associated with medicalisation '… "thingifies" persons and treats them as "defective machine[s]" …' (Szasz 1973, cited in Haslam 2006: 253). Kelman's perspective can be explored further in the context of the following scenario.

Consider the case scenario of Charlie (Box 4.15) and reflect upon whether dehumanisation is present.

> **Box 4.15 Case study of Charlie**
>
> Charlie was a patient on a general hospital ward and was in a bay with five other male patients. Charlie had some mild confusion, but was generally very sociable and friendly. Charlie had a tendency to expose his genital area inadvertently, and some patients had made comments. The staff nurse on the ward decided to move Charlie to a side room. This was announced to Charlie just prior to the move happening, as his possessions were being taken to the new room. Charlie was not involved in the decision, he was merely informed of the move, and no reasoning was given.

This might seem an everyday occurrence on the wards, where bed moves are made, but the actions of the staff nurse convey more than just a 'rational bed move'. Charlie was subject to someone else's decision about where he would spend his time; he had already adjusted to the bay he was in and enjoyed the company of the other men. The staff nurse had made the choice for Charlie; he was expected to 'do as he was told', to have no attachment to where he was located, to have no feelings, hopes, and concerns about his environment. He was not even offered time to adjust to the move, it was happening as he was told. In short, he was treated as an object to be moved around as ornaments may be moved on a sideboard. The staff nurse's view was that Charlie was incapable of making a choice, as with any object, he was not offered the capacity as a 'human' to have an input in the decision. There was no exploration of Charlie's behaviour with him, there was no consideration of what was causing him to expose himself, no effort to help him to stay in the environment he enjoyed and was settled in. This situation could be said to meet both of Kelman's dimensions of dehumanisation (1973). Firstly, Charlie was not treated as an independent individual capable of making choices, so was denied his 'identity', and secondly, his place within an 'interconnected network of individuals' was withdrawn without any opportunity for him to amend his behaviour and remain with the community he had made connections with. He was placed in a side room alone. It might be said that he was denied his 'community'.

Opotow included dehumanisation as an extreme form of 'moral exclusion', where moral values and 'fairness' are not a feature of the relationship with another (Opotow 1990: 1). Haslam (2006) has picked up on three of Opotow's processes of moral exclusion, identified as 'milder forms' but which might also be considered under the label of dehumanisation here: *psychological distance* – perceiving others as objects or non-existent; *condescension* – patronising others as inferior, irrational, and childlike; and *technical orientation* – a focus on means-end efficiency and mechanical routine (Opotow 1990, cited in Haslam 2006: 254).

Psychological distance might be seen in Charlie's situation, and condescension has been illustrated within both infantilisation but also in the scenario for Joyce. Joyce was seen as irrational for making the choice she made, and whilst her choice was respected on the surface, the health carers were dismissive of her choice, and this dismissal revealed itself within the care she received. The issue of *technical orientation* might be seen in Michael's situation (Box 4.16).

This might be seen as a technical orientation, where the mechanical routine of collecting the observations took precedence over human contact. It appeared easier and quicker to

---

Box 4.16   Case study of Michael

Michael had lung cancer and had been admitted to a general ward after an acute episode at home. As a result he had become immobile, was confined to his bed, and also found it difficult to talk, but did communicate with short phrases and plenty of non-verbal facial movements e.g. smiles, stares, raised eyebrows. One day whilst his wife and daughter were visiting, the nurse came round to do his observations. She walked in, saying 'just got to do the obs', whereupon she fitted the cuff around Michael's arm, clipped the oximeter to Michael's finger, and after this directed the thermometer into his ear. Then she tapped the results into her pocket computer and then smiled and left the room. At no point did she converse, pass the time of day, or enquire after the well-being of Michael or his family members.

---

psychologically distance herself from the people in the room, in order to speed up her process of collecting the observations. This was her task to complete before lunch and she wanted to enhance her efficiency by avoiding human contact. However, it is precisely this avoidance of human contact, and absorption in the task, the routine, which represents the dehumanising aspect of the scenario. The ordinary human interchanges of asking Michael's permission to carry out the observations – asking if he minded her putting the cuff on, letting him know the results, asking how his wife and daughter were, even just talking about the weather – were all avoided in the name of expediency. Michael was an object, a means to her end of collecting observations, he did not have feelings, fears, or hopes, and he was merely a body to operate her instruments on. This could be construed as dehumanisation through a technical orientation.

Wen *et al.* (2007) examined the perceptions of 'welcomeness' and 'unwelcomeness' experienced by 17 homeless individuals in past encounters with healthcare settings. The responses regarding 'unwelcoming' healthcare encounters suggested being 'treated as a piece of meat', or 'being made to feel like you were subhuman'. Dehumanisation was frequently noted in comments suggesting that participants 'felt treated as an object and in a manner not recognizing their worth and personhood' (Wen *et al.* 2007: 1013). An interesting analysis of these experiences of dehumanisation is offered by Wen *et al.*, who draw upon Martin Buber's (1923, cited in Wen *et al.* 2007) concept of I-Thou and I-It forms of relating to the world to understand the dehumanisation experienced by the homeless people.

'I-It' represents the way a person relates to a thing or object whereas I-Thou (or more simply, I-You) describes the way in which a person relates to a dynamic being who has a say in defining who they are. In normal human interchanges, the expectation would be that people relate to each other in the 'I-You' manner, recognising the individuality and autonomy of that person. However, Buber suggested that people sometimes relate to other persons in an 'I-It' manner rather than an 'I-You' manner, that is, they relate to people in the same way as they would an object (Wen *et al.* 2007: 1012).

Wen *et al.* suggest that where participants described unwelcoming experiences, there was a consistency with Buber's description of an 'I-It' way of relating, where the patient felt that the healthcare provider:

> reduced them to an object, was unwilling to know and empathize with them, ignored or failed to listen to them, was preoccupied with their own agenda, and made them feel disempowered.
> (Wen *et al.* 2007: 1013)

Welcoming experiences on the other hand were likened to an 'I-You' way of relating, where the healthcare provider:

> valued them as a person, was willing to know and empathize with them, truly listened, acknowledged their needs, and minimized power imbalances. (Wen *et al.* 2007: 1013)

It could be said that the welcoming, 'I-You' style relationship was more conducive to reducing vulnerability. Indeed, the literature on dehumanisation points to the value of empathy as a means to reduce dehumanisation, since empathy requires recognition of the humanness of the client and awareness of their mind (Haslam 2006, Fiske 2009). Thus, empathy forces the health carer to offer a humanised as opposed to dehumanised approach to the relationship.

Trivialisation

As the name suggests this process refers to the undermining or diminishing the importance of issues. It can operate in two main ways: firstly, by underplaying or disbelieving a significant issue, and secondly, by an over-focus on trivial issues at the expense of the wider more major concerns. Let us examine each separately.

Firstly, trivialisation occurs when individuals trivialise or downplay the real and significant concerns of an individual or group (see Box 4.17).

The clear implication of some staff was that Moira's claustrophobia was not a reason for her to be anxious, and she should understand the 'facts' of the situation and perhaps 'get a grip on her feelings'. Her behaviour was unwarranted. This suggests that her very real experience of terror as a result of the claustrophobia was not being taken seriously; it was considered a 'trivial' factor. Thus, her experience was undermined by disbelief and a lack of understanding. As a result, Moira was 'emotionally harmed' and made to feel vulnerable due to trivialisation of her condition.

Secondly, trivialisation occurs by an almost opposite *over-attention*, but to the minor and trivial aspects of a situation at the expense of the more serious and significant concerns. Thompson (2011) offers the example of whether a man should hold the door open for women in debates about sexism or gender oppression. The argument is that this issue pales

---

Box 4.17   Case study of Moira

Moira was admitted to hospital for rehabilitation following a stroke. The only wards available had side rooms rather than bays and Moira was placed in one of these rooms. Moira was unable to mobilise as a result of the stroke and needed help to move from the bed. Moira also stated that she had claustrophobia and was concerned about the room. The nurses replied that these were the only beds available; there was nowhere else for her to go. Soon after she arrived, Moira started becoming anxious and using the call bell frequently. On one occasion she was found hanging off the bed, on another, she had pushed over the table beside her bed.

At handover, some staff could not understand why she was 'acting so crazy', 'she's lucky to have a bed at all'. They commented on how ridiculous it was to be anxious when she was in the safest place, adding 'she's just getting herself worked up'. Some staff had tried to reassure Moira by saying 'you're perfectly safe, no harm's going to come to you here'.

into insignificance compared to other aspects of a woman's daily reality. As a woman, I would rather that debates focused on the underrepresentation of women in senior positions or the lower pay received by women. These issues are of greater significance in my daily life than whether a man opens the door for me or not. Here, the excessive focus on a relatively minor aspect pushes aside and almost invisibilises the debates which should be heard. Thus, the over focus on a minor issue trivialises the real experiences of sexism in women's lives.

Another example refers to the frequent stories which appear around December time in the UK. The stories refer to councils not putting up Christmas decorations, or the 'banning of Christmas', or it's renaming as 'Winterval'. These measures are reported as being due to sensitivity to other religious groups or even at the direct request of Muslims. There is considerable debate and discussion in the media on this issue and 'outrage' is commonly expressed. However, these stories are 'urban myths' (Arscott 2011) or 'scare stories' (Siddique 2011), they are not based on reality or at best very loosely based on reality. Here, the debate on a minor issue pushes aside any discussion on the significant daily reality of racism; it can also have a divisive effect within communities by suggesting that Muslims have requested the change when this is not the case (Siddique 2011). Potentially, such debates may even encourage or embolden some individuals to diminish or trivialise other more significant issues of racism.

Debates such as the one about Christmas frequently employ the phrase 'political correctness gone mad'. The term *political correctness* is one which is 'usually deployed by people with a malignant rejection of attempts to encourage equality' (Fanshawe and Sriskandarajah 2010: 14). The term tends to dismiss and trivialise efforts to encourage equality and greater inclusivity. So to suggest 'political correctness gone mad' is not just dismissive but almost contemptuous about such efforts. These phrases thus encourage a dismissal and trivialisation of any efforts at reducing oppression and thus vulnerability and may act as a cautionary disincentive for individuals.

Conclusion

This chapter has explored some of the processes which can lead to discrimination and oppression. These are everyday processes which are clearly occurring within healthcare settings and which play a key part in the creation of vulnerability for individuals receiving healthcare. Many of the processes occur without us knowing, and readers may feel shocked at the recognition that they have been involved in such processes – however, this is not the goal of the chapter. The chapter has aimed to raise awareness of the insidious nature of such processes and to enhance the scope for personal reflection. The crime is not in having been an unwitting participant; it is in not trying to avoid repeating such practises through reflection and self-development.

Links to other chapters

- Chapter 2 explores vulnerability which occurs as a consequence between different groups in society.

- Chapter 3 examines the Foucauldian concept of 'clinical gaze' in greater detail as an aspect of power.
- Chapter 6 offers a fuller account of the concept of discourse together with further attention to the role of language in vulnerability. Additionally, the links between stigma and stereotyping and the social construction of vulnerability are explained.
- Chapter 7 offers a full and detailed account of stereotyping as a psychological process.
- Chapter 8 includes some psychosocial explanations for many of the processes included in this chapter.
- Chapter 9 follows up with some suggested strategies which practitioners can use to avoid some of these processes.

References

Allen, D. and Hardin, P.K. (2001) Discourse analysis and the epidemiology of meaning. *Nursing Philosophy*, 2, 163–176.

Allport, G.W. (1988) The nature of prejudice, Reading 1. In: *Stereotypes and Prejudice* (Stangor, C. ed.), pp. 20–48. Psychology Press, Taylor and Francis Group, Hove.

Almerud, S., Alapack, R.J., Fridlund, B. and Ekebergh, M. (2007) Of vigilance and invisibility – being a patient in technologically intense environments. *Nursing in Critical Care*, 12 (3), 151–158.

Arscott, K. (2011) Winterval: The Unpalatable Making of a Modern Myth. *The Guardian*. Available from http://www.guardian.co.uk/commentisfree/2011/nov/08/winterval-modern-myth-christmas [accessed on 29 May 2012].

Balsam, K.F. and Mohr, J.J. (2007) Adaptation to sexual orientation stigma: A comparison of bisexual and lesbian/gay adults. *Journal of Counseling Psychology*, 54 (3), 306–319.

Bandura, A. (2002) Selective moral disengagement in the exercise of moral agency. *Journal of Moral Education*, 31 (2), 101–119.

Bell, K., Salmon, A., Bowers, M., Bell, J. and McCullough, L. (2010) Smoking, stigma and tobacco 'denormalization': Further reflections on the use of stigma as a public health tool. A commentary on Social Science and Medicine's stigma, prejudice, discrimination and health special issue 67(3). *Social Science and Medicine*, 70, 795–799.

Blaine, B.E. (2007) *Understanding the Psychology of Diversity*. Sage, London.

Blando, J.A. (2001) Twice hidden: Older gay and lesbian couples, friends and intimacy. *Generations*, 25 (2), 87–89.

Clark, D. (2002) Between hope and acceptance: The medicalisation of dying. *British Medical Journal*, 324, 905–907.

Cohen, M., Quintner, J., Buchanan, D., Nielsen, M. and Guy, L. (2011) Stigmatization of patients with chronic pain: The extinction of empathy. *Pain Medicine*, 12, 1637–1643.

Comas-Herrera, A., Wittenberg, R. and Pickard, L. (2001) *Projections of demand for residential care for older people in England to 2020*. Personal Social Services Research Unit Discussion Paper 1719, 21 December 2001. Available from http://www.pssru.ac.uk/pdf/dp1719.pdf [accessed on 6 June 2012.

Concannon, L. (2009) Developing inclusive health and social care policies for older LGBT citizens. *British Journal of Social Work*, 39, 403–417.

Cowling, W.R., Shattell, M.M. and Todd, M. (2006) Hall's authentic meaning of medicalization – an extended discourse. *Advances in Nursing Science*, 29 (4), 291–304.

Creel, E. and Tillman, K. (2011) Stigmatization of overweight patients by nurses. *The Qualitative Report*, 16 (5), 1330–1351.

Crisp, A.H., Gelder, M.G., Rix, S., Meltzer H.I. and Rowlands, O.J. (2000) Stigmatisation of people with mental illnesses. *British Journal of Psychiatry*, 177, 4–7.

Emslie, C., Hunt, K. and Watt, G. (2001) Invisible women? The importance of gender in lay beliefs about heart problems. *Sociology of Health and Illness*, 23 (2), 203–233.

Fanshawe, S. and Sriskandarajah, D. (2010) Thinking outside the box. *Adults Learning*, 21 (7), 12–15.

Fernandes, P.T., Snape, D.A., Beran, R.G. and Jacoby, A. (2011) Epilepsy stigma: What do we know and where next? *Epilepsy & Behavior*, 22 (1), 55–62.

Fiske, S.T. (2009) From dehumanization and objectification to rehumanisation – neuroimaging studies on the building blocks of empathy. *Annals of the New York Academy of Sciences*, 1167, 31–34.

Fleming, A.A. (1999) Older men in contemporary discourses on ageing: Absent bodies and invisible lives. *Nursing Inquiry*, 6, 3–8.

Foucault, M. (1975) *The Birth of the Clinic: An Archeology of Medical Perception*. Vintage Books, New York.

Foucault, M. (1979) *Discipline and Punish: The Birth of the Prison*. Penguin, Harmondsworth.

Goffman, E. (1968) *Stigma – Notes on the Management of Spoiled Identity*. Penguin, Harmondsworth.

Green, G., Hayes, C., Dickinson, D., Whittaker, A. and Gilheany, B. (2003) A mental health service user's perspective to stigmatisation. *Journal of Mental Health*, 12 (3), 223–234.

Gould, D. (2002) Subliminal medicalisation. *British Journal of Midwifery*, 10 (7), 418.

Gouvier, W.D., Coon, R.C., Todd, M.E. and Fuller, K.H. (1994) Verbal interactions with individuals presenting with and without physical disability. *Rehabilitation Psychology*, 39 (4), 263–268.

Hall, B. (2003) An essay on an authentic meaning of medicalization. *Advances in Nursing Science*, 26 (1), 53–62.

Hall, J.M., Stevens, P.E. and Meleis, A.I. (1994) Marginalization: A guiding concept for valuing diversity in nursing knowledge development. *Advances in Nursing Science*, 16 (4), 23–41.

Harding, J. (1997) Bodies at risk: Sex, surveillance and hormone replacement therapy. In: *Foucault, Health and Medicine* (Petersen, A. and Bunton, R. eds), pp. 134–150. Routledge, London.

Hargie, O. (2011) *Skilled Interpersonal Communication: Research, Theory and Practice*. 5th ed., Routledge, London.

Haslam, N. (2006) Dehumanization: An integrative review. *Personality and Social Psychology Review*, 10 (3), 252–264.

Hayes, J. and Hannold, E.L.M. (2007) The road to empowerment: A historical perspective on the medicalization of disability. *Journal of Health and Human Services Administration*, 30 (3), 352–377.

Illich, I. (1975) Clinical damage, medical monopoly, the expropriation of health: Three dimensions of iatrogenic tort. *Journal of Medical Ethics*, 1, 78–80.

Illich, I. (1990) *Limits to Medicine: Medical Nemesis: The Expropriation of Health*. Penguin Books, London.

Kayser-Jones, J.S. (1990) *Old, Alone, and Neglected: Care of the Aged in Scotland and the United States*. University of California Press, Berkeley.

Kelman, H.C. (1973) Violence without moral restraint: Reflections on the dehumanization of victims and victimisers. *Journal of Social Issues*, 29 (4), 25–61.

Kessler, T. and Mummendey, A. (2008) Prejudice and intergroup relations. In: *Introduction to Social Psychology – A European Perspective*, 4th ed (Hewstone, M., Stroebe, W. and Jonas, K eds), pp. 290–314. Blackwell Publishing, Oxford.

Killaspy, H. (2006) From the asylum to community care: Learning from experience. *British Medical Bulletin*, 79–80 (1), 245–258.

Kitwood, T. (1997) *Dementia Reconsidered: The Person Comes First*. Open University Press, Buckingham.

Liesener, J.J. and Mills, J. (1999) An experimental study of disability spread: Talking to an adult in a wheelchair like a child. *Journal of Applied Social Psychology*, 29 (10), 2083–2092.

Link, B.G. and Phelan, J.C. (2001) Conceptualizing stigma. *Annual Review of Sociology*, 27, 363–385.

Livingstone, D. (1990) Mentally handicapped people, community care, and the general practitioner. *Occasional Paper Royal College of General Practitioners*, 47, 2–3.

Meleis, A.I. and Im, E. (1999) Transcending marginalization in knowledge development. *Nursing Inquiry*, 6, 94–102.

Mencap. (2007) *Death by Indifference*. Available from http://www.mencap.org.uk/sites/default/files/documents/2008-03/DBIreport.pdf [accessed on 17 February 2012].

Michael, J. (2008) *Healthcare For All: Report of the Independent Inquiry into Access to Healthcare for People with Learning Disabilities*. Available from http://www.dh.gov.uk/prod_consum_dh/groups/dh_digitalassets/@dh/@en/documents/digitalasset/dh_106126.pdf [accessed on 6 June 2012].

O'Connor, B. and Rigby, H. (1996) Perceptions of baby talk, frequency of receiving baby talk and self-esteem among community and nursing home residents. *Psychology and Aging*, 11 (1), 147–154.

Opotow, S. (1990) Moral exclusion and injustice: An introduction. *Journal of Social Issues*, 46 (1), 1–20.

Philo, G., Henderson, L. and McCracken, K. (2010) *Making Drama Out of a Crisis – Authentic Portrayals of Mental Illness in TV Drama*. Available from http://www.shift.org.uk/files/media/shift_tv_research_full.pdf [accessed on 22 June 2011].

Popay, J. (2010) Understanding and tackling social exclusion. *Journal of Research in Nursing*, 15 (4), 295–297.

Price, E. (2005) All but invisible: Older gay men and lesbians. *Nursing Older People*, 17 (4), 16–18.

Pugh, S. (2005) Assessing the cultural needs of older lesbians and gay men: Implications for practice. *Practice*, 17 (3), 207–218.

Puhl, R.M. and Heuer, C.A. (2010) Obesity stigma: Important considerations for public health. *American Journal of Public Health*, 100 (6), 1019–1028.

Rogge, M.M., Greenwald, M. and Golden, A. (2004) Obesity, stigma and civilised oppression. *Advances in Nursing Science*, 27 (4), 301–315.

Rose, D., Thornicroft, G., Pinfold, V. and Kassam, A. (2007) 250 labels used to stigmatise people with mental illness. *BMC Health Services Research*, 7, 97.

Ross, C.A. and Goldner, E.M. (2009) Stigma, negative attitudes and discrimination towards mental illness within the nursing profession: A review of the literature. *Journal of Psychiatric and Mental Health Nursing*, 16, 558–567.

Ryan, E., Hummert, M.L. and Boich, L. (1995) Communication predicaments of aging: Patronizing behaviour toward older adults. *Journal of Language and Social Psychology*, 14, 144–166.

Salari, S.M. (2005) Infantilisation as elder mistreatment: Evidence from five adult day centers. *Journal of Elder Abuse and Neglect*, 17 (4), 53–91.

Sanderson, C.A. (2010) *Social Psychology*. John Wiley and Sons, Hoboken.

Scott, A. (2009) Illness meaning of AIDS among women with HIV: Merging immunology and life experience. *Qualitative Health Research*, 19 (4): 454–465.

Scullion, P.A. (2010) Models of disability: Their influence in nursing and potential role in challenging discrimination. *Journal of Advanced Nursing*, 66 (3), 697–707.

Serafini, G., Pompili, M., Haghighat, R., Pucci, D., Pastina, M., Lester, D., Angeletti, G., Tatarelli, R. and Girardi, P. (2011) Stigmatization of schizophrenia as perceived by nurses, medical doctors, medical students and patients. *Journal of Psychiatric and Mental Health Nursing*, 18, 576–585.

Siddique, H. (2011) Christmas is not Just for Christians. *The Guardian*. Available from http://www.guardian.co.uk/world/2011/dec/24/christianity-religion [accessed on 29 May 2012.

Simmonds, L. and Coomber, R. (2009) Injecting drug users: A stigmatized and stigmatizing population. *International Journal of Drug Policy*, 20 (2), 121–130.

Smith, E.R. and Mackie, D.M. (2007) *Social Psychology*. 3rd ed., Psychology Press, Taylor and Francis Group, Hove.

Szasz, T.S. (1973) Ideology and insanity. *International Social Science Journal*, 25 (4), 504–511.

Thompson, N. (2011) *Promoting Equality: Working with Diversity and Difference*. 3rd ed., Palgrave Macmillan, Basingstoke.

Van Den Tillaart, S., Kurtz, D. and Cash, P. (2009) Powerlessness, marginalized identity, and silencing of health concerns: Voiced realities of women living with a mental health diagnosis. *International Journal of Mental Health Nursing*, 18, 153–163.

Vasas, E.B. (2005) Examining the margins – a concept analysis of marginalization. *Advances in Nursing Science*, 28 (3), 194–202.

Walker, A. and Walker, C. (1998) Normalisation and 'normal' ageing: The social construction of dependency among older people with learning difficulties. *Disability and Society*, 13 (1), 125–142.

Wen, C.K., Hudak, P.L. and Hwang, S.W. (2007) Homeless people's perceptions of welcomeness and unwelcomeness in healthcare encounters. *Journal of General Internal Medicine*, 22 (7), 1011–1017.

Whitbourne, S., Culgin, S. and Cassidy, E. (1995) Evaluation of infantilizing intonation and content of speech directed at the aged. *International Journal of Aging and Human Development*, 41 (2), 109–116.

Williams, R. (2010) Poll Reveals Widespread Discrimination Against People with Learning Disabilities. *The Guardian*. Available from http://www.guardian.co.uk/society/2010/jul/14/discrimination-learning-disabilities [accessed on 1 June 2012].

Williams, A. and Giles, H. (1998) Communication of ageism. In: *Communicating Prejudice* (Hecht, M.L. ed.), pp. 136–160. Sage Publications, Thousand Oaks.

Wilson, D. and Neville, S. (2008) Nursing their way not our way: Working with vulnerable and marginalised populations. *Contemporary Nurse*, 27 (2), 165–176.

Chapter 5

Professional culture and vulnerability

Karen Cooper and Janet Scammell

Introduction

Working with people with health care needs can be challenging but also very rewarding. It is an enormous privilege but rightly brings with it certain roles and responsibilities to which they are held to account. Health care professionals belong to professional groups and learn the art and science of their work from experienced and often expert practitioners and educators. Part of this learning involves exposure to the knowledge, skills, and values that underpin their profession. Through interaction with practice and practitioners, students are socialised into the culture of that profession.

This chapter will explore the relationship between professional socialisation and the experience of vulnerability. In keeping with the ethos of the book, it is accepted that we are all vulnerable particularly when in unfamiliar or frightening situations. This may apply when experiencing a health care problem or indeed as a student on a health care course, when the fear of causing harm is very real. Both situations demand the empathetic response of a caring professional. However, the wider working environment affects the behaviour of an individual. It will be suggested that the culture of a professional group either as a whole or operating in a specific locality influences the way in which care or practice is experienced and as such can increase or decrease a person's experience of vulnerability.

The concept of professional socialisation will first be explored and linked to personal and professional values as well as public expectations of health care practitioners. The values underpinning professional codes of practice will be considered, focusing on the central importance of advocacy and empowerment in the promotion of anti-oppressive practice. Drawing upon Thompson's (2011) PCS model, it is suggested that the implementation of personally held and structurally determined anti-oppressive values depends upon the prevailing professional culture. This will be explored using examples mainly from nursing, although many of the issues are transferable to other professional groups. The impact of oppression on practitioners and students will be considered, concluding with suggestions on how to challenge oppressive working cultures and improve client care and with it job satisfaction.

Understanding Vulnerability: A Nursing and Healthcare Approach, First Edition. Edited by Vanessa Heaslip and Julie Ryden.

The influence of professional culture on vulnerability will be explored from the perspective of a health care student. It would be useful for you to think of your own experience as a student particularly as you work through the chapter activities. *Lucy's story* (Box 5.1) reflects an amalgam of different but not uncommon student experiences. Read this first before moving onto the main body of the chapter.

Box 5.1   Lucy's story

Lucy started her health care course aged 28, following several administrative jobs. She was excited, keen to learn, and looked forward to having a career where she felt she could 'make a difference' for people. The first term at university was interesting and varied, including topics such as sociology, anatomy and physiology, psychology, and communication. She learned about terms such as holism, patient-centred care, empathy, compassion, and empowerment and felt comfortable that these ideas reflected her own views about care. As her first practice placement approached, she looked forward to applying some of her learning in the classroom to practice. Prior to starting, she contacted the placement, introduced herself, and found out about the learning opportunities that might be available. Although slightly anxious about what to expect, she was looking forward to giving direct patient care and being part of a team.

During the first placement experience, Lucy enjoyed learning new skills and interacting with the patients. She respected her practice assessors and was slightly in awe of how knowledgeable they were. She had lots of positive experiences but was challenged at times by how much there was to learn, expectations of students, and at times wondered whether she would remember everything! Lucy became more aware of the demands on the staff – documentation, patient care, teaching, and assessing responsibilities. Lucy tried her best to help the staff and patients as much as possible and often felt tired at the end of a shift. Sometimes, Lucy felt that she did not have as much time as she would have liked to spend with patients because there were so many things to do. She often felt pressurised to get the jobs done.

Lucy became aware that sometimes the staff were so busy that patient care was compromised, communication was brief, and patients were asked to wait without any explanation. She noticed that some staff appeared unhappy in their role, worrying about all the tasks they had to do and would occasionally appear frustrated and unsympathetic to patients' requests. At times, she felt they were not supportive with each other or the students. Lucy felt that she therefore had to help the staff as much as possible rather than asking questions or investigating potential learning opportunities. She did not want to be labelled a 'difficult student'; she was hoping to be valued as part of the team and receive positive feedback from her assessors. She thought about the theory she had learned and accepted that at times it was not possible to achieve the best quality care and that compromises had to be made.

When Lucy returned to university, she reflected on her placement experiences and discussed some of these with her group. She thought about the differences she had observed between the mentors she had worked with and identified the key attributes that made some mentors excellent role models. She reflected on both positive and negative situations and became aware that she felt unable to challenge or question the staff about some of the things that she had seen. This surprised Lucy as her family and previous employers often discussed how Lucy constantly asked questions, was resourceful, and led others.

In her future placements, Lucy became more confident and competent in her practice skills. She started to reflect more and was able to clearly identify 'good placements' as those where the patient was at the centre of care and fully involved in decision making. She reflected on experiences where care could have been improved and began to wonder if she could have done things differently. As Lucy progressed through the course, she found she became more confident to challenge her practice assessors and others about care concerns, although sometimes felt this was not welcomed. In her final year, she enjoyed managing a caseload and teaching others. She realised that she was modelling practice she had seen from some of the excellent practitioners she had worked with and aspired to be like them.

Professional socialisation

From birth, individuals interact with others and all aspects of their environment and in so doing their behaviour is modified (Giddens 2006). This process is known as socialisation and is the mechanism through which people learn how to act within a given society. Professional socialisation has been defined as the process by which an individual learns the culture of a profession (White and Ewan, 1991). Chapter 3 introduced and explained the concept of 'culture', and here we want to further explore this issue in relation to professional cultures. For health care professions such as nursing, a key outcome of the undergraduate education programme is to gradually socialise the student into their future professional role (Fitzpatrick *et al.* 1996). According to Cohen (1981: 14) this is a

> Complex process by which a person acquires the knowledge, skills, and sense of occupational identity that is characteristic of a member of that profession. It involves the internalisation of the values and norms of the group into the person's own behaviour and self-conception. In the process a person gives up the societal and media stereotypes prevalent in our culture and adopts those held by members of that profession.

As this definition indicates, the values and norms of a specific group are central to notions of group identity and indeed group self-image. However, just as the way we talk about ourselves may not always reflect the way we act, so also is the case with professional groups. In the latter case, organisational culture has a part to play; Davies *et al.* (2000) state that colleagues shared beliefs, attitudes, values, and norms of behaviour are reflected in their shared perception of situations and this is crucial to the way organisations function. Insiders may not be fully aware of this but outsiders coming into an organisation quickly ascertain whether people are 'friendly' or 'caring', for example. Thompson (2003) acknowledges that organisational norms and values are often apparent to newcomers as 'that's the way we do things round here'. Ideally, individual practitioners will find congruence between their personal values, their professional values, and those of the organisation for whom they work. However, some may feel vulnerable if they find they are working with conflicting cultural norms. Spouse (2003) recognised that students face particular difficulties in this respect, being transient team members that move between several clinical settings for placement experience. Spouse found that students felt they had to conform to local practices or face negative consequences particularly in terms of their relationship with their practice assessor. Furthermore, Stacey *et al.* (2011) identified that having to cope with conflict over values may affect an individual's capacity to work with people in distress.

Personal values

Clearly, in order to challenge inappropriate organisational values, it is important to have a strong sense of one's own personal values. Values are culturally defined (Giddens 2006) and are held by individuals or groups. As part of our primary socialisation, we develop our values initially from those involved in our upbringing, usually families and educational institutions. Secondary socialisation involves the influence of wider society (Clouder 2003) when our beliefs are affected by other significant groups and cultures and especially by the mass media. Values are central to the way we view the world as they determine our attitudes towards what is good or bad, right or wrong and therefore impact on our behaviour.

It is likely that in selecting an occupation we will look for some match between our perception of occupational values and our own personal values. For those working in public sector occupations, for example, ideas of service are likely to predominate and in health services, compassionate care (Maben *et al.* 2010). For example, a study by Stacey *et al.* (2011) found that person-centred care was one of the core values of health care students as they entered professional education. These values were reinforced when students worked with like-minded practitioners who acted as positive role models during the programme. However, Fagermoen (1997) identified that practitioners held both other-orientated values and self-orientated values. Other-orientated values included upholding the rights, trust, and humanness of individuals and attending to the need for protection and help. Self-orientated values were linked to independence, stimulation, and achievement. A study by Mackintosh (2006) however indicated that whilst caring values were of prime importance in nursing students in the first year of their programme, lack of reinforcement in practice and an emphasis on technical tasks weakened commitment to person-centred care. She found that some students developed an 'emotional hardening' (Mackintosh 2006: 959) which was a form of self-preservation required in order to cope with the emotional challenges in the clinical setting (this is explored further in chapter 2). Pearcey (2007) also found that the structure of nursing work focused on rituals and tasks which detracted from holistic care. These findings support the work of Kelly (1998) on professional socialisation in nursing which indicated that students often experience conflict between the values they hold and develop during their education and their ability to apply them in the workplace.

Professional values

Whilst appropriate personal values are vital for aspiring practitioners, clearly this is not enough. Health care professionals (including students) in the UK are subject to the rules and policies of their professional regulatory body (see activity in Box 5.2).

Box 5.2   Activity

Early in the first year of Lucy's programme, she is introduced to the Standards of Conduct, Performance, and Ethics set down by the body responsible for regulating her health care profession. Find a web-based copy of the code related to your profession and make a list of values that you feel are embedded in this professional code.

The main institutions are the Health Professions Council (HPC) for professions allied to medicine; the Nursing and Midwifery Council (NMC) for nurses, midwives, and health visitors; and the General Medical Council (GMC) for doctors. The aims of these important bodies are largely shared: to safeguard public health and well-being and to regulate the work of health care professionals in the UK. This includes promoting good practice, setting standards for education and training, maintaining a register of appropriately qualified practitioners, and investigating practitioners whose fitness to practice is in doubt (NMC 2010a, GMC 2012a, HPC 2012a). Regulatory bodies' remits extend beyond providing a professional organisation; increasingly, service users and carers are extensively involved in the work of these organisations to ensure that public protection and meeting public expectations remain the top priorities.

The GMC and the NMC are also statutory bodies meaning that they have legally prescribed governance roles; they are accountable to Parliament and members of the public. One major way they fulfil this role is to give guidance to practitioners on matters of professional conduct, performance, and ethics. This guidance is enshrined in professional and ethical codes, and these reflect the central values that underpin the work and behaviour of health professionals.

Table 5.1   Examples of professional values apparent within professional codes for health professionals.

Professional values	NMC	GMC	HPC
Act in the best interests of service users at all times	√	√	√
Maintain trust and confidentiality	√	√	√
Maintain high standards of personal conduct	√	√	√
Be trustworthy	√	√	√
Communicate effectively and with respect	√	√	√
Gain informed consent	√	√	√
Behave with honesty and integrity	√	√	√
Keep knowledge up to date	√	√	√
Collaborate with others in care	√	√	√
Duty to raise concerns	√	√	√
Provide high standards of care	√		√
Respect dignity	√		
Treat people kindly and considerately	√		

Sources: Data from NMC (2008) *Standards of conduct, performance and ethics for nurses and midwives*; GMC (2006) *Guidance on good medical practice*; HPC (2008) *Standards of conduct, performance and ethics*.

Whilst the professional codes differ to some extent across the three regulatory bodies, many of the values that underpin the different professions are the same (Table 5.1). If you had problems identifying the values, just think about what you would want from health care professionals if you or someone you care about were a recipient of heath care. Here are some suggestions drawn from the three codes:

When things go wrong

Professional codes are essential in order to 'police' members of a profession to ensure that standards set by the professional body (which is accountable to the public) are maintained. The codes are developed by the professional body increasingly in conjunction with service users and as such generally reflect the personal values of the vast majority of practitioners. In this respect, although the professional body is obliged to take action if an individual falls below these standards, so are fellow practitioners in order to uphold the integrity of their profession. Most practitioners take pride in providing excellent care; however, sometimes practice on the ground can significantly fall short of public and professional expectations (Healthcare Commission 2009, CQC 2011, Parliamentary and Health Service Ombudsman Report 2011); Patients Association (2009, 2011) and *No Secrets* (DoH 2000). Despite clear professional standards, reflecting laudable values, why is it that 'good' people allow 'bad' things to happen?

The Parliamentary and Health Service Ombudsman (2011) presented investigations of ten complaints concerning the care of older people by the NHS in hospital and community settings. The report claimed that the NHS fell short of its published principles and values as it failed to respond to the needs of these service users with care, compassion, and sensitivity.

> There are very many skilled staff within the NHS who provide a compassionate and considerate service to their patients. Yet the cases […] confirm that this is not universal. Instead, the actions of individual staff described here add up to an ignominious failure to look beyond a patient's clinical condition and respond to the social and emotional needs of the individual and their family. The difficulties encountered by the service users and their relatives were not solely a result of illness, but arose from the dismissive attitude of staff, a disregard for process and procedure and an apparent indifference of NHS staff to deplorable standards of care.
> (Parliamentary and Health Service Ombudsman 2011: 8)

Whilst poor practice could be due to one 'bad apple that spoils the barrel', the evidence suggests that, for such failures in care to occur, there needs to be active or more often passive cooperation from many people. A number of reports focus on deficiencies in nursing (Mencap 2007, Patients Association (2009, 2011). It must be acknowledged that a lot of care described as nursing is not undertaken by professional nurses or always under the supervision of professional nurses and so is at present unregulated. Nevertheless, contrary to these reports, nurses claim to adopt a holistic approach to care enabling them to respond to individuals' physical, emotional, and spiritual needs (Fletcher 2000). However, nursing practice has had to change due to rapid technological change and new treatments, necessitating new roles and a changing skill mix. Fletcher (2000) expresses concern that despite claiming to be *the* caring professional, this cannot be taken for granted. In fact, her experience as a service user indicated that doctors were more caring than nurses. Cornwell and Goodrich (2009) claim that compassionate nursing care cannot be assumed, nor indeed caring working relationships according to Firth-Cozens and Cornwell (2009). Having professional codes where compassionate care is embedded offers a commendable aspiration for practice but for this to become a reality involves an active commitment from all practitioners. Given health professionals come into contact with people who are likely to feel very vulnerable, such care should not be 'done to' service users but rather 'done with' people in order that they feel involved in and as such have some control of their situation. This relates to Thompson's notion of 'power with' (2007) as mentioned in Chapter 3.

Advocacy, empowerment, and anti-oppressive practice

One means through which the values underpinning professional codes can be enacted in health care is through a commitment to anti-oppressive practice. This term will be discussed in greater depth in Chapter 9, but for the purpose of this chapter, it is defined as '… a way of working that is not based on bias, prejudices, discrimination, injustice or unfair treatment.' (Okitikpi and Aymer 2010: 26) It is an approach to working with people that does not 'just happen' but involves raising our personal awareness of how we interact with others and adopting a conscious effort not to be prejudiced and to challenge unfairness. Key to anti-oppressive practice is the adoption of an empowering approach, which involves working in partnership with service users in a critically reflective manner and using inclusive communication skills such as negotiation, advocacy, and facilitation (Dalrymple and Burke 2006).

Empowerment and advocacy are important values that underpin anti-oppressive practice. Whilst health care professionals are able to offer their skills and knowledge to help clients with health needs, except in certain emergency situations, they do not necessarily 'know what's best' for an individual. According to Nzira and Williams (2009: 26), 'empowerment involves addressing the imbalance of power between groups in society'; an example relating to health care could include power within health professional–client relationships. Rather than telling people what to do and expecting them to obey on the basis of authority, the health professional shares knowledge with clients in order to help them understand the options thus enabling them to act according to their choice. Essentially, this involves a process of respect for clients to self-determine providing the resources, education, and self-awareness to facilitate and increase individual's personal power (Thompson 2006: 117).

Advocacy is one major means through which a health professional may empower a client. Advocacy in simple terms is the act of pleading for. Nzira and Williams (2009: 29) define advocacy as

> the representation of a need or an idea, either by a person or group on behalf of themselves or by someone or an organisation on behalf of another person or group.

The concept is allied to political action; for example, an advocate (individual or pressure group perhaps) seeks to influence decisions through changing legislation. In terms of health care, it can be about helping people to access the means to live a good quality of life despite health issues. For example, a nursing organisation might want to promote inclusion and to recognise and act upon injustices; they may therefore advocate on behalf of older people for personal care to be funded by the state (Ford and Waddington 2006). The concept can include self-advocacy by disadvantaged groups, for example, patients with breast cancer seeking equal access to medication wherever they live in the UK.

As a health professional, advocacy usually involves acting with or on behalf of those you support in your work, using your knowledge and experience to influence positive outcomes (see activity in Box 5.3).

Empowerment and advocacy are apparent implicitly or explicitly in all the codes featured in table one. For example, nurses are required to 'act as an advocate for those in

---

Box 5.3   Activity

Turn again to your professional code and identify any elements where advocacy and empowerment are mentioned or implied. Thinking about Lucy's story, note down any examples where empowerment and advocacy were an issue in her practice placement.

---

your care, helping them to access relevant health and social care, information and support' (NMC 2008). Doctors are required to accept that 'Patients who complain about the care or treatment they have received have a right to expect a prompt, open, constructive and honest response including an explanation and, if appropriate, an apology' (GMC 2006). The concepts are more implicit within the HPC code; for example, 'You must take all reasonable steps to make sure that you can communicate properly and effectively with your patients, clients and users, and their carers and family' (HPC 2008).

Box 5.4   Case study – the 'unpopular patient' (Stockwell 1972)

Stockwell found that patients on a ward were found to be either 'popular' or 'unpopular' with the nurses.

   Patients were judged 'good' or 'bad' according to certain criteria such as how 'demanding' or 'attention seeking' they were deemed to be or about their mood and 'cooperativeness', and this then affected the way that nurses interacted, or didn't, with those patients.

   Therefore, the study found that 'good' patients were rewarded by the nurses (reward power) with attention, were more 'liked', and positive evaluations made about them as people, while 'unpopular' patients were deemed 'uncooperative' or 'demanding' and were 'punished' (coercive power) by having negative evaluations made about them; they were treated more indifferently and sometimes even ignored. Some patients deemed more 'demanding' even had their call bells disconnected.

Focusing on Lucy's story, she comments that 'patients were asked to wait without any explanation' which appears to be rather disrespectful. She also noted that at times staff seemed 'unsympathetic to patients' requests'. When discussing patient-centred care and the uniqueness of individuals, it has to be acknowledged that the notion of the unpopular patient exists within the practice setting. Russell *et al*. (2003) discussed clients who were labelled as non-compliant. These labels that are used by professionals reinforce the maintenance of power and control over clients. Nurses have known about unpopular patients for over two decades and Stockwell's study in 1972 highlighted the impact that this had (please read Case study – the unpopular patient located in Box 5.4).

   Further studies (Kus 1990, Johnson and Webb 1995) have identified the ongoing labelling of clients and the consequences of this. Terms such as 'he's a lovely man' and 'demanding', 'manipulative', and 'attention seeking' have been cited. These can be reinforced by the culture of the workplace and other staff members. Judging persons to be 'good' or 'bad' may be nothing more than a human entitlement to appreciate, indeed to prefer, those aspects of a person's behaviour or make-up which we have learned to value (Johnson and Webb 1995). However, given the vulnerability of patients and the power of the staff, these comments indicate a degree of client disempowerment.

Equally Lucy indicates that she did not challenge these behaviours as *she did not want to be labelled a* 'difficult student', which hints that she also felt disempowered. Lucy could have advocated on behalf of the patients with the support of her practice assessor. Advocacy sounds easy but sometimes a conflict of interest makes challenging others rather complex, for example, if a patient complains about a colleague. Perhaps Lucy might feel less powerful in the work team as a temporary member which is the case for all students. However, if we know something is wrong and we have a code of conduct to back us up, what prevents us from acting appropriately?

Thompson's PCS model and the influence of professional culture

Thompson's PCS model of oppression and anti-oppressive practice (Thompson 2006, 2011) has been described in detail in Chapter 3. To briefly recap, Thompson describes three inter-related levels of oppression. The *P* level relates to the *personal* experiences of oppressed people in everyday life and can include health care settings. The *C* level refers to *culture* not in the religious or national sense but in terms of groups that have a set of shared meanings about the way they see the world. This is evident in the language and imagery they use about other groups in society which in turn influences their attitudes and behaviour towards other groups. One example of culture in this sense is the work culture that is apparent in a specific health care setting or prevalent within a professional group. Finally, *S* refers to a *structural* or *society-wide* level of oppression and considers how the organisation of institutions or society can work to reinforce oppression.

Applying the PCS approach to Lucy's story, it seems that, at the *personal* level, Lucy adhered to the values underpinning concepts such as 'holism, patient-centred care, empathy, compassion, and empowerment'. She is also aspiring to become a professional who is bound by a code of conduct and ethics that advocate similar values, as indeed are her practice assessors. The code is at a *structural* level as it is a legally sanctioned mechanism that governs the behaviour of a professional group in order to ensure public protection. However, the code is *culturally* implemented; the work culture influences the way that health care is practiced and therefore how the professional code is implemented. The perception that patients have to wait without explanation and their requests are received unsympathetically by some staff indicates that a degree of oppression is operating in that particular work culture. An oppressive culture impacts on patients but it seems also to have had an impact on Lucy. Could it be that Lucy also feels oppressed and this is preventing her challenging poor practice? (The activity in Box 5.5 will enable you to explore this further.)

Box 5.5   Activity

In Chapter 4, you were introduced to nine interacting processes of discrimination and their link to inequality and oppression (Thompson 2003). To recap, the processes are stereotyping, marginalisation, invisibilisation, infantilisation, welfarism, medicalisation, dehumanisation, trivialisation, and stigmatisation. Reread Lucy's account of her first practice placement. Jot down some examples of where these processes are evident in relation to Lucy.

Thompson (2003, 2006) argues that there is a clear link between disempowerment and vulnerability because of the potential to deprive people of control over lives. This lack of control promotes feelings of marginalisation and isolation. Lucy's story indicates that *stereotyping* of students may have been part of the placement culture. It could be that permanent staff viewed all students as the same rather than judging them as individuals. Some negative stereotypes may be apparent such as 'they need to learn to get the job done', or 'students are so slow, it's easier to do it yourself'. Curtis *et al.* (2007) discussed the 'pecking order' of students where comments were made ensuring that they knew their place within the organisation. Within the hierarchy, Curtis *et al.* (2007) refer to the 'us and them' mentality, where some hospital trained nurses made negative comments about university educated nurses such as 'Uni students don't know much about "real" nursing'. Many students have commented that their assessors berate their current education, 'not like it used to be in my day'. Such attitudes may contribute to Lucy's feeling that she did not always feel supported when learning so many new skills. She may have felt somewhat *marginalised* as a student and temporary team member but may have feared being marginalised further as a 'difficult student' if she raised any concerns about the patient care. She may have considered that her concerns would have been *trivialised* and put down to her lack of experience. She tried to be helpful, aware of the power that her practice assessor had over her in terms of the placement assessment – behaviour that can be linked to *infantilisation*. Understanding the reasons for feeling disempowered is not offered as an excuse for inaction, nor is it about apportioning blame. It is however a first step to being able to challenge oppression by developing an awareness of our part in contributing to unfair practices.

Vulnerability and 'belongingness'

It has been argued that culture can prove very significant in terms of preventing oppressive practice. Even where appropriate personal and structural factors are in place, cultural issues need to be addressed in order to reduce feelings of vulnerability. A highly significant aspect of this for health care students is their temporary status as team members as they move between practice placements. We all like to belong, and good practice assessors will ensure that students are welcomed and orientated so they know their role and feel valued within the team. The desire to 'fit in' is not new. Melia (1987) conducted a study with nursing students and found that there were a number of unwritten rules with which students felt they had to comply in order to fit in. The students perceived that within placements the focus was primarily on 'getting the work done' and learning how to fit in with the 'way things were done'. It is acknowledged that health care practice has changed significantly since that time, but are some of the practices the same? More recently, in the further study of newly qualified nurses, Maben *et al.* (2007: 103) identified four 'covert' rules to guide clinical practice. These were:

- Rule 1: 'hurried physical care prevails' (to the detriment of psychological care)
- Rule 2: 'no shirking' (need to be seen to be doing a fair share of the physical and 'dirty work' especially by unqualified staff)

- Rule 3: 'don't get involved with patients' (keep an emotional distance)
- Rule 4: 'fit in and don't rock the boat' (don't try and change practice)

These findings support the earlier work by Melia (1987). Students told her of the dominance of maxims such as 'talking isn't working', 'look busy', and 'pull your weight'. Nursing students learned that the valued nurse was one who did not shirk physical labour and could get through the work as rapidly as possible. McGuire and Dewar (1995) found that nurses working on care of the elderly wards did not always feel comfortable asking for help, believing they would be 'better regarded' if they managed alone. Although such strategies of 'fitting in' are often viewed as necessary for survival, the result may be the continuation of questionable nursing practice without challenge (Mackay 1989). Gray and Smith (1999) uncovered the strong desire of student nurses to dispel their status as an 'outsider', motivating them to conform to prevailing norms within the clinical area and to do their share of the work. Indeed, Burnard (1989) argues that the socialisation of nurses may encourage conformity.

Levett-Jones and Lathlean (2009a) also discussed themes that emerged from their study regarding conformity and compliance. These included 'Don't rock the boat' and 'getting the Registered Nurses offside'. Not rocking the boat meant that they would not be viewed as an outsider and if they got the Registered Nurses 'offside' then this was felt to impede the lack of future learning opportunities. Students described how and why they adopted or adapted to the teams' and institution's values and norms, rather than challenging them, believing that this would improve their likelihood of acceptance and inclusion by the permanent staff. The importance of fitting in and being accepted dominated their thoughts through the placement experience. Let us take a moment to consider this in light of Lucy's experience; please read and complete the Time for reflection (Box 5.6).

Lucy's first placement experience was both positive and negative, and she identified that she was anxious at times. Rogers (1997) discussed the concept of situational vulnerability and linked this to the fact that everyone is vulnerable at different times in life, but notably in new situations such as practice placement experiences. Gray and Smith (1999) identified that students view going to the wards for the first time as a momentous event, but early in their first placement realise that their pre-placement expectations do not fully reflect reality.

The impact of situational vulnerability on students is usefully explored in a study by Levett-Jones and Lathlean (2009b). They investigated students' experience of 'belongingness' when undertaking practice placements and concluded that attainment of confidence is only possible after previous needs have been met (Figure 5.1).

Box 5.6   Time for reflection

Lucy could relate to Maben *et al.'s* (2007) findings reflecting back when the practice area was busy and there seemed limited time to get things done. Perhaps as a student Lucy felt more comfortable, potentially reducing her own vulnerability, by contributing to the busy workload, aiming to impress her mentors, and be a part of the team. She was also aware that this could help with her practice assessment as she wanted to achieve a pass. Have you ever felt like this? Jot down some notes about these experiences.

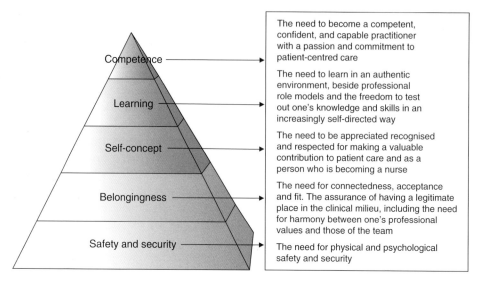

Figure 5.1   Ascent to competence conceptual framework (adapted from Maslow's Hierarchy of Needs, 1987). Source: Levett-Jones and Lathlean 2009b: 2873.

According to a study by Allan *et al.* (2008), students can experience significant stress and anxiety whilst undertaking practice placements. They identified themes such as lack of time for learning, supernumerary status not being a reality, and lack of support from mentors and the clinical team as a whole. Clearly, this would influence their ability to move beyond the base of the triangle as they may not feel safe or secure. For nursing and midwifery students, there is an additional concern that for historical reasons and due to staffing shortages students may be treated as workers rather than learners. Holland (1999) argues that this can lead to role conflict and the related stress that this would entail. Similarly, Fulbrook *et al.* (2000) found that it was common practice for students to be used as 'an extra pair of hands' at the expense of undertaking activities to meet their learning needs. It is acknowledged however that repeating tasks can facilitate the development of competence and confidence.

Many students do experience excellent practice learning environments with committed practice assessors. Donaldson and Carter (2005) discuss the impact of role models on the student experience. Murray and Main (2005) identify the importance of role models in maintaining enthusiasm for the profession. They often lead by example and enjoy teaching and caring for patients and students. When reflecting, like Lucy, on how working with good role models enhances your own practice, it is important to recognise that this will enable you to more effectively support clients who are vulnerable. Students also need to be committed to making the most of all learning opportunities. However, even in the best situations, situational vulnerability will come into play and impact to some extent on learning.

Allan *et al.* (2008) identified several factors that influence student learning such as support from mentors, staff, and peers, emotional demands of the clinical area, lack of supernumerary status, role conflict in terms of balancing assignments with family life, and not being prepared for the placement. Bradbury-Jones *et al.* (2007) highlighted that students being empowered during clinical placement can affect their learning. Being encouraged to take responsibility enables deep learning to occur and has a direct impact on the students' self-esteem. Being part of the team, nurturing, and being included in patient care also empowered students to demonstrate a sense of control. Day (2006) suggests that effective teams support each other unconditionally and proactively offer and ask each other for help as and when needed. They also voice their appreciation and feel a sense of loyalty to each other. Effective team work in the clinical area supports not only students but also the quality of care for patients.

Levett-Jones and Lathlean (2009b) also discussed that being involved and included in care delivery, where the student's input was valued along with support, all impacted on the learning. Salamonson *et al.* (2011) highlight the importance of the learning environment in providing the real life context which is essential for the knowledge, values, and skills required of a graduate nurse. It also provides the optimal environment for observing role models, to practice nursing skills and to reflect on what is seen, heard, and done. Windsor (1987) identified three phases of development apparent in nurse education:

- An initial stage of anxiety in which students are 'obsessed' with rules and tasks
- A stage of transition in which they struggle to identify the role of the nurse and reconcile their initial vision with the realities of practice
- A later phase in which students feel increasingly comfortable with their image of what nursing is really all about and explore the role more fully and with growing independence

---

Box 5.7   Activity

Reflect on Lucy's story. Later in her course she felt more able to challenge and question some of the care delivery practices encountered in her practice placement. With reference to the ascent to competence diagram and Windsor's work (mentioned earlier), what might have influenced her confidence in this respect?

Using this understanding, let us return to explore Lucy's story again (see activity in Box 5.7)

All health professional students, given the nature of their work, are likely to feel anxious about 'doing the right thing', particularly in the early stages of their programme when knowledge and skills have yet to become integrated seamlessly into the way they act in practice. Beckett *et al.* (2007) support this in relation to nursing students who they found initially become preoccupied with their perceived knowledge and lack of technical skills. Such a lack of confidence may make challenging practice more difficult as an individual may feel both unsure of their facts and also that they lack practical experience. Whilst this is understandable, nonetheless, where basic human values are not being respected, we are all experts, as professional knowledge is not the issue. We can all judge whether a person is being treated the way we would want to be treated and justifiably ask questions about this. If the culture within a placement team does not encourage questioning and perhaps rewards compliance, our need to 'belong' may outweigh the imperative to challenge practices that conflict with our personal values. The prevailing work culture is therefore a highly significant influence on us to decide to do what we know to be right.

Increasing vulnerability through ritual and routine work practices

Earlier we discussed how professional socialisation was influenced by both personal and professional values. The nature of health professions has changed over time. One key purpose of the education process for aspiring practitioners is to expose them to relevant knowledge, skills, and attitudes but to develop the critical thinking skills that will enable them to use these appropriately within contemporary practice. However, students will also come into contact with the prevailing professional culture which will be influenced by the valued expertise of experienced practitioners but may also reflect inappropriate and outdated ways of working. Jowett *et al.'s* (1991) writing about nursing highlighted an example of this; some work cultures valued routine and task-based work practices over patient-centred care. Indeed, the imperative to get the job done as quickly as possible seems to be strong in some professional groups but can have a very negative impact on patient experience.

Philpin (2002) explores the meaning of rituals in work practices; it is often referred to in the literature as unthinking actions which lack any evidence base. Rituals and task-focused care can be disempowering and increase both patients' vulnerability (because their choices are secondary to 'the way things are done') as well as the vulnerability of staff (personal values might be compromised because 'this is the way we do it here'). However, there are some positive aspects to rituals. Menzies (1960) argued that rituals of practice may protect staff from anxieties that they have in dealing with human suffering. In this way, it could be debated that rituals and task-focused care may be 'comforting' to the student, enabling them to feel useful to the team and therefore feel safe (Brennan and McSherry 2007). Freshwater and Biley (1998) also proposed that rituals can help the client feel more at ease, comfortable, and relaxed if care is aimed at maintaining their normal routine.

However, maintaining comforting routines is not the same as ritualised care, which has connotations of unthinking, production-line-type practice focused on the needs of the professional and not the patient. The seminal study of nursing by Menzies (1960) identified that focusing on tasks reduced the personal interaction between staff and patients. The effect was to depersonalise care and deny the clients' individuality. Nurses talked about patients, not by their name, but by bed numbers or their disease category. This study had a huge impact on nurse education and the organisation of nursing care, resulting in a move away from task-oriented to patient-centred care planning and delivery. Whilst much has changed for the better within nursing and health care practice more generally, regrettably 50 years later it is of note that the NHS has been criticised for a 'failure to look beyond a patient's clinical condition and respond to the social and emotional needs of the individual and their family' (Parliamentary Health Service Ombudsman 2011: 8) (please undertake the activity in Box 5.8).

Box 5.8 Activity

Ritualised work practices can lead to objectification and dehumanisation of patients. Where can you identify this from Lucy's description of her experiences in practice placement?

Horizontal violence

As an outsider looking in, it is relatively easy to identify uncaring, dehumanised practices. Despite the fact that most practitioners and students have caring values, we have argued that sometimes the culture in which practitioners work can inhibit our ability to challenge practice. Horizontal violence is a term that describes bullying and aggression involving inter-group conflict and most commonly takes the form of psychological harassment (Farrell 1997, 1999, 2001). It can include a range of covert and overt harassment; this can range from being neglected and ignored, being denied access to learning opportunities and being subjected to verbal and written threats (McKenna *et al.* 2003) or being exposed to excessive criticism, intimidation, ridicule, making excessive workload demands, and inequitable working conditions (Jackson *et al.* 2002).

The literature regarding bullying or horizontal violence cuts across the health sector and the health professions. Horizontal violence is linked to job dissatisfaction and reasons why people leave their profession, for example, in midwifery (Curtis *et al.* 2006). A study of workplace bullying in an NHS Community Trust (Quine 1999) involved a survey of a range of staff that included community nurses, occupational therapists, physiotherapists, and speech and language therapists. They found bullying to be a serious problem, linked to staff attrition as well as anxiety and depression. Stevens and Crouch (1998), cited in Curtis *et al.* (2007), adds that horizontal violence appears to be tolerated to a much higher level in nursing compared with other professions. Some writers argue that this is linked to the view that nursing as a profession is considered to be oppressed (Hendricks-Thomas and Patterson 1995) and that nurses are a disempowered group within the health care sector (Matheson and Bobay 2007).

Kelly and Ahern (2008) identified that the culture of the workplace was pivotal to the prevalence of horizontal violence. In their study of nursing, bullying could be readily identified through the presence of cliques as well as the tolerance of unfair and disrespectful behaviours and language within practice teams. This was apparent in the misuse of power, a tendency to be overly critical of new practitioners and ideas ('eating their young'), the presence of rigid hierarchies, and the tolerance of 'bitchiness'. One participant stated 'I felt like an alien. I'd walk on the ward and nobody would speak to me, acknowledge me or even say hello' (Kelly and Ahern 2008: 913). Students reported being ignored and referred to as 'the student' rather than by name. Curtis *et al.'s* (2007) study with nursing students found that they often felt this powerlessness and being invisible, sitting alone on their breaks, being ignored, for example, during handovers, and not being included in team discussions. This dismissed their individuality and is reflective of invisibilisation, one of the processes of discrimination described by Thompson (2011).

These studies indicate the negative impact that bullying has on self-esteem and ultimately the care given to clients. If individuals are concerned with their own 'survival', then the ability to respond to vulnerable clients must inevitably be affected. For health professional students, bullying can result in students withdrawing from their course which represents a considerable financial as well as personal loss. Of even greater concern, students may learn to accommodate this way of working and, because perhaps it is rewarded, adopt bullying practices themselves. Randle (2003) and Mackintosh (2006) found that whilst nursing students were initially shocked at some uncaring attitudes they encountered in some practice placements, by the time they reached the latter part of their programmes, they had come to accept this as part of the culture (Gray and Smith 1999). Unfortunately, behaviour that is reinforced is likely to be repeated (Skinner 1953). New recruits may perceive that aggression in the work place is both commonplace and accept-able and therefore unable to be challenged. Seligman (1974, 1975 cited in Gross 2010: 169), referring to animal studies, found that dogs learned that no behaviour on their part had any effect on the occurrence (or non-occurrence) of a particular event. Extrapolating these findings to humans, he drew similar conclusions in certain situations. In circum-stances involving horizontal violence, the victim may perceive that there is nothing they can do about their situation and that it is part of working life and completely out of their control. The associated disempowered behaviours including depression are termed 'learned helplessness' (Faulkner 2001). This concept has been explored in greater depth in Chapter 7.

Oppressive practices and the link to increased vulnerability of patients and health care staff is unacceptable. The first stage to challenging this is to increase our understanding of some of the issues, one of the main purposes of this chapter and the book in general. However, to stop at understanding is not enough. As Thompson (1992 cited in Thompson 2006: 15) states, when it comes to anti-oppressive practice, 'If we are not part of the solu-tion, then we are part of the problem'. We would argue that claiming we can do nothing is an attitude of mind. Even small positive changes eventually add up to making a differ-ence. Chapter 9 will examine some strategies that practitioners can use in order to work in an anti-oppressive manner and in a way that reduces vulnerability.

Conclusion

This chapter has explored the influence of routines, rituals, and oppressive practice within the practice setting and how this can influence the care given to clients who are vulnera-ble. The powerful influence of professional culture and socialisation is also discussed which highlights the need to 'belong' and how this can impact on personal vulnerability which in turn affects the ability to care for others who are vulnerable. The importance of values and the role of professional codes are identified as linking to advocacy and empow-erment which are key factors in the promotion of person-centred care and reducing clients' vulnerability.

Links to other chapters

- Chapter 2 explores how professionals can experience feeling vulnerable in more depth.
- Chapter 4 recaps on the processes of oppression and reflects on how the placement culture can influence this.
- Chapter 7 will explore the concept of 'learned helplessness'.
- Chapter 9 will explore strategies whereby vulnerability can be reduced.

References

Allan, H.T., Smith, P., Lorentzon, M. and O'Driscoll, M. (2008) *Leadership for Learning*. Centre for Research in Nursing and Midwifery Education, University of Surrey, Guildford.

Beckett, A., Gilberston, S. and Greenwood, S. (2007) Doing the right thing: Nursing students, relational practice and moral agency. *Journal of Nursing Education*, 46 (1), 28–32.

Bradbury-Jones, C., Sambrook, S. and Irvine, F. (2007) The meaning of empowerment for nursing students: A critical incident study. *Journal of Advanced Nursing*, 59 (4), 342–351.

Brennan, G. and McSherry, R. (2007) Exploring the transition and professional socialisation from health care assistant to student nurse. *Nurse Education in Practice*, 7 (4), 206–214.

Burnard, P. (1989) The sixth sense. *Nursing Times*, 85 (50), 52–53.

Care Quality Commission (CQC) (2011) *Dignity and Nutrition Inspection Programme: National Overview*. CQC, Newcastle upon Tyne.

Clouder, L. (2003) Becoming professional: Exploring the complexities of professional socialization in health and social care. *Learning in Health & Social Care*, 2 (4), 213–222.

Cohen, H.A. (1981) *The Nurse's Quest for a Professional Identity*. Addison-Wesley, California.

Cornwell, J. and Goodrich, J. (2009) Exploring how to ensure compassionate care in hospital to improve patient experience, *Nursing Times*, 105 (15), 14–16.

Curtis, P., Ball, L. and Kirkham, M. (2006) Bullying and horizontal violence: Cultural or individual phenomena? *British Journal of Midwifery*, 14 (4), 218–221.

Curtis, J., Bowen, I. and Reid, A. (2007) You have no credibility: Nursing students' experiences of horizontal violence. *Nurse Education in Practice*, 7 (3), 156–163.

Dalrymple, J. and Burke, J. (2006) *Anti-Oppressive Practice: Social Care and the Law*. Open University Press, London.

Davies, H., Nutley, S. and Mannion, R. (2000) Organisational culture and quality of health care. *Quality in Health Care*, 9 (2), 111–119.

Day, J. (2006) *Interprofessional Working: An Essential Guide for Health and Social Care Professionals*. Nelson Thornes, Cheltenham.

Department of Health (DoH) (2000) *No Secrets: Guidance on Developing and Implementing Multi-Agency Policies and Procedures to Protect Vulnerable Adults from Abuse*. HMSO, London.

Donaldson, J.H. and Carter, D. (2005) The value of role modelling: Perceptions of undergraduate and diploma nursing (adult) students. *Nurse Education in Practice*, 5 (6), 353–359.

Fagermoen, M. (1997) Professional identity: Values embedded in meaningful nursing practice. *Journal of Advanced Nursing*, 25 (3), 434–441.

Farrell, G.A. (1997) Aggression in clinical settings: Nurses' views. *Journal of Advanced Nursing*, 25 (3), 501–508.

Farrell, G.A. (1999) Aggression in clinical settings – a follow-up study. *Journal of Advanced Nursing*, 29 (3), 532–541.

Farrell, G.A. (2001) From tall poppies to squashed weeds: Why don't nurses pull together more? *Journal of Advanced Nursing*, 35 (1), 26–33.

Faulkner, M. (2001) Empowerment in policy and practice. *Nursing Times*, 97 (22), 40–41.

Firth-Cozens, J. and Cornwell, J. (2009) *The Point of Care: Enabling Compassionate Care in Acute Hospital Settings*. Kings Fund, London.

Fitzpatrick, J.M., While, A.E. and Roberts, J.D. (1996) Key influences on the professional socialisation and practice of students undertaking different preregistration nurse education programmes in the United Kingdom. *International Journal of Nursing Studies*, 33 (5), 506–518.

Fletcher, M. (2000) Doctors have become more caring than nurses. *British Medical Journal*, 320 (7241), 1083.

Ford, P. and Waddington, E. (2006) *Caring in Partnership: Older People and Nursing Staff Working Towards the Future*. Royal College of Nursing, London.

Freshwater, D. and Biley, F. (1998) Rituals: The 'soul' purpose. *Complementary Therapies in Nursing and Midwifery*, 4 (3), 73–76.

Fulbrook, P., Rolfe, G., Albarran, J. and Boxall, F. (2000) Fit for practice: Project 2000 student nurses' views on how well the curriculum prepares them for clinical practice. *Nurse Education Today*, 20 (5), 350–357.

General Medical Council (GMC) (2006) *Good Medical Practice*. Available from http://www.gmc-uk.org/guidance/good_medical_practice/contents.asp [accessed on 7 July 2012].

GMC (2012a) *About Us*. Available from http://www.gmc-uk.org/about/role.asp [accessed on 7 July 2012].

Giddens, A. (2006) *Sociology*. 5th ed., Polity, Cambridge.

Gray, M. and Smith, L. (1999) The professional socialization of diploma of higher education in nursing students (Project 2000): A longitudinal qualitative study. *Journal of Advanced Nursing*, 29 (3), 639–647.

Gross, R.D. (2010) *Psychology: The Science of Mind and Behaviour*. 6th ed., Hodder and Stoughton, London.

Health Professions Council (HPC) (2008) *Standards of Conduct, Performance and Ethics*. Available from http://www.hpc-uk.org/assets/documents/10002367FINALcopyofSCPEJuly2008.pdf [accessed on 7 July 2012].

HPC (2012a) *About Us*. Available from http://www.hpc-uk.org/aboutus/ [accessed on 7 July 2012].

Healthcare Commission (2009) *Investigation into Mid Staffordshire NHS Foundation Trust*. Available from http://www.midstaffsinquiry.com/assets/docs/Healthcare%20Commission%20report.pdf [accessed on 7 July 2012].

Hendricks-Thomas, J. and Patterson, E. (1995) A sharing in critical thought by nursing faculty. *Journal of Advanced Nursing*, 22 (3), 594–599.

Holland, K. (1999) A journey to becoming: The student nurse in transition. *Journal of Advanced Nursing*, 29 (1), 229–236.

Jackson, D., Clare, J. and Mannix, J. (2002) Who would want to be a nurse? Violence in the workplace – a factor in recruitment and retention. *Journal of Nursing Management*, 10 (1), 13–20.

Johnson, M. and Webb, C. (1995) Rediscovering unpopular patients: The concept of social judgement. *Journal of Advanced Nursing*, 21, 466–475.

Jowett, S., Walton, I. and Payne, S. (1991) *The NFER Project 2000 Research: An Introduction and Some Interim Issues*. National Foundation for Educational Research in England and Wales, Berkshire.

Kelly, B. (1998) Preserving moral integrity: A follow-up study with new graduate nurses. *Journal of Advanced Nursing*, 28 (5), 1134–1145.

Kelly, J. and Ahern, K. (2008) Preparing nurses for practice: A phenomenological study of the new graduate in Australia. *Journal of Clinical Nursing*, 18 (6), 910–918.

Kus, R.J. (1990) Nurses and unpopular patients. *American Journal of Nursing*, 90 (6), 62–66.

Levett-Jones, T. and Lathlean, J. (2009a) 'Don't rock the boat': Nursing students' experiences of conformity and compliance. *Nurse Education Today*, 29 (3), 342–349.

Levett-Jones, T. and Lathlean, J. (2009b) The ascent to competence conceptual framework: An outcome of a study of belongingness. *Journal of Clinical Nursing*, 18 (20), 2870–2879.

Maben, J., Cornwell, J. and Sweeney, K. (2010) In praise of compassion. *Journal of Research in Nursing*, 15 (1), 9–13.

Maben, J., Latter, S. and Macleod Clark, J. (2007) The sustainability of ideals, values and the nursing mandate; evidence from a longitudinal qualitative study. *Nursing Inquiry*, 14 (2), 99–113.

Mackay, L. (1989) *Nursing a Problem*. Open University Publications, Milton Keynes.

Mackintosh, C. (2006) Caring: The socialisation of pre-registration student nurses: A longitudinal qualitative descriptive study. *International Journal of Nursing Studies*, 43 (8), 953–962.

Matheson, L. and Bobay, K. (2007) Validation of oppressed group behaviours in nursing. *Journal of Professional Nursing*, 23 (4), 226–234.

McGuire, T. and Dewar, J. (1995) An assessment of moving and handling practices among Scottish nurses. *Nursing Standard*, 9 (40), 35–39.

McKenna, B., Smith, N., Poole, S. and Coverdale, J. (2003) Horizontal violence: Experiences of registered nurses in their first year of practice. *Journal of Advanced Nursing*, 42 (1), 90–96.

Melia, K. (1987) *Learning and Working: The Occupational Socialization of Nurses*. Tavistock Publications, London.

Mencap (2007) *Death by Indifference*. Mencap, London.

Menzies, I.P. (1960) A case-study in the functioning of social systems as a defence against anxiety. *Human Relations*, 13 (2), 95–121.

Murray, C.C. and Main, A.A. (2005) Role modelling as a teaching method for student mentors. *Nursing Times*, 101 (26), 30–33.

Nursing and Midwifery Council (NMC) (2008) *The Code: Standards of Conduct, Performance and Ethics for Nurses and Midwives*. Available from http://www.nmc-uk.org/Publications/Standards/The-code/Introduction/ [accessed on 8 July 2012].

NMC (2010a) *About Us*. Available from http://www.nmc-uk.org/About-us [accessed on 7 June 2012].

Nzira, V. and Williams, P. (2009) *Anti-Oppressive Practice in Health and Social Care*. Sage, London.

Okitikpi, T. and Aymer, C. (2010) *Key Concepts in Anti-Discriminatory Social Work*. Sage, London.

Parliamentary and Health Service Ombudsman (2011) *Care and Compassion? Report of the Health Service Ombudsman on Ten Investigations into NHS Care of Older People*. The Stationery Office, London.

Patients Association (2009) *Patients… Not Numbers, People… Not Statistics*. Patients Association, London.

Patients Association (2011) *We've Been Listening, Have You Been Learning*. Patients Association, London.

Pearcey, P. (2007) Tasks and routines in 21st century nursing: Student nurses' perceptions. *British Journal of Nursing*, 16 (5), 296–300.

Philpin, S. (2002) Rituals and nursing: A critical commentary. *Journal of Advanced Nursing*, 38 (2), 144–151.

Quine, L. (1999) Workplace bullying in NHS community trust: Staff questionnaire survey. *British Medical Journal*, 318 (7178), 228–232.

Randle, J. (2003) Bullying in the nursing profession. *Journal of Advanced Nursing*, 43 (4), 395–401.

Rogers, A. (1997) Vulnerability, health and health care. *Journal of Advanced Nursing*, 26 (1), 65–72.

Russell, S., Daly, J., Hughes, E. and Op't Hoog, C. (2003) Nurses and 'difficult' patients: negotiating non-compliance. *Journal of Advanced Nursing*, 43 (3), 281–287.

Salamonson, Y., Bourgeois, S., Everett, B., Weaver, R., Peters, K. and Jackson, D. (2011) Psychometric testing of the abbreviated Clinical Learning Environment Inventory (CLEI-19), *Journal of Advanced Nursing*. 67 (12), 2668–2676.

Skinner, B. (1953) *Science and Human Behaviour*. Free Press, New York.

Spouse, J. (2003) *Professional Learning in Nursing*. Blackwell Publishing, Oxford.

Stacey, G., Johnston, K., Stickley, T. and Diamond, B. (2011) How do nurses cope when values and practice conflict? *Nursing Times*, 107 (5), 20–23.

Stevens, J. and Crouch, M. (1998) 'Care' – The guiding principle of nursing? In: *Nursing Matters: Critical Sociological Perspective* (Keleher, H. and McInnerney, F. eds), Harcourt Brace & Company, Marrickville.

Stockwell, F. (1972) *The Unpopular Patient.* Royal College of Nursing, London.

Thompson, N. (2003) *Promoting Equality: Challenging Discrimination and Oppression.* 2nd ed., Macmillan, Basingstoke.

Thompson, N. (2006) *Anti-Discriminatory Practice.* 4th ed., Palgrave Macmillan, Basingstoke.

Thompson, N. (2007) *Power and Empowerment.* Russell House, Lyme Regis.

Thompson, N. (2011) *Promoting Equality: Working with Diversity and Difference.* 3rd ed., Palgrave Macmillan, Basingstoke.

White, R and Ewan, C. (1991) *Clinical Teaching in Nursing.* Chapman and Hall, London.

Windsor, A.W. (1987) Nursing students' perceptions of clinical experience. *Journal of Nursing Education,* 26 (4), 150–154.

Chapter 6

The social construction of vulnerability

Janet Scammell and Gill Calvin Thomas

Introduction

In this chapter, we will be taking a sociological perspective to explore the concept of vulnerability. Questions such as why do I 'see' things the way I do and interpret them in the way I do can be explored through sociology. Sociology concerns the study of human society, including the development of groups, their organisation, and how this has changed over time (Barry and Yuill 2008: 6). We focus upon the way our identity is constructed and the implications for how vulnerability may feature within these constructions.

The chapter firstly explores social constructionism, a major sociological perspective, which will be explained and used to explore the social construction of identity. A person's identity is complex and is influenced by our sense of who we think we are and how we see others in relation to ourselves (Dominelli 2002). This is important in the study of vulnerability because if someone is seen as vulnerable this can become *the* defining aspect of their identity, perhaps to the exclusion of most other aspects. The effects of such labelling will be considered including the impact on the power dynamic between practitioner and service user and the potential for engaging in oppressive practice. It will be argued that identity is not one-sided but multi-factorial, that it is not fixed but changing and is profoundly influenced by context. We conclude by bringing together some learning from this chapter, drawing upon a case scenario to illustrate and integrate the chapter's discussion. The chapter argues that health care practitioners need to see beyond labels such as 'the disabled', as each person is unique and should be respected and empowered by practitioners as an expert in their own life.

Social constructionism

The study of society can be viewed through various 'lenses' according to differing theoretical perspectives. It is important therefore as writers that we clearly state the way we are looking at the world when we analyse vulnerability. The theoretical perspective that we are using is known as social constructionism. According to this perspective, our view of reality and therefore what constitutes knowledge and 'truth' is constructed by

Understanding Vulnerability: A Nursing and Healthcare Approach, First Edition. Edited by Vanessa Heaslip and Julie Ryden.
© 2013 John Wiley & Sons, Ltd. Published 2013 by John Wiley & Sons, Ltd.

individuals and communities (Berger and Luckmann 1966). This means that rather than accepting that it is 'common sense' or 'natural' that things are the way they are, the social construction perspective holds that most facets of society are created by its members and subject to change over time.

Consider the concept of illness; as Clarke (2010) argues, whilst illness is a biophysical condition, it is also a social state. In other words, doctors may attach a diagnostic label to a condition, but the way the illness is experienced by the individual and perceived by the society in which that person lives is shaped and *constructed* by society itself. For example, depending on how 'genuine' the illness is perceived to be will determine how much resource is allocated to the associated care as well as how much 'sympathy' it engenders from others. Myalgic encephalomyelitis (ME), also known as chronic fatigue syndrome, prompted wide debate in UK society with attitudes ranging from 'it's all in their head' to recognition of this diagnosis as a medical condition (Scott *et al.* 1995, Burns 2012). The same collection of symptoms has moved from being 'fictitious' to 'real' as a result of changes in society's perceptions. This is of course important to those with the condition but it is also important for health practitioners to be aware that this is just one example of where decisions as to whether to allocate resources to provide clinics or to allow ME sufferers to access social care benefits are based upon society's construction of ME as an illness.

It is argued then that concepts such as illness or health are constructions, reflecting the way a given society views these issues at a specific time. Both context and time are very significant in this respect; certain mental health disorders for example are not recognised as medical conditions in some Black and Minority Ethnic (BME) societies (Regan *et al.* 2012). Clearly, this could have significant implications for those with mental health issues, including whether specific health resources are provided and whether these are accessed. Similarly, time period is important; in the nineteenth century in the UK, a disease known as hysteria was diagnosed in women who did not conform with the prevailing societal view that a 'woman's place was in the home'. This view was related to a perceived bio-logical imperative linked to gender, namely, to reproduce (Clarke 2010). Then as now, where social constructions are reinforced by powerful institutions like education, family, health professional services, and the media, such powerful constructions or 'ways of see-ing things' become so embedded that most members of that society view the prevailing perspective as 'common sense'; for example, 'it's only natural that women should want to be mothers'. It becomes difficult then to perceive that such concepts (the role of women, the nature of illness) are not facts, but rather their meaning is constructed by society.

These 'constructions' or 'ways of seeing things' are known as 'discourses', and there-fore the chapter will now examine this concept in depth. It has already been identified as a significant aspect of 'power' and power relations (Chapter 3) and also as a mechanism for 'invisibilisation' (Chapter 4), so more detailed exploration is certainly overdue.

Discourses and vulnerability

Please read Definitions of a discourse in Box 6.1.

Discourses are inherited in the sense that we learn how to view things initially through primary socialisation as a child, from parents and teachers, for example. As time goes on,

---

Box 6.1 Definitions of a discourse

- Discourses are inherited and acquired 'guides' for viewing the worlds, events, situations and objects we encounter (Allen and Hardin 2001: 166).
- A discourse provides a set of possible statements about a given area, and organizes and gives structure to the manner in which a particular topic, object, process is to be talked about. (Kress 1985, cited in Cheek 1999: 387)
- A discourse refers to a set of meanings, metaphors, representations, images, stories, statements and so on that in some way together produce a particular version of events. It refers to a particular picture that is painted of an event, person or class of persons, a particular way of representing it in a certain light. (Burr 2003: 64)

---

these guides may become modified in the light of life experience. We can only 'know' the world through the discourses we have been given; they are the means by which we construct social reality ('ways of seeing things'). To put it another way, we draw upon discourses to 'make sense' out of things. Whilst this is very similar to the concept of 'culture', the term 'discourses' reflects the fact that there are many 'ways of seeing' the same 'thing' or scene or situation, but we may be influenced to see only *one* way as a result of the particular discourses or 'guides' we have been given in our socialisation.

According to Thompson (2011), discourses have two particular characteristics. The first is that they can either shape or constrain the way that we see the world. Discourses steer us in certain directions and therefore away from others. Discourses, in effect, construct reality. According to Rolfe, '…[whilst] the world might exist independently of people, truth cannot' (Rolfe 2000: 62). Therefore, the world is created according to and through our perception of that world and by the discourse we have acquired which shapes the way we think or speak of that thing. Within a discourse is the *power* to define. To define what is *normal* as opposed to *abnormal, sick* from *healthy*, who is *deserving* from *undeserving* (Thompson 2007). Discourses therefore socially construct the reality we see; as Foucault suggests, discourses are 'practices which form the objects of which they speak to' (1969, cited in Foucault 2002: 54).

The second characteristic of discourse is that it offers powerful people the potential to present their construction of the world in a way that reinforces their position of power at the expense of less powerful individuals (Thompson 2011). Discourses make you believe that there is no question or doubt; this is 'the' way to view the world, 'it's obvious', 'it's common sense'; we take this perspective for granted. What is often hidden by discourses is that it is not *the only* version, but is a 'particular' version, possibly the version of the world preferred by powerful people. Therefore, we are not always aware we have a choice in how we see the world. Some discourses become so dominant that it is hard to resist them. Dominant discourses are:

> …taken-for-granted sets of assumptions, beliefs and practices that often reflect a privileged, oppressive understanding (Gavey 1997, cited in O'Connor 2001: 141).

Some discourses become so dominant that most of us are unaware of their influence on our attitudes and behaviour. One example could relate to attitudes towards the termination of pregnancy; in the UK, a battery of tests is available and accessed by most pregnant women to establish whether their unborn baby is developing 'normally'. If it is discovered that the unborn child has cystic fibrosis, some people might argue that whilst it is very sad, *obviously* the parents will choose to have the pregnancy terminated. This decision might be made on the basis that *naturally* everyone would, if given the option, choose to terminate a pregnancy where the unborn child that was not 'normal'. Some groups may hold that this is common sense because preserving *abnormal* genes makes the human race weaker.

This example however reflects just one view of the world from a range of possible other discourses. The championing of 'normality' is very dominant within biomedicine, and this discourse is particularly prominent within the health systems in richer, developed countries. Whilst there are alternative discourses around the sanctity of life related to religious belief systems or the intrinsic value of all human beings and their right to life, one might imagine that to resist the dominant biomedical discourse would mean setting oneself apart. The prevailing discourse might be so strong that some may not fully realise that a different choice is an option. Further, when the child is born, mainstream society reflecting the dominant biomedical discourse, will label the child as 'disabled' because they deviate from 'normal'. They may be perceived as part of a vulnerable group – 'the disabled'. Discourses about disabled people are very apparent in society; one dominant discourse constructs disabled people as a homogenous group of people to be pitied and cared for by society (Thompson 2003). Such perceptions can serve to increase the vulnerability of groups by portraying people in negative ways resulting in discrimination and oppressive practices. See Example of a dominant discourse (Box 6.2).

Discourses shape the taken-for-granted assumptions and unwritten rules that can then influence cultural norms (cultural practices), social practices, and social structures (Thompson 2007). Again the influence of discourses on the social construction of reality is clear to see, and it follows that discourses will therefore have a significant influence upon the social construction of 'vulnerability' and 'vulnerable groups'. Practitioners are rarely 'bad' people; most come into this type of work with the best of intentions. However, powerful discourses underpin professional cultures and perhaps unwittingly these can influence the way that we operate and may increase patients' vulnerability.

Language – A vehicle of discourse

Language is obviously a key aspect in communicating discourses and as such offers a significant insight into the discourse. Language is not always (or ever) innocent and innocuous (Thompson 2007, 2011). The language that we use can try to steer us towards a particular way of viewing the world and reflects a particular discourse in operation. Habermas (1984, cited in Powell 2001) and Hecht (1998) cite language as one of the principle discourses which reproduces social structure and domination. For Habermas (1971) and others who share this concept of discourse, discourse is about not just 'what does a word (or utterance or expression) mean', but what does the word 'do' to people. Simply put, words can oppress people and make them feel vulnerable (see Box 6.3). According to Burr (2003), Hecht, Habermas, Thompson, and Foucault amongst others, language is a vehicle for conveying power and shapes social attitudes, behaviour, and even social structure.

Box 6.2   Example of a dominant discourse: The biomedical model

One influential discourse is that of biomedicine in modern medicine. At the end of the Middle Ages, with the development of rational thought in Europe in the period known as the Enlightenment, the way that the body and the nature of health and illness were perceived changed completely.

Health came to be seen as 'the absence of medical disease' and illness as 'the presence of medical disease'. In this discourse, ill health is to be treated through medical intervention, treatment, and cure. The goal of treatment is to achieve biologically defined normality, through manipulation of physical and biochemical processes including the use of drugs or surgery.

The discourse ignores other possible determinants on health and illness such as poverty or workplace stress, by making both health providers and patients focus on treating illness and sickness, rather than focusing on the real social and structural determinants of ill health and 'dis-ease' (Illich 1975).

The discourse elevates the power of the medical profession to be chief agents of cure and treatment through medical means (Illich 1975). As such, the associated medical specialities achieve a high status, as do the people associated with them, both health care professionals and the clients themselves. Ivan Illich (1975) wrote an influential analysis of the power of the medical profession and the biomedical model of health and illness, and the way it may have socialised many of us to think about our own health and illness.

Our lifelong socialisation into this biomedical model might make it very difficult to say 'no' to medical and health care professionals or to ask for alternatives to traditional surgical or pharmacological treatments. Talcott Parsons (1951) in his identification of the 'sick role' described the role of 'patient' as one of passivity, dependence, and helplessness in their relationship with the doctor or health care professional. Illich (1975) argued that the medical model has turned us all into 'patients', dependent on medical practitioners and their 'quick fixes' for all our ills, and weakening our tolerance to suffering. The biomedical model merely creates new types of disease even harming us as with the side effects of medication and surgical procedures (doctor caused harm – *medical iatrogenesis*: Illich 1975, and also cited in Cooke and Philpin 2008: 114 and in Barry and Yuill 2008: 37).

The critique does not set out to undermine biomedicine completely, it is certainly very effective in acute situations (such as a broken leg) where the cause of illness can be located through clear symptoms that can be linked to a diagnosis and treated. However, it is less effective in situations where multiple pathology and complex social factors are present. People can experience symptoms but a disease may not be able to be identified and therefore treated. On the other hand, people sometimes get diseases but without symptoms and therefore treatment may be too late to be effective. Sometimes treating certain diseases does not necessarily improve quality of life because absence of disease does not necessarily equate to good quality of life. This element may not be considered because the focus is on the physical and as such this approach has much less to offer in chronic health conditions. Additionally, Illich (1975) was highly critical of the biomedical model in that it had little to do with real improvements in health and longevity during the twentieth century which had more to do with clean water, improved sewerage, and better food.

It is also important to be aware that the biomedical approach is so dominant it can exclude (or discount) the perspective of other health beliefs. This may be very disempowering for some people. In recent years, the dominance of this approach and its associated limitations have been acknowledged (Fava and Sonino 2008). Particularly in relation to chronic health conditions, there has been recognition that the normal–abnormal dyad excludes many people and increases vulnerability. This has given rise to the 'patient expert' initiative (NPCRDC 2006) which acknowledges the fact that some patients are the expert on their condition and have to be viewed as equal partners in their care, including the sharing of control that this implies. It is argued that this transforms the negativity associated with some vulnerable groups.

Box 6.3   The power of language

The following is some discussion of the possible power of words and language in conveying power relationships.

Word	Discussion
Mankind/All men	Could reinforce a view that only male humans are of significance.
'Lower' social class	Could imply that someone is of 'lower' or 'lesser' social worth or value.
Medical and nursing texts	Can reinforce gender stereotypes, through the use of words and pictures that convey that doctor is a he/male, the nurse is a she/female. (See Microsoft Word clip art representation of nurses!)
'Compliance', 'non-compliance'	More *practitioner centred* term than 'therapeutic cooperation' or 'partnership'. The term 'non-compliance' blames the patient or service user for being 'awkward and uncooperative': this can ignore the fact that the original 'demand' was unreasonable, unasked for, not fully and freely consented to, or poorly explained in the first place which is then down to the action or omission of the practitioner.

Box 6.4   Practice suggestions

Therefore, according to Thompson (2011: 83–84), we should consider the following when using language with service users, patients, and colleagues:

- Be sensitive in our use of language by remembering that it can oppress and reinforce social inequalities.
- Remember that language can alienate: just as language can bring people together, the use of jargon or complex language can drive other people away.
- The focus and attention on language can be trivialised by people who use the argument of 'political correctness gone mad' to minimise and ignore the very real oppressive impact of language. Such attempts to trivialise and dismiss the focus on language should be challenged.
- Be inclusive and sensitive in our use of language by using accessible language that can be understood, as well being sensitive to the needs and rights of others who may use sign language or not speak English as their first language.

Further examples of the ways in which language and discourse can stereotype, dehumanise, marginalise, stigmatise, invisibilise, infantilise, or trivialise are examined in Chapter 4. Practice suggestions to consider when using language are provided (Box 6.4).

Social construction of identity

The way that we understand who we are and related to this why we act as we do can be described as our social identity. Try the Activity in Box 6.5.

How did you get on? People tend to classify themselves as well as other people according to their membership of social groups. Perhaps you identified yourself with a social role such as wife or son, or from a particular country or culture? Maybe you identified yourself as belonging to a social grouping around gender, class, or age. Perhaps you

---

Box 6.5   Activity

Who am I? Write down ten responses as fast as you can!

1

2

3

4

5

6

7

8

9

10

Box 6.6   Time for reflection

Reflect briefly on your responses:

• Do they fully and accurately describe who and what you are?
• Does this list tell me everything I need to know about you?
• If you had more time, which aspects would you add and which would you remove?
• Would you be happy to present all of the descriptions mentioned earlier to everyone you meet?
• Which people would you give the whole list to, and which aspects would be restricted for others?
• Would you reveal all aspects of the list to someone you have just met?
• In which situations would you reveal the whole list?
• Are there aspects of the list that only you are aware of?

---

reflected your employment status as a worker, student, or unemployed. You might have identified a religious or political affiliation. Now move on to the Time for reflection (Box 6.6).

Canton *et al.* (2008: 48) state that

> Family, friends and nationality, alongside our work and lifestyle/leisure identities, are routinely drawn upon to construct our overarching social identities. One identity tends to overlap the others and it is in the 'mix' that we know who 'we' and 'others' are.

This suggests that the 'reality' of who we are is not residing within us as a *fixed* and *static* identity to be identified by the 'right' personality test but is evolving over time and according to the people we mix with. Mair (1977) suggested that each of us is a 'community of selves', so that we have different identities that emerge at different stages in our lives and in different situations. According to this perspective, we are a fluid 'work in progress' which is never completed. We are constantly in the process of being socially constructed according to the situations, people, and roles we encounter.

Common groupings used by individuals and the wider society include

- Social class
- Ethnicity
- Age
- Gender
- Occupation/profession
- Sexual orientation
- Religion or belief system

In order to understand how identification with certain groupings comes about, let us consider one facet of identity – gender. When choosing a sleep-suit for a new baby as a gift, would the gender of the child influence your choice of colour? Even if it would not, consider whether this influences the makers of these goods and those that choose the stock for shops. Pink for girls and blue for boys is still a common feature in British retail (Cunningham and Macrae 2011). We learn this association from a young age; indeed, we may have worn such clothes and adults around us may have reinforced this link. In the same way, other gender associations are made such as girls learn dancing and boys play football; girls wear make-up, boys do not; girls are good at English and the humanities, whilst boys are good at maths and science; and boys are logical, girls are intuitive. Children are socialised from an early age into understanding the significance of categorisations or groups. We learn to place ourselves and others into groups and then *identify* ourselves and others as belonging to these groups. In effect, therefore, our identity is constructed through group membership; in describing ourselves we often describe these groups, for example, I'm a nurse, a mother, a Christian. The groups I belong to are 'in-groups' and the ones I do not belong to are 'out-groups' (Jenkins 2008). When my security feels threatened, I tend to seek refuge with my 'in-group'. Certain behaviours are expected in the group and so in order to 'belong', a series of subtle rewards or punishments keep us acting according to the 'rules' or norms of the group. Social institutions such as the media, family, and the education system play a very important role in reinforcing these norms.

Social groupings are widely used at all levels in society, for example, by government to collect statistical information about different segments of the population, as well as by groups and individuals themselves. There is a common belief however that we all share the same understanding about what each of these group labels means. For example, if I describe myself as a nurse, this 'label' may immediately conjure up some ideas about nurses in the mind of the listener based on their *construction* of nurses: some common media stereotypes of nurses according to Summers (2010) include 'battle-axe', 'sex-toy', submissive, 'not that bright', dedicated, caring, and so on. Media images of groups can affect our attitudes and indeed help to construct them, particularly if we have no personal experience of the grouping concerned. These images then underlie the label and therefore define its meaning for each individual. Further labels can be used as a kind of 'shorthand' to encapsulate the whole person rather than one facet of their identity. These categories/groupings/labels can therefore be restrictive, inaccurate, and stereotyped, leading to a 'self-fulfilling prophecy' where an individual is viewed by society as belonging to

> **Box 6.7   Time for reflection**
>
> So does it matter how others might describe our identity?
>   Look back at the notes you made for the Activity in Box 6.5 in which you were asked to describe 'Who am I?'
>   Given what you have just read, take one 'label' and make notes on how others might interpret this label. Try to think as broadly as possible. Include all possible views, even those you do not agree with.

a particular grouping and therefore expected to act accordingly. Before we continue to explore this further – let us take a moment to consider this, please undertake Time for reflection activity in Box 6.7.

This is quite a difficult activity as you are being asked to look 'through another lens' at labels that you perhaps take for granted. For example, you may have described yourself as female and believe this gender as equal to male. Others might believe females are very different from males and therefore have particular roles because they are 'naturally' good at certain things, like cooking and childcare. If people do believe this, they might treat you accordingly, for example, they might not encourage you to go to university because you are 'not likely to need a lot of education'. Unfortunately, if treated in this way, a female may then come to believe that indeed she is not capable of going to university, resulting in a 'self-fulfilling prophecy'.

It is important to realise that others may or may not describe us as we see ourselves. Thinking about what you have written, consider how others might describe your identity. There might be some terms that others use about us that may make us feel uncomfortable, even vulnerable; the way others describe our age or our sexual orientation perhaps. There might be situations where you could feel vulnerable in disclosing your marital status, because others may make judgements based on the grouping this places us in rather than about us as a person.

Essentialist views of identity

The tendency to share a generalised view of people and their behaviour based on their affiliation to social groups is linked to an essentialist perspective of social identity. Essentialism in this context refers to the belief that people have an underlying, fixed 'essence' in contrast to social constructionism and its view of the person as an evolving work in progress always in the process of being socially created and constructed.

Essentialism privileges biological and physiological explanations of human behaviour over sociological or psychological explanations (Culley 2000). This approach, sometimes known as universalism, gives rise to generalised statements about behaviour that take little account of cultural, historical, or individual variation. An essentialist view of gender, for example, might hold that because of their role in reproduction, women are biologically suited to take on nurturing and caring roles both within the family and wider society. Such attitudes affect societal perceptions of the type of occupations to which men and women are 'suited'. The problem with essentialist attitudes according to Bilton *et al.*

(2002) is that it is assumed that some universal *essential* feature identifies the phenomenon under study, in this example that *all* women are 'naturally' able to (and want to) take on care roles and by extension 'caring' occupations like nursing and primary school teaching. In other words, *all* women share particular essential traits in common and *all* men share other essential traits in common.

An essentialist approach to identity is apparent both in everyday conversation as well as some policy documents where understandings of social groupings are being used in a unified manner. For example, a speaker or writer may describe the experiences of black women who are single parents in generalised terms, as if all people viewed as from these categories – black, female, and single parent – are homogenous. To put it another way, by virtue of such group memberships, it is assumed that all individuals will share the same experience. In reality, each person's experience is likely to be shaped by a wide range of other factors such as support networks, economic circumstances, culture, and historical context. Such groupings are therefore heterogeneous (Culley 2000). The difference between *essentialist* concepts of identity and the notion of socially constructed identities is acceptance by constructivists that identity is complex and uniquely expressed (Bilton *et al.* 2002).

The following extract is from a book written by a young woman and her husband, both of whom have cerebral palsy.

> By the way, did you know, I'm only allowed one label. And it's Cerebral Palsy, or physically disabled! The following labels have apparently dropped off: Woman, White, British, heterosexual, daughter, wife, friend, the one with brown hair and glasses and the one who loves horse riding, that's me, but other people who have physical disabilities, are denied their label of being gay, being alcoholic, or a drug addict, or having mental health issues, behavioural disabilities or learning disabilities. For example, not all facilities for people with mental health issues have wheelchair access and not all facilities that are for people who are in wheelchairs are geared up to assist people with learning disabilities. Therefore individuals don't fit in to societies boxes, which is fine, but not if it means their needs go unmet. I don't fit in my box, I want more than daytime TV. (Dykes and Dykes 2009: 89)

You can see from this extract how a young woman understands her world and the way that people view her identity. She is very clear that she is more than her label, and that when people see beyond her label they become aware of her as a unique person. They will become aware of her strengths and of what she can do rather than what she cannot do. Equally, it is clear that services and facilities have reduced her social world through a narrow vision of identity and the privileging of one aspect of identity over others.

Essentialism and stereotyping

Thompson (1994), cited in Thompson (2011) argues that *naturalisation* results from essentialist thinking. This is the perception that on the basis of biological and physiological differences, people will 'naturally' and 'inevitably' fulfil different social roles. Try the Activity in Box 6.8.

Essentialist thinking might lead us to assume that because of changing physical abilities related to ageing, this 'decline' will mean that *all* old people are *naturally* unhappy, ill,

---

Box 6.8   Activity

Quickly jot down some words or images that you have commonly heard or seen used to describe and portray the following:

• Older people
• People with learning disabilities
• Asylum-seeking people

---

dependent, and therefore vulnerable. Equally, because people with learning difficulties have different cognitive abilities, *naturally* they will *all* need to lead simple lives, because they have simple personalities and aspirations, and do not feel things as deeply as (us) 'normal' people might. Similarly, it could be assumed that most asylum seekers are not white. A discourse from the colonial period of British history, but still with some power, characterises *all* people from BME communities as from 'under-developed' countries and therefore *naturally* poorer and uneducated in comparison to Britain. Black in this scenario is perceived as different from the dominant physical 'norm' of white.

Reflecting on the aforementioned paragraph, you might identify evidence of stereotyping – as described in Chapter 4. A stereotype is also a form of essentialist thinking about people that according to Thompson (2011) represent an over-simplified and biased conception of a social group. Like all essentialist views, the term has an inflexible meaning that is applied to all group members regardless of other factors. By contrast, Nzira and Williams (2009) argue that identities are *socially constructed* and in reality are not fixed but instead are as varied as there are different individuals living in different contexts. Older people, for example, may look different from younger people but *feel* the same as younger people. Individuals may feel less able physically to do some things (play football) but more able to do new things (play golf). Nzira and Williams (2009) write that health care practitioners must avoid stereotyping because it leads to treating people from social groupings not as individuals but as a homogenous group. In this way, everyone who is disabled may be viewed as dependent, for example, when for many a high degree of independence, differently fulfilled perhaps, is perfectly possible. It is paramount to get to know individuals before using essentialist views to make assumptions about them. Some generalisations about groups based on evidence are possible as a starting point, but it must always be appreciated that these groups are made up of individuals to whom the general may not apply.

It is not simply a question of niceties 'to get to know the person' rather than act according to the assumptions commonly held about social groupings. Not to do so could lead to increased vulnerability. For example, an essentialist perception of people fails to consider black identities and white identities as diverse and changing rather than fixed. Lewis and Phoenix (2004) write that the effect of highlighting racialised identities is to set and maintain boundaries between groups. In a study of internationally recruited nurse (IRN) mentors and white nursing students (Scammell and Olumide 2012), it was found that whilst students rarely mentioned race or ethnicity nor black or white, they frequently differentiated themselves from IRNs on the grounds of 'culture'. There was a tendency to categorise IRNs as a homogenous group; the participants implied that IRNs shared the same identity position whilst other facets of identity were ignored. The IRN participants were predominantly South Asian, Filipino, or Black African, except one, a White Canadian, all diverse groups in themselves; but also whilst all Filipinos hail from the same country, this does not mean all Filipino nationals are the *same* or experience being Filipino in the same way. Fixed identity constructions ignore the complexity that reflects real people. This was the case in the findings: generally IRNs as a group were constructed as having a negative identity – for example, their training was perceived as inferior despite evidence of excellent biomedical knowledge and technical skills.

Essentialist perspectives and vulnerability

To recap, the concept of essentialism reflects a view that societal structures and identity are fixed. These often privilege the role of biology as defining the person; for example, you are a boy so you are pre-determined by your gender to act in a certain way or you are Black so you a pre-determined by your ethnicity to act in a certain way. We attach labels to people who belong to particular groups. These labels are then imbued with meanings that reflect stereotypical attributions of the qualities and value we attach to different groups (Thompson 2003). Not only do these labels give rise to societal expectations about group behaviour but they also impact on the way group members themselves perceive how they are expected to act. So society creates the identity through shared understandings of the labels rather than being based on any fixed and core quality – recognising that such identities are 'created' by society rather than being fixed at birth (and natural) reflects the social constructionist perspective. Understanding these perspectives is central to explanations of how social identities are developed and maintained.

   Whilst group membership is part of our identity, the ways that people are labelled and described by self or others could contribute to feelings of vulnerability. This is because some labels carry a negative stigma (see Chapter 4 for an explanation of the process of stigmatisation). Certain labels can stigmatise, dismiss, or marginalise people such as asylum seekers or people from gypsy traveller communities. Moreover, being given negative social identities may contribute to experiences of a self-fulfilling prophecy and lowered self-esteem and self-worth. For example, black young men might be stigmatised by society as troublemakers and anti-authority and so some may feel devalued and 'act the part' (Cushion *et al.* 2011) Whether they do or not, stigmatisation might mean that mainstream society avoid the potential problems related to the label and avoid employing young black men. Given the fact that stigma is a feature and cause of many health and social problems and leads to significant vulnerability, it is essential that health professionals learn to recognise stigma and work to militate against its impact.

Social identity, oppression, and power

According to Dominelli (2002), identity uses perceived physical, psychological, and sociological differences to mark one individual or group from another. The differences are used to distinguish one from another not simply descriptively but in an evaluative sense.

Box 6.9   Time for reflection

- Think back to the Activity in Box 6.5 and the traits you chose to characterise yourself by.
- Now try to identify the 'opposite' trait to those you have identified for yourself.
- Consider each of the 'binary oppositions' you have identified and try to suggest which might be seen as 'superior' or 'more desirable' in Western culture, in your peer group culture, or in your family group.

Identity differentiation places groups representing certain traits in binary opposition to another, for example, old–young, black–white, men–women, able–disabled. The effect of such clear oppositions is that one trait can be valued in a society as more desirable and indeed superior to another. For example, in patriarchal societies, men are placed in a position of superiority over women. With superiority comes power; the superior group becomes the elite of the society and controls the workings of that society. In so doing, it follows that the society will be structured to enable the superior group to maintain its position over the inferior group (see Box 6.9). This links with the Marxist and 'system' theories of power discussed in Chapter 3.

Identity differentiation leads to the creation of 'them–us' divisions between people. In societies where biomedicine dominates, the able-bodied and healthy will be seen as 'normal' and therefore 'insiders' because they possess the desired characteristics of that society. In contrast, people with disabilities are constructed as 'outsiders' and therefore marginalised and socially excluded. Identities are constructed through interaction and reflect where people position themselves and are positioned by others in the social world (Woodward 2004). Identity is marked by difference, be this through symbols or physical characteristics such as skin colour or accent. By using criteria that we consider, marks people as the same as 'us', has the effect of marking others as 'them' on the grounds that 'they' are different from 'us', and are therefore outsiders. Further, difference is relational; the meaning of blackness, for example, is created through its relation to and difference from whiteness and vice versa. Skin colour is associated with sets of assumptions; being black or white is not only a means of marking difference but is also used as means of asserting superiority. Some differences such as skin colour are unequally weighted in favour of white people (Lewis and Phoenix 2004). Movements such as 'Black power' are a response to this and so passive acceptance of inferiority cannot be assumed. It is important therefore to recognise that blackness as well as whiteness can be used as to compensate for different power dynamics within interactions (Lewis and Phoenix 2004).

This power dynamic, where one group is perceived as superior to another, underpins the social construction of oppression (Dominelli 2002). It is important to note however that the powerful (superior) group needs the inferior group to maintain power. The dominant group defines their social standing in relation to others; insiders are the privileged group and outsiders are the excluded, inferior, and disadvantaged group. This constitutes a process of 'othering' that serves to dehumanise the outsider group. This is a very ethnocentric or egocentric view where the majority feel that *they* are the norm or standard and it is only *others*, especially when that difference may be highly visible, who are 'other', 'abnormal', or 'outsider'. When this happens, inhumane acts can become justified, leading to brutal treatment of Jews and other outsider groups in Nazi Germany or the institutionalisation of the mentally ill in the UK in the past with the associated loss of human rights (Rogers and Pilgrim 2001). Thus, othering is not simply noting difference, instead it is a process that identifies those that are thought to be different from oneself or the majority, reinforcing and producing positions of domination and subordination (Johnson *et al.* 2004).

It is however important to note that because identity is multidimensional, people can feel oppressed whilst also oppressing others (Dominelli 2002). For example, a female surgeon may be made to feel inferior by her male peers, yet act in an oppressive manner towards the female nurses working in the surgical ward. Alternatively, people can gain insight into oppression through the holding of insider and outsider status (Merriam *et al.* 2001). For example, a black male teacher may feel that his promotion prospects are being curtailed by his identity position in white-dominated British society. At the same time, he may be aware of the vulnerability of a white unemployed teenager that he pays periodically to wash his car. This insider–outsider perspective can develop empathy with the oppressed whilst also understanding the perspective of the oppressor (Dominelli 2002).

Being part of an oppressed group is for many a very disempowering experience. This identity can be accepted, accommodated, or rejected (Dominelli 2002).

A collective type of rejectionist activity according to Anspach (1979, cited in Clarke 2010) is through identity politics. This describes a form of political activism by marginalised groups to challenge the prevailing social construction of a negative social identity. In this way, groups who have attracted a negative social label seek to redefine their situation. For example, physically disabled activists have challenged socially accepted definitions of 'normal' to create a new positive self-image. They claim that the social construction of their disability is more disabling than the disability itself (Anspach 1979, cited in Clarke 2010). Disability activists argue instead for treating disability simply as one of many factors to be accommodated when living their life.

For health care practitioners, there is an imperative to contest these disempowering identities by engaging in anti-oppressive practice. Universalist and essentialist claims by dominant groups need to be challenged to promote social inclusion rather than exclusion. Dominelli (2002: 48) writes that 'anti-oppressive practice challenges the universalised biological representation of social divisions'. Rather than viewing people in a one-dimensional way through the lens of one social grouping, she argues for identity to be perceived as multi-dimensional, fluid, and constantly changing – thus emphasising a social constructionist rather than essentialist perspective.

Multiple identities

It has been argued that a person's identity is both complex and multifactorial. According to Nzira and Williams (2009), some aspects of identity are largely beyond our control, such as the colour of our skin, but others can be chosen such as parenthood or religion. We need to be aware that the way we see ourselves is not necessarily the way others see us. Context is clearly linked to the way a person feels in a given situation and therefore how they choose to define their identity at that time. Lewis and Phoenix (2004) write that the identities we adopt and those ascribed to us by others interact, giving us a sense of who we are but may not reflect what others 'read off' from us. One just has to think that the type of joke you might tell when with your peers, with your lecturer, or with your grandmother may vary according to each context when you might be presenting yourself as 'one of the lads', a responsible student, or an ideal grandson. In the same way, an individual may be a Muslim, a mother, a lawyer, British, and middle aged. These multiple identities interact to make the person who she is; however, one aspect may come to the fore at different times, for example, in a Mosque, at the school gate, or in a law court.

An essentialist conception of identity is therefore not reflective of reality. Multiple experiences and identities related to gender, age group, social class, sexuality, and occupational role, to name a few, are dynamically interacting to represent who we are. There are several facets of multiple identities. Shifting identities is a term used by Bristow (2011) to reflect the unstable nature of identity. For example, sexuality is a moving and changing identity for all gay, lesbian, and heterosexual people through life. So that whilst someone may identify themselves as 'heterosexual' at one stage in their lives, this may later change, and equally whilst defining themselves as 'gay' an individual may have a heterosexual experience.

Dominelli (2002) describes hybrid identities to reflect the changing nature of groupings within differing contexts. Essentialist discourses view culture as fixed. In this way, if you move to the UK from Bangladesh, perhaps to others you appear to live according to Bangladeshi ways. However, in reality the UK and Bangladeshi cultures overlap: clothes, for example, are adapted to the different climatic conditions. There may be a degree of assimilation into the dominant culture, as individuals may perceive this as a way to access some of the benefits of the privileged group. Different combinations result in complex hybrid identities. Indeed, some people do not want to accept one heritage but would prefer to embrace both (Browne 2008).

Finally, Sirin and Fine (2008) describe hyphenated identities such as Muslim-American; other examples include Black-African Briton or British-Asian. It is argued that a dual group membership means that a Black-African Briton is different from being either Black African or British but constitutes a new identity. Dominelli (2002) adds that hyphenated identities like British-Asian reflect the social construction of identity through the ongoing struggle to achieve legitimate self-definition for political purposes.

Social identity and practice

Nzira and Williams (2009) note that the ability to show that you respect and value someone's identity is a vital aspect of being anti-oppressive. An awareness of how people define their own identity, and how others perceive their identity will help practitioners to appreciate certain facets of vulnerability and in turn promote empathy with individuals. Scammell and Olumide (2012) note that considerable responsibility is placed on the practitioner to ensure unbiased care is provided for individual patients. Within health care policy literature, this is frequently paraphrased as providing sensitive care. In the context of working with multicultural populations, nurses, for example, are expected to provide culturally sensitive care (NMC 2008). This can sometimes be translated within education and practice as learning about differing cultural practices and drawing upon those based on the appearance of the patient and grouping him or her accordingly. This reflects essentialist conceptions of culture that involves learning the unique characteristics of an ethnic group and results in the differentiation of self from 'other'. The approach ignores the heterogeneity and changing nature of ethnic groups and privileges ethnicity over other aspects of identity. The perception of categories of difference as fixed and bounded has been challenged as unreflective of reality and derived from ideologies that privilege White people (Gustafson 2005). As we have seen from our discussion of multiple identities, the only way to know the needs of a patient is to interact with them on an individual basis, not to practice according to stereotypes about cultural (or other) groupings.

On the other hand, as Nzira and Williams (2009) state, an anti-oppressive stance is also not simply about treating everyone the same. Practitioners need to have an informed sense of the identity of the other person; this comes from genuine interaction to determine what aspects of their identity are particularly important given the context of care. Whilst drawing upon 'factfiles' (Culley 2000) about differing cultural groups, for example, is not advocated as a substitute for getting to know the individual person, some knowledge of the culture, language, and beliefs may demonstrate respect and help to put people at ease. Through authentic interaction, the practitioner may help reduce the risk of oppression and prejudice about vulnerable people and provide support to empower them in the process.

Practitioners need a clear sense of their own identity and how it impacts on others. We need to be open to the differing ways that people live out their identities and take care not to impose our realities onto others – this requires honest reflection and also the use of peer feedback. Whilst easy to say (and write), this process can be quite uncomfortable and is therefore sometimes avoided. Thompson (2003: 102) notes:

> When long-standing taken-for-granted assumptions are challenged, we can feel that our very identity is under threat.

As mentioned earlier in the chapter, key facets of identity are formed in our early years and reinforced by authority figures. Therefore, our perception of issues such as gender, ethnicity, disability, and sexuality become embedded in our understanding of the world. If these are questioned or challenged, this may seem to be challenging our very identity. The raising of awareness therefore requires sensitivity in order for people to open their minds to differing possibilities and realities – Chapter 9 explores the skill of elegant challenge as a means to offer sensitive peer feedback. In this way, we can become aware of oppressive attitudes and practices and our own part in reinforcing these.

To conclude the chapter, we would like to draw upon the real life case study of David to illustrate some of the issues discussed (Box 6.10).

In the scenario, we see how a patient's identity was redefined within a hospital setting as his life was inexorably changing and drawing to a close. Drawing on the essentialist perspective discussed earlier in this chapter, one might suggest that the health professional viewed Mort as naturally and inevitably falling into a role shaped and constructed by an ageist society. An ageist *discourse* might suggest the *social identity* of the 93-year-old man in the scenario would be non-productive, retired – therefore of little worth in a

---

Box 6.10 Case study of David

A 93-year-old man is admitted to a general ward in a large district hospital following a series of falls. His health is visibly failing and he presents as very frail. One of his children visits him and notices that the name over his bed is different to what she would have expected. She says to the health professional:

'You know, my father has never been called David. He has always been known by his second name, "Mort".'

The health professional replies, 'You don't mind us calling you David, do you David?'

Her question was taken as a statement of fact. Nothing was going to change. She went on with the task she was carrying out ignoring the patient's relative.

The old man sinks back into his bed and smiles weakly at her. In the last week of his long and productive life his identity has been changed.

Points for Reflection

• What do you think was the impact of this brief encounter on the old man and his daughter?
• Consider issues of identity, power, and control.
• What could the health professional have done differently?

---

capitalist society, 'over the hill', needy, and disabled. However, drawing upon the concept of *multiple identities*, rather than focusing on the *essentialist* stereotype of old age, in fact the following applied: father, grandfather, great grandfather, car driver, keen gardener, and raconteur. Additionally, the *ageist discourse* would have coloured Mort's perception of himself particularly in a relatively powerless position as an inpatient and may have led to Mort becoming a more passive, dependent, and a less resilient patient. Fook (2002) suggests that people can assume a disempowered, 'victim' identity because of being assigned to a certain category, for example, 'old' or 'patient'.

It is apparent that some groups are more powerful than others depending on the context that they are found in. For example, in the scenario, a *biomedical discourse* would attribute power to the health care professional. In contrast, the inpatient or their relative would be attributed with less power. In other contexts, where power is not located within a medical model, power may shift. Imagine being Mort's relative and being ignored. Despite having a relatively powerful status outside of the biomedical discourse, the relative felt 'paralysed' by her own concept of a *socially constructed identity* as a relative of a patient. The biomedical discourse influenced her to see herself as being less powerful and therefore unable to challenge within this context. This illustrates the concept of identity being socially constructed and varying depending on the context in which people find themselves (Nzira and Williams 2009).

The role of *language* is also clearly significant here – the apparently simple choice of the word 'David' rather than 'Mort' was powerful. It conveyed a power beyond the apparent simplicity of being 'just the wrong name'. The choice of 'David' conveyed to Mort that he was now 'under the control' of health carers, that his individuality and uniqueness was now at risk. It conveyed that his autonomy was under threat and that he was less important than the health carers. It also conveyed that if they could so easily get his name wrong, then what else might they misinterpret or treat as trivial? 'You don't mind us calling you David, do you David?' was a powerful statement disguised as a practical and

> **Box 6.11** Time for reflection
>
> When you look at patients what do you see? Do you see the whole person? A person who has lived a life outside of their current care setting. Do you see someone who has a rich history, family, and friends?
> Consider a patient you may have worked with recently. Were you aware of how you may have been influenced by how their identity was socially constructed?
> What stands in your way of considering a vulnerable person holistically?
> Make a list and then think about what stops you practicing holistically.

normal suggestion. The outcome, however, was that it reinforced the power imbalance between the patient and the health care professional.

Before we move on, we would like you to undertake the Time for reflection activity in Box 6.11.

As health care professionals, we should reflect on how we can enable, and if we are not enabling, then conversely how we can disempower, vulnerable people in our care (Healey 2005). Working with vulnerable people is a privilege and indeed puts us into a privileged position. However, we can so easily 'tip over' into unintentionally being disempowering. Saleebey (1996) suggests that language can elevate and inspire or demoralise and destroy. It follows therefore that language has the power to hurt. Health care professionals have the capacity to think about the meaning of words and the impact of the words they use on the people in their care. We have a responsibility to practice in the best way that we possibly can. We should reflect on how easily we can reinforce the social construction of vulnerability and consider how much energy it takes for a vulnerable person to challenge what appears to be acceptable practice within a powerful organisation or professional culture.

Conclusion

People are a unique mix of identities. They should be judged as people first and not labelled according to perceived attributes of societal groupings. Labels give rise to societal expectations about group behaviour but they also impact on the way group members perceive they should act. The approach professionals can adopt in labelling and categorising people can give rise to the potential for inaccuracies, stereotyping, and self-fulfilling prophecies. We should beware of treating people with particular identities as a homogenous group because fixed identity constructions ignore the complexity that reflects real people. People are more than their labels – seeing beyond labels leads professionals to become aware of unique individuals.

The role of 'expert' has a powerful impact on the relationship between the professional and the patient. Patients who want to be involved in their own health care may need permission from the health professional to do so. Respecting and valuing identity and being able to convey this is an important aspect of being anti-oppressive. Each person is unique and should be respected and empowered by a practitioner who perceives the patient as an expert in his or her own life.

Links to other chapters

- Power is explained in detail in Chapter 3 and may help to clarify some issues discussed in this chapter.
- Chapter 4 explores the processes of stereotyping and stigmatisation in greater depth.
- Chapter 6 explores the role of discourse in invisibilisation, together with offering further examples of the role played by language in the various processes of discrimination.
- Chapter 8 develops the concept of 'othering' further and illustrates the concept as a psychosocial explanation for oppression and vulnerability.
- Chapter 9 identifies a number of strategies for reducing vulnerability, amongst these is 'elegant challenge', a strategy identified in this chapter and explained further in Chapter 9.

References

Allen, D. and Hardin, P. (2001) Discourse analysis and the epidemiology of meaning. *Nursing Philosophy*, 2, 163–176.

Barry, A. and Yuill, C. (2008) *Understanding the Sociology of Health: An Introduction*. 2nd ed., Sage, London.

Berger, P. and Luckmann, T. (1966) *The Social Construction of Reality: A Treatise in the Sociology of Knowledge*. Anchor Books, New York.

Bilton, T., Bonnett, K., Jones, P., Lawson, T., Skinner, D., Stanworth, N., Webster, A., Bradbury, L., Stanyer, J. and Stephens, P. (2002) *Introduction to Sociology*. 4th ed., Palgrave Macmillan, Basingstoke.

Bristow, J. (2011) *Sexuality*. 2nd ed., Routledge, Oxford.

Browne, C. (2008) *Culture and Identity*. Polity Press, Cambridge.

Burns, D. (2012) Chronic fatigue syndrome or myalgic encephalomyelitis. *Nursing Standard*, 26 (25), 48–56.

Burr, V. (2003) *Social Constructionism*. 2nd ed., Routledge, Hove.

Canton, N., Clark, C. and Pietka, E. (2008) Living Together Programme. Migrant Cities Research: Glasgow. British Council. Available from http://www.crfr.ac.uk/spa2009/Clark%20C%20-%20 Intercultural%20dialogue%20in%20Glasgow%20-%20Migrant%20Cities%20Report%202008. pdf [accessed on 8 July 2012].

Cheek, J. (1999) Influencing practice or simply esoteric? Researching health care using postmodern approaches. *Qualitative Health Research*, 9 (3), 383–392.

Clarke, A. (2010) *The Sociology of Healthcare*. 2nd ed., Pearson Education, Harlow.

Cooke, H. and Philpin, S. (2008) *Sociology in Nursing and Healthcare*. Churchill Livingstone/ Elsevier, Edinburgh.

Culley, L. (2000) Working with diversity: Beyond the factfile. In: *Changing Practice in Health and Social Care* (Davies, C., Finlay, L. and Bullman, A. eds), pp. 131–142. Sage, London.

Cunningham, S. and Macrae, C. (2011) The colour of gender stereotyping. *British Journal of Psychology*, 102 (3), 598–614.

Cushion, S., Moore, K. and Jewell, J. (2011) *Media Representations of Black Young Men and Boys*. Report of the REACH media monitoring project. HMSO, London.

Dominelli, L. (2002) *Anti-Oppressive Social Work Theory and Practice*. Palgrave, Basingstoke.

Dykes, K. and Dykes, J. (2009) *Don't Give Up*. Roman Group, Bournemouth.

Fava, G. and Sonino, N. (2008) The biopsychosocial model thirty years later. *Psychotherapy and Psychosomatics*, 77, 1–2.

Fook, J. (2002) *Social Work, Critical Theory and Practice*, Sage, London.

Foucault, M. (2002 [1969]) *The Archaeology of Knowledge* (trans. Sheridan Smith, A.). Routledge, London.

Gustafson, D. (2005) Transcultural nursing theory from a critical cultural perspective. *Advances in Nursing Science*, 28 (1), 2–16.

Habermas, J. (1971) *Knowledge and Human Interests*. Beacon Press, Boston.

Healey, K. (2005) *Social Work Theories in Context, Creating Frameworks for Practice*. Palgrave Macmillan, Basingstoke.

Hecht, M. (ed.) (1998) *Communicating Prejudice*. Sage, London.

Illich, I. (1975) *The Limits of Medicine – Medical Nemesis: The Expropriation of Health*. Penguin, Harmondsworth.

Jenkins, R. (2008) *Social Identity*. 3rd ed., Routledge, Oxford.

Johnson, J., Bottorff, J., Browne, A., Grewal, S., Hilton, B.A. and Clarke, H. (2004) Othering and being othered in the context of healthcare services. *Health Communication*, 16 (2), 253–271.

Lewis, G. and Phoenix, A. (2004) 'Race', 'ethnicity' and identity. In: *Questioning Identity: Gender, Class, Ethnicity* (Woodward, K. ed.), 2nd ed., pp. 112–129. Routledge, London.

Mair, J.M.M. (1977) The community of self. In: *New Perspectives in Personal Construct Theory* (Bannister, D. ed.), pp. 1–29. Academic Press, New York.

Merriam, S.B., Johnson-Bailey, J., Lee, M.-Y., Kee, Y., Ntseane, G. and Muhamad, M. (2001) Power and positionality: Negotiating insider/outsider status within and across cultures. *International Journal of Lifelong Education*, 20 (5), 405–416.

National Primary Care Research & Development Centre (NPCRDC) (2006) *The National Evaluation of the Pilot Phase of the Expert Patients Programme*. Final Report. NPCRDC, London.

Nursing and Midwifery Council (NMC) (2008) *The Code: Standards of Conduct, Performance and Ethics for Nurses and Midwives*. NMC, London.

Nzira, V. and Williams, P. (2009) *Anti-Oppressive Practice in Health and Social Care*. Sage, London.

O'Connor, D. (2001) Journeying the quagmire: Exploring the discourses that shape the qualitative research process. *AFFILIA*, 16 (2), 138–158.

Parsons, T. (1951) Illness and the role of the physician: A sociological perspective. *American Journal of Orthopsychiatry*, 21 (3), 452–460.

Powell, F. (2001) *The Politics of Social Work*. Sage, London.

Regan, J., Bhattacharyya, S., Kevern, P. and Rana, T. (2012) A systematic review of religion and dementia care pathways in black and minority ethnic populations. *Mental Health, Religion & Culture*, 1, 1–15.

Rogers, A. and Pilgrim, D. (2001) *Mental Health Policy in Britain: A Critical Introduction*. 2nd ed., Palgrave, Basingstoke.

Rolfe, G. (2000) *Research, Truth and Authority*. Macmillan, Basingstoke.

Saleebey, D. (1996) The strengths perspective in social work practice: Extensions and cautions. *Social Work*, 41 (3), 296–305.

Scammell, J. and Olumide, G. (2012) Racism and the mentor–student relationship: Nurse education through a white lens. *Nurse Education Today*, 32 (5), 545–550.

Scott, S., Deary, I. and Pelosi, A. (1995) General practitioners' attitudes to patients with a self-diagnosis of myalgic encephalomyelitis. *British Medical Journal*, 310, 508.

Sirin, S. and Fine, M. (2008) *Muslim American Youth. Understanding Hyphenated Identities Through Multiple Methods*. New York University Press, New York.

Summers, S. (2010) The image of nursing: Does nursing's media image matter? Available from http://www.nursingtimes.net/nursing-practice/clinical-zones/educators/the-image-of-nursing-does-nursings-media-image-matter/5019099.article [accessed on 09 October 2012].

Thompson, N. (2003) *Promoting Equality: Challenging Discrimination and Oppression*. Palgrave Macmillan, Basingstoke.

Thompson, N. (2007) *Power and Empowerment*. Russell House, Lyme Regis.

Thompson, N. (2011) *Promoting Equality. Working with Diversity and Difference*. 3rd ed., Palgrave Macmillan, Basingstoke.

Woodward, K. (2004) *Questioning Identity: Gender, Class, Ethnicity*. 2nd ed., Routledge, London.

Chapter 7

Psychological perspectives of vulnerability

Nikki Glendening and Sid Carter

This chapter will explore the concept and experience of vulnerability from a psychological perspective both in terms of clients' and practitioners' own vulnerability and experiences. In doing so, it will offer a coherent link between the ideas explored in the previous and subsequent chapters using a range of narratives to explore and illustrate the theoretical explanations offered. For example, it will show how unconscious bias within cognitive appraisal and personal perception of situations, rather than the situation itself, can create and perpetuate vulnerability.

This chapter will therefore draw on theoretical concepts related to perceptual defence, attribution theory, and learned helplessness as a way of exploring and explaining these often unconscious psychological processes and the subsequent impact they can have on the lived experience of vulnerability.

Understanding how prejudice comes about is also argued within this chapter to be extremely helpful in explaining why people are discriminated against and oppressed. This chapter then utilises the evidence base surrounding this together with an understanding of resilience and hardiness to offer help to practitioners in reducing vulnerability and oppression in their own practice. As such, this chapter aims to raise practitioner self-awareness about their own behaviour and to show how an informed psychological understanding can help individuals adopt a more anti-oppressive approach in the future (see Chapter 9 for further explanation of this term).

Definition: Psychology

Psychology can be conceptualised as 'the scientific study of human behaviour' and the thoughts, feelings, and ideas that influence it (Rungapadiachy 1999). Psychology therefore seeks to explain and understand human beings and in particular their behaviour and the many individual and internal characteristics that influence this, including thoughts, feelings, beliefs, and ideas. In the case of social psychology, the influence of

Understanding Vulnerability: A Nursing and Healthcare Approach, First Edition. Edited by Vanessa Heaslip and Julie Ryden.
© 2013 John Wiley & Sons, Ltd. Published 2013 by John Wiley & Sons, Ltd.

the external social environment and the presence of other people, whether real, imagined, or implied, are also studied.

Psychology advocate or detractor?

Psychology, nonetheless, has many advocates and detractors. Indeed, you may start reading this chapter positioned somewhere along such a continuum. For example, advocates tend to place value on the application various psychological insights can have in understanding health, happiness, and how to promote a less discriminatory and oppressive society in which to live. In contrast, detractors tend to see psychology as misleading, deluded, and that its findings, at times, running counter to their intuitive experiences.

Interestingly, Butler-Bowdon (2007: 2), himself drawing on the writing of the early psychological researcher Ebbinghaus, described psychology as having 'a long past, but a short history'. What Ebbinghaus was alluding to is that people have tried to solve many of the human problems they encounter daily by thinking about and trying to understand human behaviour and its influences for hundreds of years. However, psychology as a scientific discipline only emerged in the nineteenth century, with the aim of subjecting such 'people watching' assumptions and speculations to more careful and systematic research enquiry and scientific study.

It is here perhaps that some of the tension arises between advocates and detractors. If people have been 'amateur psychologists' for aeons studying the behaviour of others and arriving at their own personal conclusions and explanations, they may see no need for a more formal discipline. They might expect psychological research findings to always match their own speculations. After all, understanding ourselves and others is 'common sense', so the line of reasoning goes. However, Hayes and Orrell (1998) point out that as human beings much of our everyday behaviour and thought processes are unconscious, fallible, and primarily self-centred; the latter being a survival technique that enables us to cope with and adapt to the world we encounter (see the discussion of 'survival' within practice settings in Chapter 5). Nonetheless, psychologists often argue that this 'natural' lack of awareness and a rather egocentric stance is prone to error, can easily be misleading, and can go on to cause us to make multiple judgement errors and mistakes, many of which we are likely to be totally unaware of (for example, Rungapadiachy 1999). Based on our own experiences alone, what we might believe with certainty about why we or others behaved as we or they did may not actually be 'true' when more rigorously and carefully investigated. This difference and potential dichotomy can lead some people to become detractors and dismiss the value of psychology. Interestingly, this very human reaction is explored further within this chapter under attribution.

To make the most of the learning opportunity that psychology, its findings, and ultimately this book has to offer, therefore, requires a degree of open-mindedness and honest self-reflection in which past certainties are suspended and new ideas are considered with the same respect afforded to existing beliefs and ideas. Try therefore not to just skip over the reflective activities or dismiss out-of-hand ideas that at first seem counterintuitive but instead engage with them and see where this leads and what new personal insights you gain.

What can psychology offer practitioners committed to reducing discrimination and oppression?

The simple answer to this question is 'plenty'. For example, and as already mentioned, psychology has the potential to help us make better sense of our own and others' behaviour. It can help provide us with answers about why people react and behave as they do, even when such behaviour appears to cause harm and at times self-defeating. It can also offer us explanations as to why *we* react as we do in similar or differing situations. Such understandings can go on to help us make more informed and conscious choices in the future about how we behave to both others and to ourselves.

For health and social care practitioners in particular, psychological understanding can help us facilitate more helping and caring relationships with clients, their friends and family as well as colleagues, and the wider community that we live and work in. It can also help us, as this chapter will go on to demonstrate, feel more in control of the events going on around us and as a consequence help ameliorate against any stress we experience as well as better cope with the demands placed upon us. Indeed, the more we feel a sense of control, the less vulnerable we ourselves can feel, as explored in Chapter 2. Psychological understanding therefore has the potential to reduce our own sense of vulnerability.

Subjective perception

A key assumption within psychology is that subjective perceptions, and the judgements that follow directly from these, provide a guide to understanding our own and others' behaviour, not necessarily the 'objective reality' of a situation. Indeed, Ornstein (1975, cited in Gross 2010) argues that instead of perceiving objective reality, we perceive only our own individual *construction* of that reality.

A distinction is therefore commonly made between sensation and perception (Malim and Birch 1998). For example, sensation relates to the collection of information (data) from the environment through our senses, whether these be the five traditional senses identified by Aristotle of sight, hearing, taste, smell, and touch, or the more recently recognised, albeit not by all, senses of temperature, kinaesthetic, pain, balance, and acceleration (Figure 7.1).

Conversely, perception relates to our *individual interpretation* of that (sensory) data. It enables us, via this interpretative process, to make sense of and interact with the world around us. Perception is thus a more individual construct. How we each interpret sensory information (i.e. perceive events around us) will nonetheless depend on many factors. For example, how much we attend or focus on something can influence how much sensory information is captured ready for interpretation, rather than being immediately filtered out before interpretation can take place. Equally, how we feel (emotional state), how much we desire and are willing to expend energy in achieving a goal (motivational state), our expectations and beliefs as well as the context in which the sensation occurs, and past experiences have all been found to influence perception.

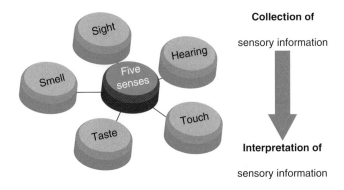

Figure 7.1 Subjective perception.

Perception is therefore selective. For example, much of the information received by our senses is never perceived and we consequently remain unaware of it. Indeed, individuals are constantly bombarded by sensory information from the world we live in but we only take in a very small amount of this information at any one time. If we did, we would easily and quickly become overwhelmed and could not attend to and concentrate on what we were doing or wish to do. We would consequently become unable to think, reason, and make decisions with any degree of clarity as well as fairly rapidly experience some form of stress. For example, trying to talk on the telephone or watch television when someone nearby is trying to simultaneously talk to you or when in lectures when others are chatting beside you while you try to listen to the invited speaker can both be stressful experiences for many. Thus, while the ability to selectively attend and, for example, block out much sensory information is in many ways desirable, it also has its limits and can lead to missed opportunities to understand the world around us as well as inadvertent judgement errors being made (activity in Box 7.1).

Box 7.1 Activity

This is a picture of Rubin's Vase designed by Danish psychologist Edgar Rubin. Spend some time looking at both pictures.

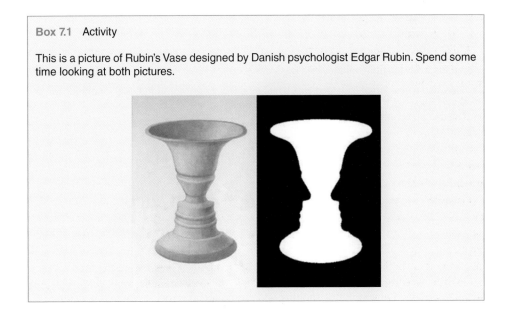

Do you see two pictures of a vase, one in colour and one in black and white? The likelihood is, if you have never seen these pictures before, if you only spent limited time attending to the picture, you were prompted to look for the vase (for example, title of the picture), so you did see a white vase on a black background in the picture on the right.

However, the picture on the right offers you two differing interpretations, each of them valid. For example, if you focused your attention more on the white, the likelihood is you saw a vase. However, if you have seen this picture before, you switched your attention to focus more on the black and were prompted to look for faces and/or attended to it closely, the likelihood is you also saw two people facing each other in silhouetted profile, albeit not at the same time as the vase.

This activity helps illustrate a number of key psychological concepts related to perception. For example, we tend to find it easier, and more readily attend to, familiar information than unfamiliar. Thus, if you have experienced Rubin's Vase before or the next time you are exposed to it, you are more likely to be able to switch your attention between the two differing images and perceive both. This can equally be applied to the perception of discrimination and oppression. If you are unfamiliar with the nature and concepts of these processes, it can be more difficult to recognise and perceive them. However, if you are aware that they exist, you can begin to notice and perceive evidence of them in your working life. This is particularly true for oppressive practices which are often, by definition, more complex and hidden and thus require a degree of active attention and awareness (see Chapter 9).

The influence of context on perception is also arguably illustrated by the Rubin Vase activity. For example, the black and white image was positioned next to an unambiguous image of a vase on the left. Gross (2010) argues that there is often an interaction between context, past experience, and expectation that lead to unconsciously misplaced, inappropriate, and/or misleading interpretations. He goes on to suggest that this is because we tend to interpret sensory information in keeping with how we normally construe or have previously understood the world (see activity in Box 7.2).

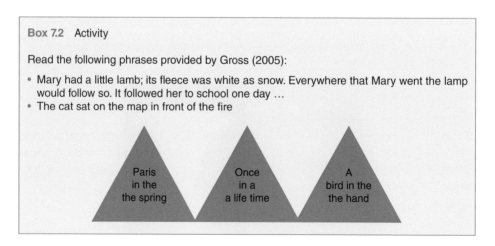

Box 7.2   Activity

Read the following phrases provided by Gross (2005):

- Mary had a little lamb; its fleece was white as snow. Everywhere that Mary went the lamp would follow so. It followed her to school one day …
- The cat sat on the map in front of the fire

Paris
in the
the spring

Once
in a
a life time

A
bird in the
the hand

Did you spot the typing errors? Did you read what you expected to read or what was actually written? Do you notice spelling and grammatical errors in your own writing?

Malim and Birch (1998: 272) highlight the central concept of *set* within such perceptual interpretations, describing it as 'a general term for a wide range of emotional, motivational, social and cultural factors which influence how we interpret and explain the world around us', that is, how we perceive it. Gross (2010) defines it further as 'perceptual biases or readiness to perceive or notice some aspect of the available sensory information while ignoring others'.

According to Gross (2010), factors that induce a perceptual set include:

- Content
- Instructions
- Expectations
- Motivation
- Emotion
- Past experience
- Individual differences
- Cultural factors
- Reward and punishment

For example, in terms of feelings and emotions that induce a perceptual set, it is argued that 'perceptual defence' is a term used to describe the widespread predisposition not to perceive something which may have unpleasant and/or unwanted emotional consequences (Malim and Birch 1998). Vulnerability, whether our own or others, discrimination, and oppression can all be subject to widespread perceptual defence biases. In the activity in Box 7.3, you will explore the links between perceptual defence and vulnerability.

Possible consequences include oppressive practices going unchallenged and unrecognised.

Gross (2010) also explores the closely related concept of schema, describing a schema as a group of persistent, deep rooted, and highly resistant ideas and assumptions, often subconscious, based on past reactions and experiences that are then used to interpret and process future sensory information and thus direct behaviour. As such, schemas influence attention and what people actually notice so that they are more likely to attend to information and perceive more easily that which fits into their existing schema, while at the same time interpreting as 'unusual, an exception, or unique' any information that appears to contradict it. Equally, schemas have a tendency to remain largely unchanged, even when contradictory information is presented, and the possibility that a schema may be 'faulty' is often not considered by individuals.

In terms of vulnerability and oppression, therefore, if clients are labelled as 'difficult', then the likelihood is clients will be perceived by practitioners as 'difficult' and only those behaviours that fit with this schema will be noticed, while other contradictory behaviours will be ignored (see, for example, the concept of the 'unpopular patient' discussed in Chapter 5).

Box 7.3   Activity

What might be the consequences of perceptual defence on the experience of vulnerability and oppression within your practice?

That subjective perceptions are prone to distortion is thus widely recognised by psychologists and has clear implications for practitioners wishing to practice in an anti-oppressive manner. The need for a critical and analytically reflective approach to interpretation of our perception is therefore paramount.

Making judgements and attributions

Many psychologists (for example, Hayes and Orrell 1998) would argue that we all regularly make judgements of others (see the activity in Box 7.4).

Box 7.4   Activity

Spend a few minutes considering whether you have a tendency to judge people and whether you might describe yourself as a judgemental person. Consider the reasons for your answer also.

Indeed, many psychologists would argue that as human beings we dislike uncertainty and incoherence (that is, lack of clarity or order) in our lives. For example, students often appear to dislike feeling uncertain about what a specific assignment task requires of them, rather than the hard work that might be involved in actually completing the task. Instead, it is argued that as human beings we have a basic and universal desire, albeit unconsciously:

- To make sense of and understand the world
- To predict what will happen next
- To feel in control in order to cope and reduce anxiety

Crisp and Turner (2010) propose that making judgements and 'attributions' is one way people try to meet this need by working out 'cause and effect'. Attribution theory thus tries to explain how we think about ourselves and other people, but as with perceptions, difficulties can arise when we make errors and/or we pre-judge a situation and/or others' behaviours. For example, prejudice or being prejudicial in essence means 'to pre-judge' someone or something and is defined by Eysenck (2002: 185) as an 'attitude and feelings (usually negative) about the members of some group solely on the basis of their membership of that group'.

> an assumption or preconceived judgement (usually unfavourable) made about someone or something before having adequate knowledge to be able to do so with any degree of certainty.

Attribution theory can thus help understand how we make judgements about the behaviour of others as well as ourselves. An attribution itself can be considered a claim about the cause of our own and others' behaviour and is thus a type of explanation we offer ourselves, albeit often unconsciously. According to attribution theory, we attribute (seek to explain) the cause of our own or other people's behaviour in one of two (main) ways, namely:

Internal or dispositional attribution – explains the cause of the behaviour as being internal to the person (for example, personality, mood, abilities, attitudes, effort)

Box 7.5   Activity

Imagine you meet a colleague for the first time on the first day of a new job or placement and you say 'hello' in a polite and friendly manner. Your colleague, who you don't really know yet, looks at you as if you've just hurled the world's worst insult at her. She then walks off without saying a word. You in turn are left wondering what on earth has just happened. What are you likely to think?

External or situational attribution – explains the cause of the behaviour as being external to the person (for example, the actions of others, nature of the situation, social pressures, luck)

The attributions we make will have important implications for the way we respond to others. For an example of this please undertake the activity in Box 7.5.

Crisp and Turner (2010) argue that when things like this happen to us, we naturally wonder why and speculate on and seek to explain what just happened. The likelihood is that we might decide that our new colleague is 'rude and not a nice person'. In other words, we offer an internal attribution as to the cause of the behaviour which in this case is perceived to be due to the personality or disposition of the colleague who is 'rude and has a rude personality'. However, these types of situations can cause us to make what is termed 'fundamental attribution errors'.

Box 7.6   Activity

Can you think of any examples from practice of prejudice when this type of Actor–Observer bias might have happened?

For example, think back to the last time you were rude to someone and ask yourself whether you also are a rude and unpleasant person just like the aforementioned colleague? According to Crisp and Turner (2010), whose example has been adapted here, you probably would not. You probably consider yourself to be a nice person who was rude because of a specific (external) and 'justifiable' reason (for example, stress from pressure of work). In other words, you offer yourself an external attribution in contrast to your colleague who you afforded an internal attribution. A key issue within attribution theory is that the attributions and judgements we make about ourselves are often quite different from those that we make about other people. This type of fundamental attribution error is known as 'Actor–Observer bias'. It is the tendency to attribute (explain) other people's negative behaviour (that we 'observe') to internal causes but our own negative behaviour (that we 'act') to external causes (see activity in Box 7.6).

Examples of fundamental attribution error (Actor–Observer bias) provided by Walker *et al.* (2007) include:

- If a client is anxious, we may attribute their anxiety to their personality (internal attribution). Yet if we are anxious, we may attribute our anxiety to specific causes and outside pressures (external attribution).
- If I am anxious about an illness symptom, I am likely to believe there is a physical cause, even if the doctor cannot find it (external attribution). If a client is worried about an

illness symptom for which there is no apparent cause, health professionals may believe the client is a hypochondriac and the cause is psychological (internal attribution).

Walker *et al.* (2007) also suggest that decisions about attribution take place on three separate dimensions, namely:

Locus – Internal (self) or External (other)
Stability – Stable (always) *or* Unstable (just on this occasion)
Globality – Global (in all situations) *or* Specific (just in this situation)

There is consequently a pervasive tendency to make judgements about ourselves as (for example) 'being rude', based on:

• External (situational causes)
• Unstable (just on this occasion)
• Specific (just in this situation)

Yet other people's rudeness attributed to:

• Internal (dispositional/personality)
• Stable (always – all occasions)
• Global (in all situations)

In such situations, people also often draw on stereotypes when making attributions, and stereotypes themselves, by definition, tend to be perceived as internal, stable, and global. Moreover, one possible result from such attribution errors includes 'victim blaming', defined by Crisp and Turner (2010) as 'holding the "victim" of a prejudice/ oppressive act to be entirely or partially responsible for the transgressions committed against them'. It is thus about often incorrectly holding individuals responsible for their own personal distress or difficulties instead of attributing responsibility to the transgressors who caused it. Such behaviours can also lead to secondary victimisation which can be considered the re-traumatisation through the responses of individuals and institutions.

The psychological concept of cognitive bias arguably offers one possible explanation of the victim-blaming behaviours. Indeed, cognitive biases, of which there are many, can help explain behaviour related to vulnerability and oppression. For example, cognitive bias is described as 'an unconscious human tendency to draw incorrect conclusions, often based on individual preferences and beliefs and regardless of the evidence and/or contrary information'. One such example relevant to 'victim blaming' is the 'just-world phenomenon' which reflects one way of feeling safer and protecting one's own self-esteem (as with all attribution distortions). Thus, if the potential victim avoids the behaviours of the past victims then they themselves will remain safe and feel less vulnerable. This is particularly true for people who believe that the world has to be fair as they often can find it hard or impossible to accept a situation in which a person is unfairly treated. This leads to a sense (distorted line of reasoning) that, somehow, the 'victim' must have surely done 'something' to deserve their fate.

Other cognitive biases commonly but unconsciously used include:

Confirmation bias

A tendency to only seek out information that matches what one already believes, rather than what the evidence might suggest.

In-group bias

In psychology, an 'in-group' refers to the group that we feel/believe we belong to, while an 'out-group' is a group of other people which we do not feel the same sense of belonging. In group bias, we tend to evaluate people within our 'in-group' more favourably than those in the 'out-group' (This is explored further in Chapter 8).

Out-group homogeneity effect (see also in-group bias)

The tendency to perceive people in an 'out-group' as homogeneous (same), while acknowledging the differences (heterogeneous) in the 'in-group'. For example, people with disabilities judged to be the same/have similar needs by someone without disabilities or impairments.

Interestingly, one explanation of why we as humans make such cognitive biases is the notion of heuristics (etymology is from Greek for 'find' or 'discover') which are conceptualised by Crisp and Turner (2010: 386) as 'timesaving mental shortcuts that reduce complex judgments to simple rules of thumb'. Heuristics thus save people time and effort in making judgements but are themselves prone to error. They are typically used when people face complex problems, incomplete information, and when they perceive themselves to be short of time. However, for practitioners working with people who may be vulnerable, accurate judgements may be preferable to quick, easy, and false ones. A number of different types of heuristics have been identified by psychologists, including the 'availability heuristic'.

Availability heuristic

The available heuristic is a tendency to rely upon information that is frequently and recently presented to us and thus more easily available as an explanation, rather than examine other alternatives or possibilities. Thus, because an explanation is repeatedly offered to us as 'true', it is mentally 'available' and easily brought to mind. Consequently, it can take on the illusion of being highly significant and valid. Let us explore this further by considering the case study of Alice (Box 7.7).

Box 7.7   Activity

Consider the case study of Alice (Case study 2.4 Chapter 2) who shortly after admission asked for a brown ham sandwich, was told this was not possible, and as a result went without supper. Now imagine how this experience might be reported in the nursing handover the following morning as well as in subsequent handovers.

What if the nurse reporting on this experience to his/her colleagues described Alice in emotive and prejudicial terms? For example, as 'difficult', 'fussy' 'cantankerous', and/or 'unreasonable' and these descriptors were then repeated at each subsequent handover. What impact do you think this may have on how the rest of the team and how they approach and interpret Alice's behaviour from then on? Consider also how this might be reinforced by the presence of the team during handover by also reviewing the Asch experiments explored in Chapter 8.

According to the available heuristic, the greater the frequency and intensity of information provided the more significant and valid it is likely to become in terms of others' perceptions. This also results in people becoming less likely to seek alternative explanations. Since nursing handover often occurs and is repeated at the start of each shift, any prejudicial information provided can therefore easily *appear* both significant and 'true' descriptors of clients' personalities, including Alice's in the example mentioned previously.

According to the available heuristic, this results in people becoming less likely to seek alternative explanations, for example, why Alice was declined supper. Moreover, nursing handover is often conducted in groups, and the Asch (1951, cited Hogg and Vaughan 2011: 239) experiments outlined in Chapter 8 illustrate how people will conform to incorrect judgements when these are made by a numerical majority of others. These findings draw attention to how people have a psychological tendency to want to 'fit in' and 'go along with the crowd', even when they feel the judgements are incorrect and are aware that going along with these will cause some degree of personal anguish (see, for example, the need to 'fit in' identified in Chapter 5). Let us consider this further in the activity in Box 7.8.

Box 7.8 Activity

Imagine you are involved in the nursing handover of Alice (see Box 7.7) in which the nurse in charge does in fact describe Alice as 'difficult' and 'cantankerous' for declining the ham sandwich offered following her admission. These comments subsequently go unchallenged by your colleagues but you feel they are unfair, discriminatory, and oppressive. However, when the handover is finished and you speak to a colleague, they too feel the same. Yet they said nothing.

List reasons why the practitioners involved, including yourself, may find it difficult to challenge the oppressive behaviours of others.

The likelihood is that you have identified numerous possible reasons. For example, you may feel that as a student or a junior member of staff, it is not your place to challenge more senior colleagues; colleagues themselves may believe there's no point as it would not change anything; a person may fear being isolated from the group (look back at the example of 'Lucy' Box 5.5 in Chapter 5). While these and other possible reasons may appear very distinct, many of these explanations can relate to the concept of control.

So far in this chapter, we have explored how cognitive and social psychology offer us many explanations of how and why we discriminate against each other. A set of theories and research which have contributed enormously to our understanding of the human propensity to treat each other badly is the psychology of prejudice.

> **Box 7.9** Activity
>
> Consider the following questions and answer them based on your current knowledge, experience, and beliefs.
>
> - Are we bound to be prejudiced in some way, whatever we do?
> - Can prejudice be a good thing?
> - Are some individuals more likely to be prejudiced than others?
> - Can we become more or less prejudiced depending on the situation we find ourselves in?
> - Can we 'catch' prejudice, become 'infected' with it?
>
> We will come back to them after you have considered the psychological evidence.

Prejudice: Psychological perspectives

Understanding how prejudice comes about is extremely helpful in explaining why people are discriminated against and oppressed but also offers an evidence base of how to combat prejudice and thus reduce vulnerability. Before we continue to consider the evidence base, we shall start by exploring your perspectives in the activity in Box 7.9.

How has prejudice been defined and explained by psychology?

Attribution theory is a well-established explanation of how we steer ourselves through complex social interactions generally, and false attributions in everyday life are often fleeting and have little impact on people's lives. However, we have seen the harm that can be done when our attributions are wrong, and negative, in the more intense world of health and social care, as they can lead to prejudice.

Psychologists have also studied prejudice as a separate entity. The motivation for most of the early findings sprang from horror at the atrocities of the Holocaust in World War II and a growing movement to end the oppression of African Americans in the USA in the same period. As a result, although the foundations of social psychology had already been laid, the 1940s and 1950s saw a huge addition to this body of knowledge. The framework for our current understanding of prejudice was created during this period, and the most notable psychologist in that enterprise was Gordon Allport. His 1954 treatise *The Nature of Prejudice* is still the model that the psychology of prejudice is based on today. A lot of Allport's writing is very quotable, but the following definition of prejudice is one that he appeared to like; he suggested that prejudice is

> thinking ill of others without sufficient warrant (Allport 1979: 6)

Allport acknowledged that prejudice can be positive, but his particular interest was racial or 'ethnic' prejudice, which he believed had no positive elements. Since then, psychologists have studied a much wider range of attributes that are discriminated against in addition to race, for example, gender, age, sexual orientation, and disability. Of these, though, research indicates that gender, race, and age are the primary bases for stereotyping (Mackie *et al.* 1996). There is an important feature of prejudice contained in the definition from Allport, which is reinforced in the findings of the various psychological approaches to prejudice, namely, that prejudice is most powerful when it is based on ignorance. Paradoxically, the less the prejudiced person actually knows about the object of their prejudice, the stronger that prejudice is likely to be. This reinforces again the importance of avoiding assumptions and having a strong evidence base for our practice.

Another popular definition of prejudice came from Rupert Brown, who built on Allport's thinking, stating that prejudice is

> the holding of derogatory social attitudes or cognitive beliefs, the expression of negative affect, or the display of hostile or discriminatory behaviour towards members of a group on account of their membership of that group (Brown 1995: 8)

Brown attempted to condense a sophisticated collection of theory and research into this phrase, some of which we will be exploring in this chapter. There are some key points about prejudice contained in his definition. One is that prejudice starts with negative attitudes that may in themselves not be directly harmful, but they can escalate into active harm under certain conditions. Hogg and Vaughan (2011) illustrate this through the example of attitudes towards a group of students doing a certain course. In their example it was engineering students, but let us consider nursing students. Students doing other courses may have some generalised beliefs about what student nurses are like, which may be partly complimentary or at worse might be irritating. In social psychological terms, this is the cognitive component. If a negative emotional element is added to this, known as the affective component, and then an intention to do something about it, known as conation, then an irritating generalisation has become a prejudice and might become more serious. Hogg and Vaughan (2011) then speculate if individuals who shared this prejudice joined together in an organisation, they might well be more likely to act on their prejudice. If that organisation then gained power in a university, they might segregate student nurses and deny them resources, and taking the scenario to its conclusion, ultimately it might end in violence. As Hogg and Vaughan point out, there are strong pressures in place to prevent such a prejudice and its consequences arising in reality, but it demonstrates how when certain conditions apply, practically any identifiable group of people could experience extreme prejudice.

Psychology has approached explaining prejudice in many ways, amongst the most significant are – prejudice as a personality trait, social categorisation, stereotyping, and intergroup relations. These will now be explored in turn.

Prejudice as a personality trait

There have been several attempts to explain prejudice as a feature of the individual, but the best known is Adorno *et al.* (1950) theory of the authoritarian personality. Their programme of research was motivated directly by revulsion at the extermination of Jews and other minorities by the Nazi regime, and their work actually commenced during the

Holocaust in 1944. Adorno and his co-researcher Frenkel-Brunswik were themselves both Jewish and had escaped from Hitler's Europe (Hogg and Vaughan 2011).

The work of Adorno and his colleagues was a combination of Marxism, Freudian psychoanalysis, and psychometric personality psychology. Their work proposed several personality 'syndromes' that could lead to a person being prejudiced, but the most prominent was the authoritarian syndrome. Put simply, this syndrome emerges from a harsh and punitive upbringing, particularly from the father, as this leads to the person 'displacing' their aggression away from their father (the real target) on to minority out-groups. Adorno *et al.* (1950) suggested that the key element of their findings was the production of personalities *susceptible* to prejudice. When many individuals have this susceptibility, and this was combined with strong social movements, such as Hitler's Nazism, mass prejudice could occur and lead to fascism.

Personality approaches to prejudice can be very persuasive, and the work of Adorno and his colleagues led to a great deal of further research. However, this approach contains several weaknesses, the primary one being that it does not take enough account of the powerful situational and sociocultural forces that are exerted on us. The alternative explanations of prejudice covered in the following sections amply demonstrate the power of these social forces.

Social categorisation

From Allport's (1979) early writings about prejudice to more current discussions about diversity (Blaine 2007), psychologists largely agree on the cognitive necessity of categorisation. From moment to moment we take in vast amounts of information, which is made much more manageable by sorting into categories. One of the authors of this chapter has worked with a couple of people who placed every file they had on the 'Desktop' of their computers. Work documents, letters to their bank managers, links to websites, it all went on the Desktop, not even in alphabetical order. Unsurprisingly, these individuals wasted a huge amount of time 'looking for things'. Imagine how their lives would have been transformed by applying even a very simple structure, or set of categories, to their files, such as 'work', 'home', and 'weblinks'.

Thankfully, we are primed to categorise information, so are much more efficient than the people described. Social psychologists propose that we deal with the enormous amount of information that we absorb about other people in the same way – we place people into simple categories. It takes up a lot less time and processing power to reduce the actual rich diversity of every person into a few simple categories, such as tall, middle class woman.

There are some categories that we are more likely to use than others, known as the primary social categories, which are age, gender, and race (Blaine 2007). Ito and Urland (2003) measured attention through brain activity when pictures of black and white men and women were presented to participants. The race of the person presented was noticed in approximately a tenth of a second, and participants noticed the person's gender shortly after that. Thus, it seems likely that the primary social categories are beyond our control. We use other social categories to add to our primary appraisals, these are guided by what

> **Box 7.10   Activity**
>
> It is interesting to reflect on this feature of categorisation in the context of health care. Imagine that you tend to categorise those around you in practice as either staff or service users. This means that you would tend to place greater emphasis on the differences between staff and service users. It would also mean that you tend to regard the staff as having similar characteristics to each other and that service users likewise share many characteristics. The staff/service user categorisation is a very likely one to make; do you see these predicted effects in yourself or in others?

attracts our attention, plus we tend to group people with similar attributes together. We also use categories that we are familiar with, and our cultures provide categories (Blaine 2007).

An important feature of categorisation noted by social psychologists is that once a categorisation has been established, differences **between** the groups tend to be emphasised even more. In addition, similarities **within** groups are accentuated (Brown 1995) – see the activity in Box 7.10.

Social categorisation is an important feature in the production of stereotypes, which are known to have an influence on an individual's vulnerability and the experience of oppression.

Stereotyping

Social psychologists tend to view social categorisation as relatively benign or neutral; it is simply a way of dealing with a large amount of information more efficiently. However, to efficiently place people in social categories, we have to discard a lot of detail, some of this detail can be replaced with a more generalised set of information called a stereotype. The notion of the stereotype within social science is more complex than it may appear. Though he was not the first, Walter Lippman, a political journalist in the early twentieth century, is credited with giving the concept of the stereotype the importance that it has today (Pickering 2001). An element of Lippman's writing about stereotypes that may help our understanding of the concept is his describing them as 'pictures in our heads' of any group of people (Allport 1979: 191). Lippman's imagery conveys some of what social psychology has since discovered about stereotypes. The consensus view is that stereotypes have the difficult job of conveying some important information about a social category as a whole, which is then applied to individuals within that category. Stereotypes are usually over-generalised and exaggerated accounts of the personalities, behaviours, and motivations of a group of people. Stereotypes also have the job of conveying how we ought to feel about, and react to, a certain group (Blaine 2007).

An example of how the process of stereotyping works could be the social category of individuals who earn their living in the construction, home delivery, maintenance, and light engineering industries. This is a neutral social category or even positive if a person in those industries has just done a good job for you. However, a potential stereotype emerging from that social category is 'white van man'. Many individuals familiar with mainstream UK culture would without hesitation be able to produce a fairly long list of individual attributes for that stereotype and also be aware that it conveys a clear negative image to us. Extending this to a health and social care context, practitioners may well have no difficulties with the social category of people with mental health problems, but what about if a service user is presented as a 'self-harmer'?

Clearly health and social care practitioners need to be wary of stereotypes, as they can be precursors of prejudice. From early on in the study of prejudice, it was noted that there may be a 'kernel of truth' in any stereotype (Allport 1979: 190), but no stereotype could apply accurately and equally to each and every member of a group that has been stereotyped.

Intergroup relations

How different groups interact with each other provides a convincing explanation for prejudice but is also one of the key ideas within social psychology. The intergroup behaviour theory suggests that though we are all individuals, our individual perceptions, thoughts, and behaviour can arise from our recognition that we belong to a distinct social group (Hogg and Vaughan 2011). From the intergroup behaviour view, how we think, feel, and act is heavily influenced by our membership of groups. We belong to our in-groups, meaning that the members of other collections of people belong to out-groups.

Campbell (1965) is credited with collating ideas from several disciplines and proposing that much social behaviour can be understood more clearly if the goals of different groups are compared. If the goals of two groups are compatible or complementary, then there is likely to be harmony between the groups. For example, in the UK in the 1980s and 1990s, due mainly to scandals and rising costs, the Government introduced policies to close large institutions for people with mental health problems and learning disabilities. Service users, their representative organisations, and professionals largely had this same goal as the Government, so relations between these 'groups' were relatively harmonious. Since then, these two groups have been more in conflict, with claims that the Government should allocate more resources to people with mental health problems and people with learning disabilities, and attitudes have changed accordingly.

Campbell (1965) named this feature of intergroup relations Realistic Group Conflict Theory: the attitudes and behaviour between groups will tend to reflect their respective, very real, interests. When two groups are fighting for the same scarce resources, hostility and prejudice are more likely to occur. When we hear prejudiced views expressed towards particular groups on radio, TV, in pubs, and so on, how often do we hear phrases such as 'they' are taking our jobs/decent housing/good school places/car parking spaces/sun loungers by the pool, the list goes on! Sherif (1966) was a significant proponent of this view, and conducted well-known experiments providing evidence that prejudice is exacerbated when intergroup goals are in conflict with each other.

Sherif's most famous experiments involved groups of boys on summer camp, chosen to be stable and from non-deprived backgrounds, to ensure that their behaviour was due to group effects, not their personality or social status. In the various versions of the experiment, the groups of boys were initially kept apart and then put into competitive situations. Changes were found when the groups were in competition: the boys showed in-group bias, hostility towards the out-group, and friendships became much more limited to the in-group. This applied even when in one condition friends were put in different groups.

Subsequent research has demonstrated that inter-group relation is a robust theory to explain how groups can become prejudiced towards each other.

Reducing prejudice

The psychology of prejudice has always contained some element of how to reduce it, a principle established early on by Allport. Following are some prejudice reduction interventions which are supported by research (Blaine 2007).

Contact hypothesis – the earliest approach, proposing that contact between groups can reduce intergroup prejudice. There is support for this, but certain conditions apply: contact should be with an out-group member of equal status, the interaction needs to be cooperative, and contact needs to be with out-group members who are typical of that group.

Self-regulation of prejudiced behaviour – stereotypes often contain positive and negative elements, leading to inconsistencies. Pointing out the negative elements can lead to shame, which motivates a more consistently positive view.

Stereotype inhibition and substitution – though stereotypes are automatic, they are amenable to change. Consistent positive associations or cognitive training can lead to a reduction in negative stereotypes.

Cross-categorisation – social categorisation can lead to over-simplified views about other groups. When individuals from opposing groups find they have joint membership of other groups, hostility tends to reduce; perceived differences are lessened.

Empathy – when individuals are encouraged to feel empathy for negatively stereotyped groups, their attitudes towards those groups improve.

To summarise, social psychology's approach of studying individuals as members of groups reveals much about prejudice. There are no absolutely right or wrong answers, but if you go back to the questions in Box 7.9, you should now be able to give more informed responses. Brown (1995) makes a very important point about the study of prejudice and how it impacts on social inequality. Social psychology continues to make an important contribution, but a full understanding of prejudice requires knowledge of the historical, political, economic, and social structures that surround a person as well.

A summary of some other psychological approaches pertinent to vulnerability

We have explored attribution theory and psychological approaches to prejudice and discovered that they offer us a great deal in terms of understanding how any of us can become vulnerable. There are other areas of theory and research in psychology that are pertinent to an appreciation of vulnerability and oppression, perhaps not as immediately obvious, but they extend our understanding of how these harmful processes operate. The concepts we will be exploring are control and resilience.

Lack of control

Control itself relates to the belief in our own ability to influence the direction of or to be able to restrain something if needed, in this case the nurse's prejudicial descriptions. The extent to which a practitioner believes they can control oppressive behaviours is therefore likely to influence whether they will try and challenge such behaviours or not. A sense of control is also central to coping and a lack of perceived control can result in stress, mental anguish, and vulnerability, in contrast to similar situations where a sense of control is achieved do not induce feelings of stress and vulnerability. Indeed, as Walker *et al.* (2007) point out, gaining control over new or difficult situations can lead to increases in self-confidence and self-esteem through a greater sense of personal mastery.

Learned helplessness

Nonetheless, the concept of learned helplessness relates to a sense of helplessness or hopelessness that people can often experience when they do not feel they are able to exert control over the situations they face. According to Seligman (1975), who first proposed this concept, this sense of helplessness leads to changes in the way people then think about their ability to control (influence) similar situations in the future, leading them to become inappropriately passive in the face of unpleasant, harmful, or oppressive situations, even when they actually do have the ability to improve the situation.

Learned helplessness has therefore been defined as the perception – not necessarily the reality of a situation – that one's own actions will have little or no influence on events and that it will therefore be futile to keep trying, both now and in the future (Taylor 1995). It is a response to perceived uncontrollability and helps describe what happens when a person gradually comes to believe that they have no control or influence over their situation and therefore whatever they do will not alter the outcome.

Learned helplessness therefore develops over time and has the potential to develop from any and all experiences people find difficult or challenging. However, it will only occur in situations where people *perceive* they cannot exert any control or influence over what is going on. For example, because they lack the necessary interpersonal skills to challenge elegantly (see Chapter 9 for more details) as exemplified within Box 7.8.

Process of learned helplessness

- Repeated exposure to situations in which a person perceives they have little or no influence or control over the situation and/or outcome (perception of uncontrollability).
- Lack of perceived influence/control leads people to feel a sense of helplessness and a reinforced belief that they can do nothing to change the situation they face and/or the outcome they desire.

- This sense of helplessness in turn increases the mental anguish and emotional response already felt, further sapping motivation while at the same time increasing a sense of physical and psychological fatigue.
- Combined these beliefs and the resulting emotional anguish and fatigue change the way people then think about their ability to control (influence) similar situations in the future so that they convince themselves that they can do nothing to change similar situations in the future, irrelevant of whether they could or not (generalisation).
- Person remains passive in the face of future unpleasant, harmful, or oppressive situations, even when they actually do have, or could develop, the ability to improve the situation.
- Person therefore 'learns to be helpless'.

People exhibiting learned helplessness therefore tend to make situational, stable, and global attributions to justify their apparent inaction in the face of oppressive and discriminatory behaviours. Further highlighting perhaps the concept of mutual vulnerability discussed earlier in Chapter 2. Indeed, failure to understand the process of learned helplessness and in particular the tendency of people to generalise a sense of hopelessness to future situations can lead to inadvertent victim blaming and an ongoing cycle of oppression.

Nonetheless, the concept of learned helplessness, by its very nature, also implies the potential for 'unlearning'. Therefore, since personal perception and cognitive appraisal, rather than the reality of situation itself, are all deemed influential in perceptions of hopelessness, active listening responses and elegant challenging of attribution errors are all potential strategies worthy of consideration. Equally, the need to actively promote a sense of personal control and guarding against undue dependence by adopting an empowering approach that includes emotional and esteem support, mastery opportunities, and encouragement is also likely to be effective.

Resilience and hardy personality

Resilience refers to an individual's psychological tendency to cope effectively with stress and repeated adverse experiences. Resilience thus has the potential to ameliorate and mitigate against emic experiences of vulnerability. Interestingly, Ungar *et al.* (2007) identified a number of interdependent and cross-cultural influences upon resilience, all arguably relevant to practitioners wishing to reduce vulnerability. For example, resilience can be increased by enabling and facilitating

- Access to resources
- Meaningful social relationships and support (for example, provision of emotional, informational, instrumental, and affiliation support)
- Valued personal and social identity
- Sense of control and personal power
- Awareness of cultural values, beliefs, and practices
- Experience of social justice and acceptance
- Affiliation and a sense of cohesion with others

Correspondingly, Kobasa (1979) coined the term 'psychological hardiness' to describe a pattern of personality characteristics closely associated with effective coping in response to potentially vulnerable and challenging situations. According to Kobasa (1979), a hardy personality consists of three personality characteristics including positive perceptions of

- *Commitment–*
  an active involvement and commitment to achieving desired goals
- *Control –*
  a high sense of personal control and belief in the ability to positive influence and overcome the demands and potential barriers encountered in achieving desired goals
- *Challenge –*
  a positive perception of change and challenge as normal and potentially leading to greater personal and professional development

Conclusion

The psychological concepts explored in this chapter reveal a great deal about how vulnerability comes about, but also how it can be tackled. Cognitive science informs us that perception is a constructive process; we use simplified 'rules of thumb' to make sense of our world, to save our precious cognitive resources. This can lead to important information being lost, which may be vital to a full and meaningful understanding of a service user's situation. The constructive nature of perception also leads to selective attention, basing our perception on what we expect, which leads to us giving greater attention to anything unusual in our environment, opening up the possibility of discrimination.

Attribution theory builds on this, providing an insight into how we can get 'differentness' very wrong, these misinterpretations potentially turning into oppressive behaviour. Without self-awareness, our attributions will almost always be in our favour.

The specific consequences of false beliefs about other people have been studied by psychologists through research into prejudice. The psychology of prejudice reveals how negative attitudes are an important root of this pernicious phenomenon. We naturally place what we perceive into categories to make our thought processes more efficient. However, when these categories become negative stereotypes based on characteristics such as race, age, and gender, they can lead to harm. Being aware of belonging to a particular group can also cause prejudice, particularly if your group and another are in competition with each other for scarce resources.

Psychology contributes to our knowledge of vulnerability by also investigating the personal resources we possess that are protective against becoming vulnerable. It is possible for us as individuals to build up a resilient approach to adversity. Ensuring that service users retain as much control as possible will also help towards preventing their vulnerability.

To return to the question asked at the beginning of the chapter, you will see by now that psychology certainly has 'plenty' to offer our understanding of vulnerability. It can appear that prejudice and discrimination are inevitable to some extent, as our minds are tuned to pick up difference, identify it, and label it. These are processes that mostly ensure our well-being but become more ominous when applied to contentious labels such as race, age, or gender.

Alternatively, psychology also teaches us that we are not necessarily trapped by these processes. Under the right conditions, ill-informed prejudice can be turned into a celebration of diversity, harmful stereotypes can be rejected, we can look to ourselves first as the potential cause of a misunderstanding, and we can actively ensure that service users retain as much control as possible. By actively applying psychology to our practice, we can become partners with service users to combat vulnerability and oppression.

Links to other chapters

- Chapter 4 discusses stereotyping and includes specific examples of the ways in which health and social care clients may be made to feel vulnerable through this process
- Chapter 5 explores the concept of the 'unpopular patient' and also the role of group culture in increasing the need to 'fit in'.
- Chapter 6 identifies the social construction of labels and the role of essentialism in encouraging the use of labels.
- Chapters 6 and 8 explore the role of labels in the process of 'othering' and 'in-group', 'out-group' behaviour which leads to discrimination and vulnerability.
- Chapter 8 explores the processes of conformity and compliance and how these group pressures might prevent an individual taking action against observed vulnerability.

References

Adorno, T.W., Frenkel-Brunswik, E., Levinson, D.J. and Sanford, S.N. (1950) *The Authoritarian Personality*. Norton, New York.

Allport, G.W. (1979) *The Nature of Prejudice*. 25th Anniversary ed., Addison-Wesley, Massachusetts.

Blaine, B.E. (2007) *Understanding the Psychology of Diversity*. Sage, Los Angeles.

Brown, R. (1995) *Prejudice: Its Social Psychology*. Blackwell, Oxford.

Butler-Bowdon, T. (2007) *50 Psychology Classics*. Nicholas Brealey, London.

Campbell, D.T. (1965) Ethnocentric and other altruistic motives. In: *Nebraska Symposium on Motivation* (Levine, D. ed.), pp. 283–311. University of Nebraska Press, Nebraska.

Crisp, R.J. and Turner, R.N. (2010) *Essential Social Psychology*. 2nd ed., Sage, London.

Eysenck, M. (2002) *Simple Psychology*. 2nd ed., Psychology Press, Hove.

Gross (2005) *Psychology: The Science of Mind and Behaviour*. 5th ed., Hodder Arnold, London.

Gross, R. (2010) *The Science of Mind and Behaviour*. 6th, Hodder & Stoughton, Abingdon.

Hayes, N. and Orrell, S. (1998) *Psychology: An Introduction*. 3rd ed., Pearson Education, Harlow.

Hogg, M.A. and Vaughan, G.M. (2011) *Social Psychology*. 6th ed., Pearson Education, Harlow.

Ito, T. and Urland, G. (2003) Race and gender on the brain: Electrocortical measures of attention to the race and gender of multiply categorizable individuals. *Journal of Personality and Social Psychology*, 85, 616–626.

Kobasa, S. (1979) Stressful life events, personality, and health – inquiry into hardiness. *Journal of Personality and Social Psychology*, 37 (1), 1–11.

Mackie, D.M., Hamilton, D.L., Susskind, J. and Roselli, F. (1996) Social psychological foundations of stereotype formation. In: *Stereotypes and Stereotyping* (Macrae, C.N., Stangor, C. and Hewstone, M. eds), pp. 41–78. Guilford Press, New York.

Malim, T. and Birch, A. (1998) *Introductory Psychology*. Macmillan, Basingstoke.

Pickering, M. (2001) *Stereotyping: The Politics of Representation*. Palgrave, Basingstoke.

Rungapadiachy, D. (1999) *Interpersonal Communication and Psychology for Health Care Professionals: Theory and Practice*. Butterworth Heinemann, Oxford.

Seligman, M.E.P. (1975) *Helplessness*. W.H. Freeman, San Francisco.

Sherif, M. (1966) *Group Conflict and Co-Operation: Their Social Psychology*. Routledge and Kegan Paul, London.

Taylor, S. (1995) *Health Psychology*. 3rd ed., McGraw-Hill, New York.

Ungar, M., Brown, M., Liebenberg, L., Othman, R., Kwong, W., Armstrong, M. and Gilgun, J. (2007) Unique pathways to resilience across cultures. *Adolescence*, 42 (166), 287–310.

Walker, J., Payne, S., Smith, P. and Jarrett, N. (2007) *Psychology for Nurses and the Caring Professions*. 3rd ed., Open University Press, Maidenhead.

Chapter 8

Psychosocial experiences and implications of vulnerability

Chris Willetts, Gill Calvin Thomas and Vanessa Heaslip

Introduction

This chapter builds on Chapters 6 and 8 and adds a psychosocial perspective, where sociological and psychological concepts and understandings can be combined together, to explore how vulnerability, discrimination, and oppression can be caused, created, and experienced. This approach has been termed *psychosocial* as it combines both psychological and sociological approaches.

Psychosocial is defined as 'relating to the interrelation of social factors and individual thought and behaviour' (Oxford English Dictionary (OED) 2012). Martikainena *et al.* (2002) who use an OED definition of psychosocial argue that it is about the interrelationship between the individual (psychological understandings of people and their behaviour) and their social environment. They give the example of health and disease as being a psychosocial process which may be a product of the interplay between the individual's perception, reaction, and response to stress, together with a presence or absence of social and environmental stressors and stressful life events. The interplay of factors at both levels can give us a better insight into who may experience good health or less than good health.

This psychosocial approach will be used to explore vulnerability in that although some more purely sociological concepts will be used to explore the causes of vulnerability, many of them, such as an individual's reaction to peer pressure to conform and go along with oppression as illustrated in the experiments of Milgram (1974) and Asch (1951, cited in Hogg and Vaughan 2010) discussed later in this chapter, clearly illustrate the interplay between the individual's choice of how to behave mixed with the presence of peer pressure and authority figures. These psychosocial phenomena such as obedience and conformity to peer and authority figure pressure can have devastating effects in terms of the extremes of dehumanising behaviour and indifference towards others that can be induced in subjects when certain sociological and psychological conditions are present. The chapter will ultimately seek to raise awareness of how these

Understanding Vulnerability: A Nursing and Healthcare Approach, First Edition. Edited by Vanessa Heaslip and Julie Ryden.

psychosocial factors can contribute to the experience of vulnerability for patients, service users, and healthcare professionals.

What is sociology and its possible use in exploring vulnerability and oppression?

The last chapter defined the term 'psychology'. So if a psychosocial approach involves combining psychological and sociological understandings, a good starting point for this chapter is to define what sociology is. Although a standard definition is offered here, you could look in any other sociology textbook in order to see how it is defined.

According to British sociologist Anthony Giddens,

> sociology is the scientific study of human life, social groups and whole societies. It's … subject matter is our own behaviour as social beings. The scope of sociological study is extremely wide, ranging from the analysis of passing encounters between individuals on the street, to the investigation of international relations (Giddens 2009: 6)

However, for Fulcher and Scott, in one simple sense, sociology could enable us to 'understand the world we live in but also to understand ourselves for we are the products of the world' (Fulcher and Scott 2011: 4). They argue that we are products of a variety of influences throughout our lives, from the socialisation that we experience in our earliest days in the family, school, and peer group right up to the influence on us as adults from mass media, wider culture, and experiences gained through employment and leisure, which can all exert a continuing influence on our attitudes and behaviours.

Bilton *et al.* (2002: 442–443) argued that the value of sociology is to look beyond 'common sense', 'taken for granted', or 'partial or incomplete understandings of society' … 'we should aim for a disciplined understanding of society', to expose those 'taken for granted assumptions' that people often make (Bilton *et al.* 2002: 442–443).

In this chapter, we will use sociological and psychosocial theories and concepts to look for both wide-scale social processes that might cause or create situations in which vulnerability or oppression may occur but also at some of the smaller scale but no less damaging processes that can occur even on a small social scale. This includes what happens in teams or groups so that in some situations, abuse, vulnerability, and oppression can flourish. In a short book chapter, we will only be able to scratch the surface of all the possible psychosocial factors which can lead to vulnerability and oppression. However, the chapter authors hope that this will stimulate some thinking and reflection about how when certain psychological and social factors come together, abuse, vulnerability, and oppression are more likely to occur.

Many sociological and psychosocial concepts, which when acted out can lead to vulnerability, discrimination, and oppression, such as labelling, stereotyping, and stigma, have already been discussed, particularly in Chapter 4 which looked at these Processes of Discrimination. This chapter will now begin by looking at other more wide-scale sociological explanations which might help explain *why* this discrimination and oppression

---

Box 8.1 Theories to explain possible causes of discrimination and oppression

1 Historical explanations
2 Exploitation explanations
3 'In and out group' (the Othering of others) explanations

---

occur (Box 8.1), and *why* and *how* some people may have been made to feel vulnerable and will then move on to more psychosocial explanations.

Historical explanations

Much prejudice, oppression, and even violence could be said to have its roots in history. Examples are in the long standing inter-racial and inter-ethnic tensions and conflicts in Afghanistan, Iraq, Syria, the genocide in Rwanda in 1994; the civil war around the Congo basin in Africa fought almost continuously since 1996; the 'ethnic cleansing' genocide in Sudan and Darfur; and the inter-ethnic conflict that has happened in Europe in the past 30 years in Bosnia-Herzogavina and Kosovo, and which has even occurred in the north of Ireland (Sun 1993, Gaines and Reed 1995, Malim and Birch 1998, Stephan 2008, Nzira and Williams 2009, Thompson 2012).

Some of the most historically enduring inter-racial and ethnic tensions include general anti-Semitism against Jewish and Arab peoples and Islamaphobia, which may have long histories, but multiple causes (Falk 2008, Cohen *et al.* 2009, Iqbal 2010, Bleich 2011). Recently, the rise of radical Islamic fundamentalism may be a reaction to perceived oppression by the West in Somalia, Afghanistan, Pakistan, Egypt, and the Palestinian homelands (Ansari 2000, Abu Sway 2005, Freeman 2008). There is also a long-standing worldwide prejudice and discrimination towards the Roma and gypsy community, which in its extreme form led to the extermination of hundreds of thousands of Roma and gypsies in Nazi Germany (Tyrnauer 1991, Bársony and Daróczi 2007) as well as the on-going discrimination experienced by these communities today in Britain and across Europe (Cudworth 2008, Ignățoiu-Sora 2011, O'Nions 2011).

Box 8.2 Time for reflection

Identify a long-standing inter-racial or inter-ethnic conflict which might have resulted in warfare and conflict at some point in the past.

• Reflect on what might have been the root causes of this conflict or violence?
• List any causes you can think of.

Critics of an historical approach, although acknowledging the often long-standing nature of these tensions, would want to explore the causes of such inter-group conflict in the first place (Sun 1993, Gaines and Reed 1995, Stephan 2008). No matter how long standing that suspicion or hatred, the reasons for the existence of the prejudice towards the 'hated' group in the first place still needs identification (see Box 8.2).

It is important to avoid using historical precedent and the long-standing nature of any inter-group or inter-ethnic conflict as a justification or legitimation as to why it should exist or be accepted (Rosado 1998, Ardil 2009). If one seeks to be anti-oppressive and to challenge discrimination and vulnerability, it is important to look for the real causes of any prejudice, discrimination, and oppression, whether that is a long-standing or recent phenomenon. Therefore, we may need to look for other possible sociological and psychosocial explanations for inter-group tensions and conflicts.

Exploitation explanations

Institutional and structural racism

Many authors have suggested that inter-group tensions and conflicts are based on the exploitation of a powerless group by a more powerful one. Prejudice and negative attitudes are used as a justification for the exploitation of the weaker or powerless group by the more powerful. An exploiting class stigmatises some group as inferior, so that it offers a 'justification' so that they (as slaves), or their resources, may be exploited by the dominant group. This could describe the Colonialism and Imperialism practised by the European powers during the 1500s in Asia, Africa, and South America, and the use of slaves within various societies throughout history (Cox 1948, cited in Allport 1958, Pelaez 1976, Foreman-Peck 1989, Fanon 2004, Samir 2012). Some authors when considering racism in modern society (Carmichael and Hamilton 1968, Mason 1982) coined the term 'institutional racism', defined as the subordination of a racial group or groups, and maintaining control over those groups, often covertly by the active and pervasive operation of 'anti-black' attitudes. Macpherson used the term in his report into the racist murder and subsequent mishandling of the investigation by the Metropolitan Police who were accused of not taking the investigation seriously or treating it as a hate crime (Macpherson 1999: Clause 6.34). See Chapters 3 and 4 for further discussion of oppression and the creation of vulnerability through cultural and structural processes.

The exploitative nature of capitalism

Another sociological explanation for the possibility of oppression and vulnerability is linked to living within a capitalist society. Capitalism exerts a double exploitative influence, in that firstly the system is inherently exploitative and oppressive but also that welfare is only offered 'generously' to people deemed to be 'economically productive' and hence useful to the capitalist class (Harbert 1988, Finkelstein 1990, cited in Oliver 1990, and Thompson 2003, 2006, Oliver and Barnes 2012). This structural aspect of power and oppression was explored in Chapter 3.

The requirement within capitalism for a compliant, pacified workforce who will sell their labour for a lot less than the value of the goods or services they produce in order to generate profit for the capitalist class is the motor driving the capitalist system. According to the critics of capitalism, beginning with influential economist and sociologist Marx (1858) and later Marx and Engels (1887, 1893, 1894 and 1863 over four volumes of *Das Kapital*), they described what they believed to be the exploitative nature of capitalism. In their view, capitalism has an inherent conflict of interest between the interests of the capitalist ruling class (*the owners of wealth and production, the bourgeoisie*) and the interests of the worker class (*the proletariat who only have their labour to sell in return for wages*), which produces two opposing and competing class interests.

Fixed structural inequalities, i.e. the exploitation of the *proletariat* class by the *bourgeois* class and their control over production and the 'masses', not through force but through 'indoctrination' into the dominant capitalist ideology, are the only ways to make the system pay for the capitalist class. Marx and Engels (1845–1846) argued that although the proletariat are paid (low) wages for their labour, they described the role of a ruling ideology as a way of co-opting the proletariat into accepting their oppression through mystification of the 'real' nature of the system, which Engels described as 'false consciousness' (Engels 1893). This works when workers are induced to believe that their 'best interests' are served by supporting capitalism which brings them employment and wages. They are encouraged to believe that they may be 'best off' under capitalism, despite low wages, exploitation of their labour, and the threat of unemployment and poverty. According to Marx (1844), in the nineteenth century capitalism, religion served a purpose in reinforcing this illusory (or false consciousness), whereby the proletariat through church attendance were encouraged to accept their 'lot' (suffering and all) in this life in the hope of a better time in the 'after-life'. Hell was the threatened consequence for 'wrong doing'.

The Christian hymn 'All Things Bright and Beautiful' is a possible illustration of this (Box 8.3) with its exhortation in *Verse 3* to accept that God made and ordered the world

---

Box 8.3   Extract: Words to Christian hymn 'All Things Bright and Beautiful' (Words by Alexander 1848)

All things bright and beautiful,
All creatures great and small,
All things wise and wonderful,
The Lord God made them all.

Verse 2
Each little flower that opens,
Each little bird that sings,
He made their glowing colours,
He made their tiny wings.
All things bright…

Verse 3
The rich man in his castle,
The poor man at his gate,
God made them high and lowly,
And ordered their estate.
All things bright…

Verse 7
He gave us eyes to see them,
And lips that we might tell,
How great is God Almighty,
Who has made all things well.
All things bright…

with 'the rich man in his castle and the poor man at his gate'. Angus (2009) decries the Christian God described in this popular Victorian hymn as the creator of the world and of *social stability*.

More contemporary critics of capitalist society argued that the mass media (Dahrendorf 1959, Marcuse 1964, Postman 1985, Chomsky and Hermann 1988, Chomsky 2002) and other social institutions such as the education system (Gramsci 1968, Althusser 1971, Illich 1971, Gatto 2005) through indoctrination and the 'hidden curriculum' in school serve the purpose of reinforcing the 'acceptance' of capitalist social relations by the 'exploited' class.

Marxist critiques of welfare (welfare payments and free welfare services such as healthcare) are that, on the surface, welfare appears to support workers and their families during temporary times of need or hardship (for example, ill health or unemployment) (Dahrendorf 1959). However, he also suggested that the welfare state helps take the rougher edges off of capitalism. A starving and desperate citizenry might be more likely to revolt against the social system and capitalism than a partially satisfied population who were 'looked after' through welfare when times were hard. To simplify, for Dahrendorf (1959) and others (Miliband 1969, 1982, Pierson 2006) the welfare state could be seen as preventing any revolution against exploitative and oppressive capitalism. In other words, the welfare state both hides capitalist exploitation whilst propping it up at the same time.

Other right wing critics of welfare and the welfare state (Friedman 1993, 2002, Hayek 1994, 2011, Murray 1996, 2001) see welfare as being 'expensive' and a 'drain' on resources away from the needs of the capitalist economy. They question why hard-working people are required to pay taxes to support people deemed to be undeserving or irresponsible. These authors recommend the rationing, means testing, and stigmatising of welfare, especially towards people who may be deemed as a 'burden' on society, who are economically unproductive and undeserving, such as 'work-shy', 'feckless', and 'amoral' individuals who do nothing but conceive children to get welfare 'entitlements' and sit at home watching endless episodes of the 'Jeremy Kyle Show'. Jones, in his book *Chavs: The Demonisation of the Working Class* (2012), shows how working people, particularly those seen to be 'benefit scroungers and work-shy loafers', have been demonised through the media and popular culture over the past 20 years. An example is the portrayal of the character of the chav 'Vicky Pollard' in the BBC TV Comedy series 'Little Britain'.

Others (Harbert 1988, Finkelstein 1990, cited in Oliver 1990: 25–42, Thompson 2003, Oliver and Barnes 2012) argue there is an oppressive welfare value that operates in a capitalist society like Britain that when the 'adult labourer' is no longer required or becomes economically unproductive, their purpose and value is greatly, if not totally, diminished to the owners of capital. Therefore, many of the oppressed groups are those who are less economically productive as actual or potential workers for the capitalist class, i.e. older people, unemployed people, people with disabilities or mental health problems, students, and anyone deemed 'uneconomic'. Not paying for welfare is a cheap option for 'right-of-centre' governments who can then reduce taxation on the middle and upper social classes.

Gender exploitation

Radical and socialist feminists such as Sylvia Walby (1990a) suggested that gender inequality and oppression are systematic and structural. Walby explained the term

---

Box 8.4   Equal pay: The facts (Fawcett Society 2010)

- The full-time gender pay gap between women and men is 14.9%.
- The pay gap varies across sectors and regions, rising up to 55% in the finance sector and up to 33.3% in the City of London.
- Interruptions to employment due to caring work account for 14% of the gender pay gap.
- Sixty-four per cent of the lowest paid workers are women, contributing not only to women's poverty but to the poverty of their children.
- There are almost four times as many women in part-time work as men. Part-time workers are likely to receive lower hourly rates of pay than full-time workers.
- Nine out of ten single parents are women. The median gross weekly pay for male single parents is £346, while for female single parents it is £194.4.
- For every £100 men take home, women are typically earning about £85, though the gap varies between regions and sectors. In London, the pay gap stands at 23%.

---

patriarchy as the systematic oppression and exploitation of women by men for gain. Walby (1990a, 1990b) notes this can be sexual, financial, and economic exploitation such as through the expectation that free domestic work, including unpaid child and adult care at home, falls to women. She also describes the exploitation of women by the capitalist class as employers rarely pay women the same as men for the same job: evidence for a 'pay gap' by the Fawcett Society (2010) suggests that the pay gap between men and women still exists today (Box 8.4).

However, the Office for National Statistics (ONS, 2011) is slightly less pessimistic suggesting that 'the gender pay gap has fallen below 10 per cent for the first time. Standing at 10.1 per cent in April 2010, the gap between men's and women's median full-time hourly earnings excluding overtime was down to 9.1 per cent in April 2011'. However, this still suggests a significant pay gap over a year after the Equality Act (2010) came into force which sought to end that pay gap.

Another area of possible exploitation and inequity is differences in 'who does the housework'. Oakley (1974), Beechey (1987), Warde and Hetherington (1993), and Sullivan (2000) found that over the last 40 years women still do disproportionally more housework and child care than men although they also found men are taking on more housework than previously. This is described as women doing a 'double' or 'second shift': doing paid work and then coming home to do unpaid domestic work (Hochschild and Machung 1989). However, Warde and Hetherington (1993) did find that although women still on the whole did more domestic work at home, there is a distinct gender division of labour where men took on chores often outside of the home such as car maintenance, decorating, DIY, and gardening.

Dunscombe and Marsden (1993) argued that women do more than a double shift, but carry a 'triple burden', as they often take on the burden of providing the demanding emotional care and support of other family members. This could include visiting sick family members in hospital or if a patient themselves, carrying the worry of who is taking care of the family and home while they are ill. What is more, Oakley (1974: 87) found that women reported housework and their domestic burden to be more monotonous, soul destroying, and lonely than factory production line work!

Other authors have identified the material and physical exploitation of women in other domains. Coy (2009) describes the exploitation of young and adult women through the systematic and widespread grooming and abuse of 'looked after children' in care and care leavers which hit the headlines in the UK with the exposure of this abuse of vulnerable young women in Rochdale and the North West (Williams 2012). There is also the serious exploitation of women through people trafficking and the coercion of women in the sex industry (Lozano 2011) and through pornography and the degrading media objectification of women such as in the *Daily Star* and the *Sun* (Russo 2001).

The reader may want to reflect that although exploitation, discrimination, and oppression of people because of their race or ethnicity, gender or social class may exist, which can contribute to their vulnerability, is the motive to exploit alone sufficient or adequate as an explanation as to why these exist?

'Othering'

Othering is a process which was described in Chapter 6 and refers to a competitive 'them and us' process whereby others (them) are treated or made to feel different, 'unwelcome outsiders' and subordinate in order to make the 'In' group (us) feel better about themselves (Dominelli 2002: 44–48). *It is* sometimes referred to as the 'In Group' and 'Out Group' phenomena as described in Chapter 7. This can lead to marginalisation, stigmatisation of the 'out'/'other' individual or group, and even dehumanisation, and a denial of their personhood, so that discrimination and even violence can take place against the targeted group. For further detailed study of the concept, you are directed to Chapter 6 and these sources: Dominelli (2002), Thompson (2003, 2006), Nzira and Williams (2009), Krumer-Nevo and Benjamin (2007), Maccullum (2002), Canales (2000, 2010), Johnson *et al.* (2004), Beisel (2010), and Hodson and Esses (2005). This chapter will focus on the concept as a psychosocial explanation for vulnerability.

Box 8.5   Activity

Think back over your experiences of healthcare either as a patient or a member of staff. What attributes do you associate with the term 'patient'?

If we see and define ourselves in relation to others, it can be argued that othering is unavoidable. Johnsen (2010) agrees and argues for a need for respectful othering in which we see the other in an objective but respectful way. If we consider this in the context of healthcare, it can be argued that as professional practitioners there is a need to objectively view patients in order for assessments to be systematic and rigorous in the context of professional practice and therefore we naturally see patients as others. For example, let us stop for a moment and consider the label we assign to people when they enter healthcare, in that they become 'patients'; this simple process can be argued as othering in that we are highlighting a difference between them as patients and ourselves as staff, and this difference does denote a power differential. Many of us may not consider labelling patients as patients problematic; however, we do have to question whether there are potential problems with assigning people with such a label (activity in Box 8.5).

Box 8.6   Oxford English Dictionary

Patient (adjective)

* able to accept or tolerate delays, problems, or suffering without becoming
* annoyed or anxious: be patient, your time will come, a patient and painstaking approach

Patient (noun)

* person receiving or registered to receive medical treatment: many patients in the hospital were more ill than she was

Pearsall (2002) *Concise Oxford English Dictionary*. 10th ed, Oxford University Press, Oxford.

In this activity, you may have written words such as ill, frail, needing assistance, compliant, hospital, unwell, patient, and accepting help and assistance. It is really interesting when we examine in the dictionary (Box 8.6) the word patient, as it is associated with receiving healthcare (noun) whilst the adjective links to being patient. It is useful to consider how many of the words you identified in Box 8.5 were linked to attributes we expect a patient to have (grateful, not demanding). We have to consider the implications if patients behave in a way that challenges our perceptions of what a patient should do or should be.

For example, have you ever heard patients being referred to as demanding, challenging, or difficult, but why were they labelled in such a way, was it perhaps because they did not confirm to our perceptions of what a patient should be? You may wish to go back to Chapter 5 to revisit the work presented there on the unpopular patient. This demonstrates some of the difficulties with assigning the label 'patient' to another and constitutes a possible psychosocial reason for the vulnerability of patients, clients, or service users.

The label of patient and nurse denotes a difference between us, asserting our professional dominance over them. This dominance is perpetuated through language (using medical terms that patients may not understand) as well as culture (wearing uniforms, as well as hospital systems that are geared towards the needs of the staff - for further exploration of this please see Chapter 2)). However, Johnsen (2010) would argue that this objectification can be managed in a way that respects the patient as a person as opposed to reducing them to a list of biomedical conditions. However, the predominance of the biomedical discourse in healthcare has led to patients being seen by their current clinical condition, rather than seeing them as a person. Just take a moment to consider the labels we assign to patients, for example, bariatric, MI, stroke patient, demented, and acopia, to name a few. The common practice within healthcare to focus more exclusively upon the medical condition rather than the person has been heavily criticised recently due to its links to poor quality care being delivered to patients (Department of Health (DoH) 2008, Parliamentary and Health Service Ombudsman 2011, Department of Health 2012). This demonstrates the real negative impact of othering on healthcare. Ultimately, as professionals, we must acknowledge our initial opinion of patients whilst remaining sensitive and flexible in our perceptions to challenge them which Johnsen (2010) refers to as respectful othering.

Shapiro (2008) identified that the most extreme form of othering is scapegoating, in which the person is somehow blamed for their condition/illness as if they are responsible. During the early 1980s and the early days of the AIDS epidemic, individuals infected were highly scapegoated and AIDS was seen and often referred to as 'the gay plague' in which homosexual men were somehow blamed for contracting HIV. Currently, within society and healthcare, politicians often refer to the 'obesity time bomb', and people who are obese are often scapegoated for their condition, in that they are seen as greedy and irresponsible for being overweight. Another example is people who have chronic obstructive pulmonary disease (COPD) are often scapegoated for their breathlessness due to the links between smoking and COPD. There are implications of this in that we know that people who have a negative experience of accessing healthcare are less likely to access it in the future and seek appropriate healthcare (Bowes 1993, cited in Johnson *et al.* 2004), thereby increasing their vulnerability to ill health.

Canales (2000) offers an alternative perspective by seeing othering as both an exclusionary and inclusionary process. Exclusionary othering uses the power within relationships for domination and subordination; here one group seeks to have power over another resulting in one group being marginalised, oppressed, and excluded (see Chapter 3 on Power, discrimination, and oppression). An example of this has been written about by Chakraboti (2010) who described an annual village bonfire celebration where the burning of a mock gypsy caravan was used to symbolise the purging of gypsy travellers from the village. This extreme view of othering identifies that in the case of the village the gypsies are not seen as part of the community but somehow as outsiders that must be eradicated. This is an extreme case of othering; however, I know from my research with gypsies and travellers that many have experienced subtle forms of exclusionary othering on a daily basis. One example is an older Romany gypsy who has lived in a village for 30 years but has never been invited to any of the village dances or activities and had even had a petition by the village community against her purchasing some land within the village. The implications of this was that she never felt valued or wanted in the village in which she lived, and she did not feel a close connection with the other people who lived in the village and preferred to undertake her shopping some six miles away. This directly impacted upon her sense of belonging and feeling valued within her community which could lead her to being vulnerable to social exclusion.

In contrast, inclusionary othering attempts to utilise the power within relationships to build bridges, a sense of community, shared power, and inclusion (Canales 2000). In the context of healthcare, this is achieved through nurses valuing the expertise that individuals bring regarding their own health, a focus upon the individuals' wishes and desires, and a true commitment to working together enabling individuals to make their own decision and facilitating access to healthcare through empowerment. This can occur at a one-to-one level by healthcare staff working with clients, supporting them to identify goals and action, rather than the practitioners thinking they know what is best for the individual. This could also be achieved at a community or service level through a commitment by healthcare staff to ensure that service users and carer's voices and experiences are used in the process of service development through direct engagement or through patient forums.

Box 8.7   Case study of Zoe

Taking part in a 'sleep out' in order to raise money for a well-known homeless charity, Zoe found herself sitting on hard ground outside a parish church at midnight. She and her friends were wrapped up in sleeping bags. They were uncomfortable and getting cold but they had brought a picnic and were chatting together and feeling reasonably cheerful. They were also feeling virtuous because they were trying to make a difference by raising money to help those who were less well off than themselves.

A group of people approached them and asked them what they were doing. The group were homeless and their response on learning the reason for the 'sleep out' was one of anger. What could this group of happy, chatting people possibly know about the reality of how it felt to be homeless? Zoe never forgot the experience. It brought home to her how safe she felt in her own life and led her towards a greater empathy for people who found themselves homeless.

Most people live with some connection with the place where they make a world for themselves. It is a state of being human that we make meaningful connections with people, that we build relationships. To not have a home and meaningful connections can lead us into a state of alienation (please read Case study of Zoe in Box 8.7).

Box 8.8   Time for reflection

Take a few moments to visualise how it might feel to become homeless.

Imagining the experience of living on the streets, what sort of words does this conjure up for you?

In the narrative, although Zoe had seen homeless people as 'other', she had attempted to use 'respectful othering' (Johnsen 2010) in order to redress the balance in some way. However, the response from the homeless group of people was one of anger which at the time she found ungrateful and hard to understand. It could be argued that by turning the 'sleep out' into something of a party in order to do good, Zoe and her friends had reinforced their position as the majority and disempowered the homeless group by making them feel subordinate (Johnson *et al.* 2004). Imagine now, what it feels like to be without a home – that is, to be truly homeless (Box 8.8).

You may have thought of words such as cold, uncomfortable, frightened, unhappy, and hopeless. There are many reasons why people may find themselves to be homeless – for example, relationship breakdown, ill health, domestic abuse, job loss, lack of affordable housing and housing arrears, leaving prison, mental health services, or some other form of care (Quilgars *et al.* 2008, Smith *et al.* 2008, McDonagh 2011).

The consequence of becoming homeless can mean that homeless people no longer feel part of a community. They may lack social support and lose contact with friends and relatives. Being unable to wash and change clothes frequently can lead to infestation and ill health. Using shelter services can feel threatening and can lead to people being labelled.

Turning to drugs and/or alcohol may feel like a way of forgetting, and it becomes a way of surviving. It is no surprise therefore that alcoholism and other types of substance misuse have been found to affect larger numbers of homeless people than the general population (Dietz 2009). Homeless people may engage in unprotected sex or become sex workers (Eyrich-Garg *et al.* 2008), in addition the risk of hepatitis and HIV are increased through sharing drug paraphernalia (Kane *et al.* 2010). Substance abuse inevitably will affect homeless people's health and in some instances may be life threatening. Some homeless people can find themselves engaging in criminal activities in order to provide for themselves. All this can inevitably lead people to feel they have no way out, to feeling overwhelmed and hopeless.

Box 8.9   Time for reflection

Spend a few moments reflecting on how you may feel as a health professional when a homeless person is admitted as an emergency. The homeless person may smell of alcohol and may be dishevelled and appear dirty.

Earlier on in this chapter, you were asked to consider your own experience and the attributes you associate with the word 'patient'. It was suggested that you might use words such as ill, frail, and needing assistance. Next, we would like you to reflect on how you may feel as a health professional looking after someone who is homeless (Box 8.9).

Box 8.10   Case study of Clare (student in the emergency department)

I was told that John frequently appeared in the emergency department. The nurse in charge was very brusque with him. John appeared angry and upset. When I spent some time with him trying to understand his situation, he calmed down and told me why he was so angry. He was used to being looked on as 'something other' because of his homeless life style. He lived with HIV. One of the reasons he was angry was because he could see a bin that had not been emptied and he feared infection. John became a different person when I talked to him and valued him. All he wanted was for us to show him some respect. I learned a lot that day. Fear of people who live an alternative lifestyle can lead to poor practice and increase people's vulnerability. In fact, there was nothing to fear, all John wanted was to be treated as a fellow human being.

Kane *et al.* (2010) suggest that there are few healthcare options available for homeless people and accommodation can be difficult to sustain. Therefore, homeless people are more likely to present themselves to emergency healthcare providers where unfortunately they may be viewed as being less worthy of care, in other words, of being 'other'. Cougnard *et al.* (2006) found that emergency service professionals perceived homeless people presenting themselves to emergency services as looking for respite from living on the streets rather than being in need of services (see Case study of Clare in Box 8.10).

Reducing fear of contact and anxiety are important goals to ensure that professionals are willing to work with homeless people (Kane *et al.* 2010). It can be argued that the staff in the emergency department really demonstrated exclusionary othering (Canales 2000), as it was evident that they had power over John resulting in John being marginalised and not valued, which can lead to poor care being experienced. In contrast, inclusionary othering would have occurred if the staff viewed John as a fellow human being and developed a professional relationship with John informing him of some of the services that may have been available to him as well as valuing him and listening to his concerns regarding the bin and subsequent fear of infection.

You have already read in this chapter – comparing ourselves with others is a way of us defining ourselves. Othering is a process that identifies those who are different from the majority (Johnson *et al.* 2004). A healthcare professional may work with patients who may feel lost and alienated and who may speak very little English. It is important to try to understand how homeless people may feel within an alien world. Drawing on the Case study of Clare (Box 8.10), the student could have made assumptions about John but instead entered into a conversation and started building a relationship that led to improved healthcare for John. Where people may be hurt, lost, frightened, and not speak fluent English, health professionals need to think about other resources, for example, pictures, sign language, or they may need to insist on an interpreter being present to provide the best possible care for that person. Doing so demonstrates a commitment to valuing the individual, as well as a desire to build a relationship with them, both of which are elements of inclusionary othering.

Having looked at all of these explanations for the existence of prejudice, discrimination, and oppression, it is suggested that one way of summarising these differing explanations can be categorised as a means to:

- Keep people *down* – through exploitation and domination, as described earlier
- Keep people *in* – through norm enforcement and inclusionary 'othering', again as described earlier
- Keep people *away* – fear of contamination, disease, infection, or infestation such as with exclusionary 'othering', scapegoating, and marginalisation as described earlier in this chapter and in Chapter 5

Phelan *et al.* (2008)

The organisational level

We started by looking at some sociological theories and have moved towards a theory which whilst being sociological also has a psychosocial element, in that 'othering' explores the interrelationship between individual thought and behaviour and the social environment. These have all had a 'macro focus', looking for society-wide explanations of oppression and vulnerability. However, each on its own, and even collectively, cannot explain all instances of oppression and vulnerability. Therefore, we will now turn to some smaller-scale, but no less damaging, psychosocial processes. We will be exploring two theories which might explain what is happening at an organisational level such as care settings, and which can contribute to vulnerability and oppression.

Care work as stressful work

Box 8.11   Why is care work so emotionally demanding which can lead to so many healthcare professionals developing emotional difficulties?

(Menzies 1960, Menzies-Lyth 1988).

- Constant contact with people who are acutely suffering.
- Working with people for whom recovery and ultimate prognosis is not always hopeful all positive.
- Carrying out of tasks which may sometimes be repulsive, disgusting, dangerous, and threatening.
- Caring for and about others can be emotionally draining and demanding, and emotional attachments to patients and clients can cause pain when they either move on or may die.
- The work is physically demanding.
- Care work is not well paid and is under resourced.
- We work in ever increasingly busy and stressful environments.

Isabel Menzies (1960) who later published as Menzies-Lyth (1988) was a psychotherapist who had a lot of nurses and healthcare professionals come to see her for therapy. She was interested and concerned about why so many of her patients experiencing real trauma and distress were healthcare professionals and set about exploring and theorising why this might be. She outlined a number of factors which make care work particularly stressful (see Box 8.11).

Given this cocktail of factors, Menzies was not surprised why so many nurses found it difficult to cope and often experienced high levels of stress, this links with the Mutual vulnerability explored in Chapter 2. Some nurses succumbed to this emotional pain and needed time off work or the help of a therapist. However, in her study, she found that other healthcare professionals used other means of 'coping' that may on one level help them cope, yet could be potentially damaging and create vulnerability in patients and clients. She identified a number of psychological defence mechanisms used by nurses and healthcare professionals to help them cope with the stressful nature of the work (see Table 8.1). These psychological defences are used because of the stressful social situation that the nurses or health professionals find themselves in.

If Menzies was accurate in describing some of the defensive behaviours displayed by healthcare professionals to protect themselves from psychological distress, it is possible to identify the possible impact on patients and clients. Please undertake Time for reflection (Box 8.12).

This defensiveness might explain why some patients are treated as unpopular patients as described in Chapter 5 or why they might be labelled and scapegoated and stigmatised as described in Chapter 4. Therefore, in order to help nurses or healthcare professionals avoid showing these behaviours, it shows the importance of providing more resources, more training, and more emotional support and care for nurses. Debriefing at the end of the shift especially when there has been a difficult situation or maybe a death on the ward could be useful. Giving nurses less people to look after might help them develop more meaningful relationships with the patients or clients they are looking after. Either way,

Table 8.1   Psychological defence behaviours to deal with the anxiety of health work (Menzies 1960, Menzies-Lyth 1988).

Social defence	Example and consequences
Keeping detached and distant from patients and clients	Task fixation; treating all clients alike; listing duties and tasks; restrictions on the closeness in caring relationships; 'friendships' and friendliness with clients strongly discouraged.
Depersonalisation, categorisation, and dehumanisation	Clients seen as a condition or diagnosis; uniformity of care plans and care management advocated; 'professional' performance and 'professional' attitude seen as preferable to being creative or being really client centred.
Denial of feelings	Staff expected to control their own feelings and show no emotion; involvement feared; control replaces care.
Ritual task performance	Anxiety that can occur when a healthcare professional's freedom of choice is replaced by systems of procedure, policy, protocol, and bureaucratic systems; decisions shelved until new policies and procedures formed; questions and questioning discouraged.
Avoidance of decisions	Decisions pushed upwards to senior managers or medics; blame pushed downwards onto 'juniors'.
Avoidance of change	Full consent sought before change can take place in order to avoid change; progress only as fast as slowest team member; fear of facing new situations because of need to restructure existing psychological defences.
Checks and counter checks	Everything has a tendency to be obsessionally recorded; trust of others and their skills a rarity; fear of failure a constant concern; mistakes and shortcomings not admitted.

Box 8.12   Time for reflection

What are the implications for the vulnerability and general experience of patients and clients if nurses do show any of the psychological defence behaviours as described by Menzies/ Menzies-Lyth?

- Make a list describing how any of those psychological defence behaviours described by Menzies might make a client or patient feel vulnerable.
- For each item on your list, identify what could be done to make a patient or client feel less vulnerable.

---

changes in the care environment and the organisation of the work will make a significant improvement in the emotional well-being of nurses and ultimately patients and clients (Menzies 1960, Menzies-Lyth 1988).

Compliance, conformity, and obedience

Another phenomenon which is relevant to vulnerability and oppression within healthcare settings, just as it might be in any other setting, is why sometimes well-meaning and well-intentioned staff sometimes turn a blind eye or fail to recognise that poor practice or even abuse is occurring and report it, or sometimes even go along with it. Whether looking at

---

Box 8.13   The Milgram experiment (Milgram 2006)

The participants were told that they were to take part in a learning experiment. The 'subjects' were seated, one at a time, at a console with clearly labelled switches, ascending from 10 to 400 V. They were shown a person in another room, a confederate of the experimenter. They were told that he was the real experimental subject. They saw him strapped into an electric chair. The fake subject was able to communicate with the person working the console by a microphone. Each time the confederate made a mistake, the participant was told to administer an electric shock of ever increasing strength.

The confederate made appropriate noises and complaints as the voltage was raised. Nearly two thirds of the people randomly selected from the telephone directory were persuaded to go up to the 400 V maximum, even when the confederate had eventually fallen silent after calling out about his weak heart.

Whenever a participant queried the dangers, Milgram or one of his assistants reassured them with the words 'You may continue. I assure you there will be no tissue damage.'

Many of those involved became upset and wanted to leave the experiment all together. They were more or less bullied into continuing.

The participants had also been told that what they were doing was for the general good, a programme designed to improve the techniques of teaching and learning.

---

the catalogue of abuse of adults with learning difficulty in the Winterbourne View Care Home (CQC 2011), or the systematic neglect and poor care given in Mid-Staffordshire Hospital (Department of Health 2010), or in the neglect and even abuse as described in Care and Compassion Report into Elder Care (Parliamentary and Health Service Ombudsman 2011), what is striking is that so many people were involved in this neglect and abuse. It is not just the active perpetrators that we should be interested in, but why so many other healthcare workers either went along with the neglect or abuse or failed to recognise it and report it.

Elsewhere in this book, such as in Chapter 5, the problems of professional culture and professional socialisation means that sometimes the desire to 'fit in' and to 'please' one's supervisor or manager, means that it can be scary and intimidating to challenge a colleague or someone in authority. Additionally, there are some well-known experiments carried out by social scientists which illustrate why it can be so difficult to stand up and either report abuse or say no to participating in something if it goes against our principles and values. These famous experiments in social science illustrate social processes that can make it difficult to challenge others, even when we know we are right and we believe that the other person or people are doing something wrong.

One famous experiment on obedience and compliance was carried out by Stanley Milgram (1974) who was interested in why so many ordinary people in Nazi Germany and Nazi-occupied Europe went along with, or failed to object to, the systematic genocide and murder of so many (please read about this further in Box 8.13).

Milgram (1974, cited in Hogg and Vaughan 2010: 242–244) identified that certain factors enhanced the likelihood of the 'teachers' administering 'lethal or near lethal shocks'. These factors were identified as:

- The experiment starts innocuously with seemingly 'trivial shocks': once the teacher has committed themselves to administering small shocks, it is difficult for them to subsequently change their minds and stop.

- The presence of the lab-coated 'expert' urging them on.
- The greater the social distance between 'teacher' and the person being punished, the greater the likelihood that 'lethal shock levels' will be administered.
- Obedience and compliance was increased when other 'obedient peers' were present, urging the teacher on along with the white-coated expert.

A second experiment into obedience and compliance was carried out by Solomon Asch (1951, cited in Hogg and Vaughan 2010: 239–240) who found that subjects will conform to incorrect judgements when made by a numerical majority of other people (see Box 8.14).

Asch claims that this demonstrated people's desire to 'fit in' and go along with the crowd, even when they believe they were right and the others in the group are wrong.

These two experiments of Asch and Milgram might be able to explain why some people go along with situations or actions (the neglect, abuse, oppression of others) that they may disagree with because of the peer group pressure to conform or through the urging on of an authority figure. Let us consider these two experiments and their potential application to practice (please undertake Time for reflection in Box 8.15).

The pressures to conform and go along with things which we do not agree with can be incredibly powerful as these two experiments show. The first thing that is needed is to be aware of the potential vulnerability of a healthcare professional to go along with neglect,

---

Box 8.14 The Asch Experiment into Conformity to the Group (Asch 1951, described by Shuttleworth 2008).

For the experiment, eight subjects were seated around a table, with the seating plan carefully constructed to prevent any suspicion. Only one participant was actually a genuine subject for the experiment, the rest being confederates carefully tutored by Asch to give certain pre-selected responses. The experiment was simple in its construction; each participant, in turn, was asked to answer a series of questions, such as which line was longest when shown a card with 3 straight lines. It was very obvious on the card which was the longest or shortest line. The test attempted to place a varying amount of peer pressure on the individual test subject to see if they could be influenced to go along with the majority confederates, even when it was obvious the confederates were wrong about the length of the lines shown. This would allow Asch to determine how the answers of the subject would change with the added influence of peer pressure. When surrounded by other people (the confederates) giving an incorrect answer, over one third of the subjects also voiced an incorrect opinion. At least 75% of the subjects gave the wrong answer to at least one question…There was no doubt, that peer pressure can cause conformity.

Box 8.15 Time for reflection

- Have you ever been in a situation, either at work or outside, where you have felt the pressure to conform to go along with something that you do not agree with?
- Describe what sort of pressure was there to make you conform?
- Did anyone else in that situation feel pressured to go along with something?
- What would it have taken to help you to resist that pressure and to say no or disagree with something that you felt uncomfortable with?

abuse, or poor practice, which will then make other people vulnerable. Saying no or standing up to disagree is very hard. In the next chapter, we will look at practical strategies that can help us challenge oppression and reduce vulnerability and to resist such pressure.

Remembering our moral and professional responsibilities and obligations, which might be laid out in a professional code of conduct, as well as remembering our legal obligations such as those required through the Human Rights Act 1998 or the Equality Act 2010 might help to give us courage to stand up for what we believe is morally and professionally right. The next chapter will also talk about skills and strategies such as elegant challenging that might help us to stand up respectfully yet assertive for what we believe and know to be right.

Conclusion

This chapter has attempted to explore a few of the psychosocial explanations as to why discrimination and oppression can occur at both the societal level and organisational level. In a word-limited chapter, it is difficult to cover every psychosocial process that might be relevant to understanding vulnerability and oppression. What we hope we havedone is at least offered a couple of areas for consideration which will help the healthcare practitioner to understand the wider causes of discrimination, oppression, and vulnerability, which can still be resisted or challenged in our everyday practice. The next chapter looking at strategies may help identify those practical actions that can address vulnerability and oppression where it exists.

Links to other chapters

- Chapter 2 explores the notion of Mutual Vulnerability in more depth.
- Chapter 4 discusses related psychosocial processes of discrimination, such as stigmatisation, dehumanisation, and stereotyping.
- Chapter 5 explores the role of professional culture in causing compliance and a lack of challenge against oppressive behaviour. Additionally, the concept of the 'unpopular patient' is explained here.
- Chapter 6 identifies and explains the phenomenon of 'othering'.
- Chapter 7 discusses the psychology of attribution, in–out groups, stereotyping, and prejudice.
- Practical suggestions of how to minimise or address the factors that can lead to oppression and vulnerability are covered in Chapter 9.

References

Abu Sway, M. (2005) Islamophobia: Meaning, manifestations, causes. *Palestine–Israel Journal of Politics, Economics & Culture*, 12 (2/3), 15–23.

Alexander, C. (1848) *Words to Hymn 'All Things Bright and Beautiful'. Cyber-hymnal.* Available from http://www.cyberhymnal.org/htm/a/l/allthing.htm [accessed on 14 October 2012].

Allport, G. (1958) *The Nature Of Prejudice.* Doubleday, Garden City.

Althusser, L. (1971) *Lenin And Philosophy And Other Essays*. New Left, London.

Angus, I. (2009) Marx and Engels...and Darwin? The essential connection between historical materialism and natural selection. *International Socialist Review*, (65). Available from http://www.isreview.org/issues/65/feat-MarxDarwin.shtml [accessed on 14 October 2012].

Ansari, H. (2000) Negotiating British Muslim identity. In: *Muslim Identity in the 21st Century: Challenges of Modernity* (Bahmanpour, M. and Bashir, H. eds), pp. 89–102. Institute of Islamic Studies, London.

Ardil, A. (2009) Sociobiology, racism and Australian colonisation. *Griffith Law Review*, 18 (1), 82–113.

Bársony, J. and Daróczi, Á. (2007) *Pharrajimos: The Fate of the Roma During the Holocaust*. International Debate Education Association Press, New York.

Beechey, V. (1987) *Unequal Work*. Verso, London.

Beisel, D. (2010) Building the Nazi mindset. *The Journal of Psychohistory*, 37 (4), 367–374.

Bilton, T., Bonnett, K., Jones, P., Lawson, T., Skinner, D., Stanworth, M., Webster, A., Bradbury, L., Stanyer, J. and Stephens, P. (2002) *Introductory Sociology*. 4th ed., Palgrave Macmillan, Basingstoke.

Bleich, E. (2011) What is Islamophobia and how much is there? Theorizing and measuring an emerging comparative concept. *American Behavioral Scientist*, 55 (12), 1581–1600.

Canales, M. (2000) Othering: Toward an understanding of difference. *Advances in Nursing Science*, 22 (4), 16–31.

Canales, M. (2010) Othering: Difference understood? A 10-year analysis and critique of the nursing literature. *Advances in Nursing Science*, 33 (1), 15–34.

Care Quality Commission (CQC) (2011) *Review of Compliance: Winterbourne View*. Available from http://www.cqc.org.uk/sites/default/files/media/documents/1-116865865_castlebeck_care_teesdale_ltd_1-138702193_winterbourne_view_roc_20110517_201107183026.pdf [accessed on 5 October 2012].

Carmichael, S. and Hamilton, C. (1968) *Black Power: The Political Liberation in America*. Cape, Boston.

Chakraboti, N. (2010) Beyond 'Passive Apartheid'? Developing policy and research agendas on rural racism in Britain. *Journal of Ethnic and Migration Studies*, 36 (3) 501–517.

Chomsky, N. (2002) *Media Control: The Spectacular Achievements of Propaganda*. 2nd ed., Seven Stories, New York.

Chomsky, N. and Hermann, E. (1988) *Manufacturing Consent: The Political Economy of the Mass Media*. Vantage Press, London.

Cohen, F., Jussim, L., Harber, K. and Bhasin, G. (2009) Modern anti-semitism and anti-Israeli attitudes. *Journal of Personality and Social Psychology*, 97 (2), 290–306.

Cougnard, A., Grolleau, S., Lamarque, F., Beitz, C., Brugère, S. and Verdoux, H. (2006) Psychotic disorders among homeless subjects attending a psychiatric emergency service. *Social Psychiatry & Psychiatric Epidemiology*, 41 (11), 904–910.

Coy, M. (2009) 'Moved Around Like Bags of Rubbish Nobody Wants': How multiple placement moves can make young women vulnerable to sexual exploitation. *Child Abuse Review*, 18, 254–266.

Cudworth, D. (2008) 'There is a little bit more than just delivering the stuff': Policy, pedagogy and the education of gypsy/traveller children. *Critical Social Policy*, 28 (3), 361–377.

Dahrendorf, R. (1959) *Class and Class Conflict in Industrial Society*. Stanford University Press, Stanford.

Department of Health (DoH) (2008) *Confidence in Caring*. Department of Health, London.

DoH (2010) *Robert Francis Inquiry Report into Mid-Staffordshire NHS Foundation Trust*. Available from http://www.dh.gov.uk/en/Publicationsandstatistics/Publications/PublicationsPolicyAndGuidance/DH_113018 [accessed on 5 October 2012].

DoH (2012) *Commission on Dignity in Care*. Department of Health, London.

Dietz, T. (2009) Drug and alcohol use amongst homeless, older adults. *Journal of Applied Gerontology*, 23, 235–255.

Dominelli, L. (2002) *Anti Oppressive Social Work Theory and Practice*. Palgrave Macmillan, Basingstoke.

Dunscombe, J. and Marsden, D. (1993) Love and intimacy: The gender division of emotion and emotion work: A neglected aspect of sociological discussion in heterosexual relationships. *Sociology*, 27 (2), 221–241.

Engels, F. (1893) *Letter From Engels to Franz Mehring*. Marx and Engels Internet Archive. Available from http://www.marxists.org/archive/marx/works/1893/letters/93_07_14.htm [accessed on 13 October 2012].

Eyrich-Garg, K., Cacciola, J., Carise, D., Lynch, K. and McLellan, A. (2008) Individual characteristics of the literally homeless, marginally housed, and impoverished in a US substance abuse treatment-seeking sample. *Social Psychiatry & Psychiatric Epidemiology*, 43 (10), 831–842.

Falk, A. (2008) *Anti-semitism: A History and Psychoanalysis of Contemporary Hatred*. Praegar, Westport.

Fanon, F. (2004 [1961]) *The Wretched of the Earth*. Grove, New York.

Fawcett Society. (2010) *Equal Pay: Where Next? A Report of the Discussions and Conclusions From the 2010 Equal Pay Conference, Marking the 40th Anniversary of the Equal Pay Act*. Available from http://www.fawcettsociety.org.uk/documents/Equal%20Pay,%20Where%20Next%20Nov%202010.pdf [accessed on 13 October 2012].

Foreman-Peck, J. (1989) Foreign investment and imperial exploitation: Balance of payments reconstruction for nineteenth-century Britain and India. *Economic History Review*, 3, 354–374.

Freeman, M. (2008) Democracy, Al Qaeda, and the causes of terrorism: A strategic analysis of U.S. policy. *Studies in Conflict & Terrorism*, 31 (1), 40–59.

Friedman, M. (1993) *Why Government Is the Problem*. Hoover Institution Press, Stanford.

Friedman, M. (2002) *Capitalism and Freedom*. University of Chicago Press, Chicago.

Fulcher, J. and Scott, J. (2011) *Sociology*. 4th ed., Oxford University Press, Oxford.

Gaines, S. and Reed, E. (1995) Prejudice: From Allport to DuBois. *American Psychologist*, 50 (2), 96–103.

Gatto, J. (2005) *Dumbing Us Down: The Hidden Curriculum of Compulsory Schooling*. New Society, Gabriola Island, British Columbia.

Giddens, A. (2009) *Sociology*. 6th ed., Polity Press, Cambridge.

Gramsci, A. (1968) *Prison Notebooks*. Lawrence and Wishart, London.

Harbert, W. (1988) Dignity and choice. *Insight*, 25th March, 12.

Hayek, F. (1994) *The Road to Serfdom*. University of Chicago Press, Chicago.

Hayek, F. (2011) *The Constitution of Liberty: The Definitive Edition* (Hamowy, R. ed.), vol. 17, *The Collected Works of F A. Hayek*. University of Chicago Press, Chicago.

Hochschild, A. and Machung, A. (1989) *The Second Shift: Working Parents and the Revolution at Home*. Viking Penguin, New York.

Hodson, G. and Esses, V. (2005) Lay perceptions of ethnic prejudice: Causes, solutions, and individual differences. *European Journal of Social Psychology*, 35, 329–344.

Hogg, M. and Vaughan, G. (2010) *Social Psychology*. 6th ed., Prentice Hall, London.

Ignătoiu-Sora, E. (2011) The discrimination discourse in relation to the Roma: Its limits and benefits. *Ethnic and Racial Studies*, 34 (10), 1697–1714.

Illich, I. (1971) *Deschooling Society*. Marion Boyars, London.

Iqbal, Z. (2010) Understanding Islamophobia: Conceptualizing and measuring the construct. *European Journal of Social Science*, 13 (4), 574–590.

Johnsen, H. (2010) Scientific knowledge through involvement – how to do respectful othering. *International Journal of Action Research*, 6 (1), 43–74.

Johnson, J., Bottorff, J., Browne, A., Grewal, S., Hilton, B.A. and Clarke, H. (2004) Othering and being othered in the context of healthcare services. *Health Communication*, 16 (2), 253–271.

Jones, O. (2012) *Chavs: The Demonization of the Working Class*. 2nd ed., Verso, London.

Kane, N., Green, D. and Jacobs, R. (2010) Perceptions of students about younger and older men and women who may be homeless. *Journal of Social Service Research*, 36, 261–277.

Krumer-Nevo, M. and Benjamin, O. (2007) *Contesting Othering and Social Distancing in Critical Poverty Knowledge*. Conference Paper Presented at American Sociological Association.

Lozano, S. (2011) Feminist debate around trafficking' in women for the purpose of sexual exploitation in prostitution. *Desafíos*, 23 (1), 217–257.

Maccullum, D. (2002) Othering and psychiatric nursing. *Journal of Psychiatric and Mental Health Nursing*, 9, 87–94.

Macpherson Report. (1999) *The Inquiry into the Murder of Stephen Lawrence*. TSO. Available from http://www.archive.official-documents.co.uk/document/cm42/4262/sli-06.htm#6.6 [accessed on 14 October 2012].

Malim, T. and Birch, A. (1998) *Introductory Psychology*. Macmillan, Basingstoke.

Marcuse, H. (1964) *One Dimensional Man: Studies in the Ideology of Advanced Industrial Society*, Routledge Classics, London.

Martikainena, P., Bartley, M. and Lahelmac, E. (2002) Psychosocial determinants of health in social epidemiology. *International Journal of Epidemiology*, 31 (6), 1091–1093.

Marx, K. (1844) (2009 online). A contribution to the critique of Hegel's philosophy of right, preface. In: *Marx and Engels Collected Works: September 1844–November 1845*. (Marx, K. and Engels, F. eds), Lawrence and Wishart, London. Available from http://www.marxists.org/archive/marx/works/1843/critique-hpr/intro.htm [accessed on 13 October 2012].

Marx, K. (1858) (publ 1993, 1997 online). *The Grundrisse: Outlines of the Critique of Political Economy (The 'Grundrisse')*. (Trans. Nicolaus, M.) Penguin, London. Available from http://www.marxists.org/archive/marx/works/1857/grundrisse/ [accessed on 12 October 2012].

Marx, K. and Engels, F. (1845–1846) *The German Ideology*. Prometheus Books Publications, New York. 1999. Full text in The Marx–Engels Archive. Available from http://www.marxists.org/archive/marx/works/1845/german-ideology/index.htm [accessed on 12 October 2012].

Marx, K. and Engels, F. (1863) (1999 online) *Capital: A Critique of Political Economy Volume 4: Theories of Surplus-Value*. The Marx–Engels Archive. Available from http://www.marxists.org/archive/marx/works/1863/theories-surplus-value/ [accessed on 12 October 2012].

Marx, K. and Engels, F. (1887) (1999 online) *Capital: A Critique of Political Economy Volume 1: The Process of Production of Capital*. The Marx–Engels Archive. Available from http://www.marxists.org/archive/marx/works/1867-c1/ [accessed on 12 October 2012].

Marx, K. and Engels, F. (1893) (1999 online) *Capital: A Critique of Political Economy Volume 2: The Process of Circulation of Capital*. The Marx–Engels Archive. Available from http://www.marxists.org/archive/marx/works/1885-c2/index.htm [accessed on 12 October 2012].

Marx, K. and Engels, F. (1894) (1999 online) *Capital: A Critique of Political Economy Volume 3: The Process of Capitalist Production as a Whole*. The Marx–Engels Archive. Available from http://www.marxists.org/archive/marx/works/1894-c3/ [accessed on 12 October 2012].

Mason, D. (1982) After Scarman: A note on the concept of institutional racism. *Journal of Ethnic and Migration Studies*, 10 (1), 38–45.

McDonagh, T. (2011) *Tackling Homelessness and Exclusion: Understanding Complex Lives*. Joseph Rowntree Foundation. Available from http://www.jrf.org.uk/sites/files/jrf/homelessness-exclusion-services-summary.pdf [accessed on 14 October 2012].

Menzies, I. (1960) *The Functioning of Social Systems As Defences Against Anxiety*. Tavistock Publications, London.

Menzies-Lyth, I. (1988) *Defence Systems as Controls Against Anxiety*. Tavistock Publications, London.

Milgram, S. (1974) *Obedience to Authority*. Harper and Row, New York.

Milgram, S. (2006) *Key Thinkers in Psychology*. Available from http://www.credoreference.com/entry/sageuktp/stanley_milgram_1933_84 [accessed on 14 October 2012].

Miliband, R. (1969) *The State in Capitalist Society: The Analysis of the Western System of Power*. Weidenfeld and Nicolson, London.

Miliband, R. (1982) *Capitalist Democracy in Britain*. Oxford University Press, Oxford.

Murray, C. with Lister, R. (ed.) With additional commentaries by Field, F., Joan, C., Brown, J., Alan Walker, A., Nicholas Deakin, N., Alcock, P., David, M., Phillips, M. and Slipman, S. (1996) *Charles Murray and the Underclass: The Developing Debate*. Institute of Economic Affairs, London. Available from http://www.civitas.org.uk/pdf/cw33.pdf [accessed on 14 October 2012].

Murray, C. (2001) *Underclass + 10: Charles Murray and the British Underclass 1990–2000*. CIVITAS, London. Available from http://www.sociology.org.uk/as4p6.pdf [accessed on 14 October 2012].

Nzira, V. and Williams, P. (2009) *Anti Oppressive Practice in Health and Social Care*. Sage, London.

Oakley, A. (1974) *The Sociology of Housework*. Martin Robertson, Oxford.

Office for National Statistics (ONS). (2011) *Gender Pay Gap Falls Below 10 Per Cent in 2011*. Available from http://www.ons.gov.uk/ons/dcp29904_244634.pdf [accessed on 14 October 2012].

Oliver, M. (1990) *The Politics Of Disablement*. Macmillan, Basingstoke.

Oliver, M. and Barnes, C. (2012) *The New Politics of Disablement*. Palgrave Macmillan, Basingstoke.

O'Nions, H. (2011) Roma expulsions and discrimination: The elephant in Brussels. *European Journal of Migration & Law*, 13 (4), 361–388.

Oxford English Dictionary. (2012) Psychosocial, Definition. Available from http://www.oed.com/view/Entry/153937?redirectedFrom=psychosocial& [accessed on 24 October 2012].

Parliamentary and Health Service Ombudsman (2011) *Care and Compassion?: Report of the Health Service Ombudsman on Ten Investigations into NHS Care of Older People*. Available from http://www.ombudsman.org.uk/_data/assets/pdf_file/0016/7216/Care-and-Compassion-PHSO-0114web.pdf [accessed on 5 October 2012].

Pearsall, J. (2002) *Concise Oxford English Dictionary*. 10th ed., Oxford University Press, Oxford.

Pelaez, C. (1976) The theory and reality of imperialism in the coffee economy of nineteenth-century Brazil. *Economic History Review*, 29 (2), 276–290.

Phelan, J., Link, B. and Dovidio, J. (2008) Stigma and prejudice: One animal or two? *Social Science & Medicine*, 67, 358–367.

Pierson, C. (2006) *Beyond the Welfare State*. Polity Press, Cambridge.

Postman, N. (1985) *Amusing Ourselves to Death: Public Discourse in the Age of Show Business*. Penguin, London.

Quilgars, D., Johnsen, S. and Pleace, N. (2008) *Youth Homelessness in the UK: A Decade of Progress?* Joseph Rowntree Foundation. Available from http://www.jrf.org.uk/sites/files/jrf/2220-homelessness-young-people.pdf [accessed on 14 October 2012].

Rosado, C. (1998) The multiple futures of racism beyond the myth of race through a new paradigm for resolution in the third millennium. *Critical Multicultural Pavilion: Research Room*. Available from http://www.edchange.org/multicultural/papers/caleb/futures_of_racism.html [accessed on 12 October 2012].

Russo, A. (2001) *Taking Back Our Lives: A Call to Action for the Feminist Movement*. Routledge, London.

Samir, A. (2012) The surplus in monopoly capitalism and the imperialist rent. *Monthly Review: An Independent Socialist Magazine*, 64 (3), 78–85.

Shapiro, J. (2008) Walking a mile in their patients' shoes: Empathy and othering in medical students' education. *Philosophy, Ethics, and Humanities in Medicine*, 3 (10).

Smith, J., Akpadio, S., Bushnaq, H., Campbell, A., Hassan, L. and Pal, S. (2008) *Valuable Lives: Capabilities and Resilience Amongst Single Homeless People*. Crisis. Available from http://www.crisis.org.uk/data/files/publications/Valuable_Lives.pdf [accessed on 14 October 2012].

Stephan, W. (2008) Viewing intergroup relations in Europe through Allport's Lens Model of Prejudice. *Journal of Social Issues*, 64 (2), 417–429.

Sullivan, O. (2000) The division of domestic labour: Twenty years of change? *Sociology*, 34 (3), 437–456.

Sun, K. (1993) Two types of prejudice and their causes. *American Psychologist*, 48 (11), 1152–1153.

The Equality Act (2010) The National Archives at legislation.gov.uk. Available from http://www.legislation.gov.uk/ukpga/2010/15/contents [accessed on 5 October 2012].

Thompson, N. (2003) *Promoting Equality: Challenging Discrimination and Oppression*. 2nd ed., Macmillan, Basingstoke.

Thompson, N. (2006) *Anti Discriminatory Practice*. 4th ed., Palgrave Macmillan, Basingstoke.

Thompson, N. (2012) *Anti Discriminatory Practice: Equality, Diversity and Social Justice*. 5th ed., Palgrave Macmillan, Basingstoke.

Tyrnauer, G. (1991) *Gypsies and the Holocaust: A Bibliography and Introductory Essay*. 2nd ed., Concordia University and Montreal Institute for Genocide Studies, Montréal.

Walby, S. (1990a) *Theorizing Patriarchy*. Blackwell, Oxford.

Walby, S. (1990b) From private to public patriarchy: The periodisation of British history. *Women's Studies International Forum*, 13 (1/2), 91–104.

Warde, A. and Hetherington, K. (1993) A changing domestic division of labour? Issues of measurement and interpretation. *Work Employment Society*, 7, 23–45.

Williams, R. (2012) Rochdale Police and Council 'Repeatedly Warned' About Sex Abuse Risk in Town, *The Guardian*. Available from http://www.guardian.co.uk/uk/2012/sep/27/rochdale-police-sex-abuse-girls [accessed on 13 October 2012].

Chapter 9

Working to reduce vulnerability

Chris Willetts, Julie Ryden and Gill Calvin Thomas

Introduction

Reducing the vulnerability of health and social care service users and carers is a key aim of this text. Strategies for reducing vulnerability have been alluded to throughout the preceding chapters; however, this chapter seeks to collate and offer a more detailed exposition of these strategies. It will address the question, 'how can you work in such a way as to reduce the vulnerability people may experience?' We will introduce the concept of 'anti-oppressive practice' and develop this as a set of specific strategies that practitioners can adopt. The strategies will be clearly aligned to the book's focus upon vulnerability as a socially constructed phenomenon and thus will consider strategies at the personal, cultural, and structural levels. A starting point for the strategies will be Thompson's anti-oppressive strategies (2011), but these will be developed to incorporate wider issues relating to communication skills and therapeutic relationships.

What is anti-oppressive practice?

A key focus of this book has been on the contribution of discrimination and oppression to the vulnerability of individuals. Therefore, any strategy which seeks to reduce vulnerability and the harm experienced as a result will need to address these issues. In doing this, it is possible to draw upon the concepts of 'anti-discriminatory practice' and/or 'anti-oppressive practice'. These are approaches to practice which seek to 'reduce, undermine, challenge and eliminate discrimination and oppression, and to promote equality' (adapted from Thompson 2011, 2012). Thompson refers to such practice as 'emancipatory practice' (2011: 51), thus emphasising the liberating nature of this practice, freeing people from the shackles of oppression and discrimination. Such practice seeks to promote and enhance the unique individuality of the client without constraining it by stereotypes, stigma, invisibilisation, marginalisation, and other processes of oppression. For Okitikpi and Aymer (2010: 26), it is:

> ... a way of working that is not based on bias, prejudices, discrimination, injustice or unfair treatment.

Understanding Vulnerability: A Nursing and Healthcare Approach, First Edition. Edited by Vanessa Heaslip and Julie Ryden.
© 2013 John Wiley & Sons, Ltd. Published 2013 by John Wiley & Sons, Ltd.

However, in line with Thompson's PCS model (2011), it is important to recognise that anti-oppressive practice is not just focused on development of the 'self', but that it requires a commitment to challenge and influence cultural, institutional, and structural development as well. Dominelli is explicit about this multi-layered approach required:

> Anti-oppressive practice addresses the whole person and ...... takes on board personal, institutional, cultural and economic issues and examines how these impinge on individuals' behaviour and opportunities to develop their full potential as persons living within collective entities. (Dominelli 2002: 36)

Thus, anti-oppressive practice requires 'both introspection and a pro-active approach' (Okitikpi and Aymer 2010: 24). This chapter offers suggestions for how the health care practitioner can develop these skills and implement anti-oppressive practice at the personal, cultural, and structural levels.

It is important to be clear at the outset that there are clear moral, professional, and legal responsibilities requiring all those who work within human care services to be working in an anti-oppressive manner. Thompson indeed poses a clear challenge to all practitioners and workers in health and social care or indeed any other part of human service:

> ... practice which does not take account of oppression and the discrimination which gives rise to it, cannot be seen as good practice, no matter how high its standards may be in other respects. (Thompson 2006: 15, Thompson 2012: 9)

For Thompson, the standard and quality of care are inextricably linked to the degree to which the practitioner recognises, challenges and reduces oppression. This includes not just our own practice, but the practice of others around us. If we do not prevent or challenge oppression where it occurs, no matter what the original intentions, we could be said to be contributing to the discrimination or oppression or adding to the vulnerability of those individuals or groups who are experiencing it (Thompson 2006: 15 and 176, Thompson 2012: 190).

He argues that there is no place for fence sitting or doing nothing if we become aware that there is something in our area of practice that is contributing to the vulnerability or oppression of others. There is no middle ground because if we ignore or do nothing to address any factors which might be adding to the vulnerability or oppression of others, we are either condoning or sharing in that oppressive practice. According to both Thompson (2012) and Nzira and Williams (2009), we have a moral responsibility to act to address the situations or the causes of that discrimination or oppression, no matter how uncomfortable that might be. The stark choice is:

> ... if you're not part of the solution, you must be part of the problem. (Thompson 1992, cited in Thompson 2012: 9)

This moral duty of care which includes addressing anything which oppresses others or adds to their vulnerability should be accepted by all who choose a career in health and social care, and it places a responsibility upon all health and social care professionals.

It should also be noted that this is *not just* a moral responsibility but is also a professional obligation for registered practitioners in health and social care. Indeed, the NMC states:

> Speaking up on behalf of people in your care and clients is an everyday part of your role, and just as raising genuine concerns represents good practice, 'doing nothing' and failing to report concerns is unacceptable. NMC (2010: 5)

The professional codes of practice and ethics for registered nurses (NMC 2008) and for other registered health and social care professionals such as social workers and professionals allied to medicine (HCPC 2012a) place a range of requirements on practitioners to work in an anti-oppressive manner as explored in Chapter 5. These responsibilities apply not just to all registered nursing, midwifery, or health and social care practitioners, but even to all students in training on pre-qualification programmes regulated either by the NMC (2011) or the HCPC (2012b) (see Activity in Box 9.1).

The guidance and support offered by the councils is a clear indication of the expectation that practitioners should seek at all times to challenge and question practice. The raising concerns procedures have several levels ranging from highlighting the issue internally with support to reporting the matter for external review. The first level should be an expectation and not viewed negatively, in order that issues are addressed in a timely fashion and learning can result to improve care in future. Clearly, it is easier to say (or write) such expectations, the practice can be a more complex and demanding process (as explored in Chapter 8); however, it is a key element of being a professional and the responsibility that goes along with the entitlement to call yourself a professional. Whistleblowing is not an optional activity, but a duty demanded of you by your regulatory body.

In addition to being a moral and professional responsibility to practice in an anti-oppressive way, it is also a legal requirement for all British citizens. These legal responsibilities will be discussed in greater depth within the Structural level strategies section towards the end of the chapter.

We will now turn our attention to using Thompson's PCS model as a framework for exploring the strategies available for reducing vulnerability (Thompson 2011, 2012). As explored earlier, the model consists of three interconnected levels or layers of factors

---

Box 9.1   Activity

Access the guidance for practitioners (including students) on raising and escalating concerns issued by your professional regulatory body:
Nursing and Midwifery Council
http://www.nmc-uk.org/Documents/NMC-Publications/NMC-Raising-and-escalating-concerns.pdf

Health and Care Professions Council (2012c)
http://www.hpc-uk.org/registrants/raisingconcerns/

General Medical Council (2012)
http://www.gmc-uk.org/guidance/ethical_guidance/raising_concerns.asp
How might you use such documents to challenge concerns about practice?

contributing to discrimination and oppression and these include the *personal, cultural,* and *structural* levels. This model can also be used to address these contributing factors through attention to each of the three levels of practice, the personal level, the cultural level, and / or the structural level. The authors hope to show that a combination of interventions from each of the three levels of the PCS model is available and may be required in order to more effectively reduce vulnerability. Please note some strategies overlap several levels, so we have chosen one level in which to explore the strategy whilst aware of the overlaps.

Personal level strategies

This section will explore

- Interpersonal communication skills
- Developing a therapeutic relationship
- Taking a 'strength-based approach'
- Critical reflection, introspection, and self-awareness
- Elegant challenging
- Minimal intervention
- Having a clear and explicit theory base

Interpersonal communication skills

The personal level of anti-oppressive practice requires a focus upon the intra- and inter-personal dimensions of communication. The 'intra-personal' refers to aspects of communication such as feelings, attitudes, beliefs, and thoughts occurring *within* the individual, whilst 'inter-personal' communication occurs *between* people and refers to both verbal and non-verbal communication between two or more people. The importance of both these levels to efforts to reduce vulnerability is clear from the definition of communication offered by Condon:

> Communication is not just a process of 'bits' of information travelling between people: it is as much an overreaching domain of trust and distrust; the multitudinous and subtle ways by which people love and hate, praise and blame, accept and reject - themselves as well as others. As such they affect the inner being of others, there to aid or hinder, with greater or lesser consequences on that inner life. (Condon 1980: 63)

This definition identifies how communication is not just about 'words' travelling between two people, but that feelings, attitudes, prejudices, and status are wrapped up in those words and also the non-verbal accompaniments to the words. Communication can deliver many messages all at once, and the individual receiving the messages is left to interpret them 'intrapersonally'. It is at this level that harm can be caused to the individual receiving the messages; the 'inner life', as Condon refers to it, is the 'intrapersonal' level at which harm can be caused by communication. The inner being of an individual refers to their social identity, self-esteem, and self-concept, all of which can either be harmed or helped through communication. Let us consider this further in Box 9.2.

Box 9.2   Time for reflection

Think about conversations you have had with another person where the conversation;

1   Aided or improved your inner being
2   Harmed your inner being

Choose one conversation from (1) and one from (2).

Now, drawing from both conversations, make a list of the aspects of that communication which affected your inner being in terms of:

1   Verbal aspects (the words spoken)
2   Non-verbal aspects (tone of voice; gestures; eye contact; body and facial movements/appearance; standing, sitting, or invading space; dress; and use of touch)
3   Intrapersonal aspects (the role your inner being played in how you interpreted the message)

It is likely that as the 'recipient' of communication you are far more aware of the non-verbal aspects of the messages being sent than the person delivering the message (Hargie and Dickson 2004). The phrases 'actions speak louder than words' and 'a picture speaks a thousand words', suggest that a listener is more sensitive to non-verbal cues than the speaker and that the non-verbal elements of inter-personal communication have a powerful effect on the messages received by the listener. Thus, for patients or clients, their 'intrapersonal' sense of vulnerability is affected by both the verbal and non-verbal aspects of health care practitioner communication.

On top of this, the individual's intrapersonal interpretation of the messages received adds another layer to those messages. Burton and Dimbleby (1995) point to the process of 'decoding' that individuals undertake when they receive messages. This process is affected not just by the senders' verbal and non-verbal messages, but also by personal needs and motivations, personality factors, and personal attitudes, beliefs, and values. Thus, the individual adds their own intrapersonal slant on the message according to their own unique make-up. For example,

> … people who experience discrimination are sensitive about the views they believe others hold about them. They therefore look to see and try and get a sense of whether the practitioner understands 'where they are coming from' and whether the practitioner is attuned to or understands their experiences in society. (Okitikpi and Aymer 2010: 105)

This suggests that people who are vulnerable are already listening to a message from a particular intra-personal stance. Any inter-personal communication will be passed through this intra-personal filter before an interpretation is gained. Devito (2008) adds further intra-personal dimensions in his concept of 'noise' which disrupts the communication of a message between two people (Box 9.3). He identifies four different types of noise disruption, only one of which refers to the physical sound of noise:

Of these four types of noise, it is physiological, psychological, and semantic which clearly refer to intrapersonal dimensions. These three dimensions further complicate the

Box 9.3 Four types of 'noise' disruption (Devito 2008)

Physical noise – For example, traffic noise, small font, illegible handwriting
Physiological noise – For example, feeling cold/hungry, hearing loss, visual impairment
Psychological noise – For example, preconceived ideas, biases and prejudices, closed mindedness, emotionalism
Semantic noise – For example, language differences, jargon, ambiguous terms

process of communicating a message between one person and another – interpersonal communication. Therefore, the idea of a 'clear and simple transfer of a message from one person to another' is hopefully being laid to rest. In fact, communication is a process fraught with side alleys and detours where the 'true meaning' is constantly up for grabs and interpretation. This has clear implications for health carers who wish to reduce the vulnerability experienced by clients if as Spiers suggests interpersonal communication is a key method for reducing vulnerability:

> Vulnerability is a feature of interpersonal interaction…there may be an intrapersonal sense of vulnerability, [but] it is only within the interpersonal encounter that these claims can be negotiated. (Spiers 2005: 344)

We are therefore constrained within the limitations of interpersonal communication when we attempt to reduce vulnerability. However, this is not to suggest that the process is impossible, but that the health carer who does not recognise and address the complexities is likely to fall short in their efforts. To more fully exploit the tool of interpersonal communication when, in Spiers's terms, 'negotiating vulnerability' (Spiers 2005: 344), health carers must take account of and try to counter the complexities identified earlier. For example, reducing the level of 'noise disruption'; understanding more of the intrapersonal factors affecting both the client's and carer's understanding of messages being sent; checking the verbal and non-verbal elements of the communication for understanding and interference. The issues discussed in the following section will build upon these ideas and enhance the effectiveness of interpersonal communication.

Developing a therapeutic relationship

For Carl Rogers, the relationship which is constructed between two people is of greatest importance in interpersonal communication, and it is the pre-requisite for all the other skills. Paying attention to the relationship and building a constructive therapeutic relationship is crucial – it is the environment within which communication takes place and determines the quality of communication. At a minimum, the relationship requires some degree of 'psychological contact' between two people, for example, the health carer and the patient (Rogers 1957). Rogers (1957: 221) goes on to identify three particular qualities required of the 'helper' in the relationship, i.e. the nurse, the health carer (Box 9.4).

If these qualities are evident to the client even to a minimal degree, then for Rogers the relationship will be constructive, beneficial, and helpful for the client. How simple could

> **Box 9.4**   Carl Roger's core conditions for a therapeutic relationship (Rogers 1957: 221)
>
> • *Unconditional positive regard and total acceptance*
>   An attitude of warmth and interest towards the other; respect for the other; prizing the other person for ALL that they are, not just parts of them; understanding without pre-conditions or judgement; open mindedness.
> • *To feel and communicate a deep empathic understanding*
>   The effort to understand another's world as they see it, not as you would see it if you were them; to be 'inside' the other's private world sensing their meanings and feelings accurately; letting the other know how much you understand whilst also recognising that understanding will always be partial and frail.
> • *Genuineness or congruence*
>   Being honest and open; being a real and authentic person rather than hiding behind a façade or a 'professional' mask; being perceived as trustworthy and dependable by the other.

it be – instead of agonising over the 'right' words to use or a mechanical performance of memorised step-by-step processes, all we need to do is 'be' these three qualities; we need to 'live' these qualities and embed them in our daily lives, and if we do so, we will increase our likelihood of being helpful to others, not just patients but relatives, friends, and others. However, whilst apparently simple there is greater complexity and nuance within each quality which is beyond the scope of this text, and readers are urged to look at the original work of Rogers for greater depth of understanding (Rogers 1957, 1980, 2003; Kirschenbaum and Henderson 1990).

Taking a 'strength-based approach'

Approaches that focus on strengths were first developed by practitioners working with people living with severe mental ill health (Saleebey 1996). Itzhaky and Bustin (2002) suggest that a pathology-orientated perspective highlights problems and the pathology of the individual. In contrast, a strengths perspective focuses on revealing the individuals strengths and abilities within a therapeutic process (Itzhaky and Bustin 2002). This is not to say that the practitioner denies ill health but works in a strength-focused way to assess people's capacities and what may be possible, in addition to what may be causing problems. Thus, each person becomes a unique individual who is respected and empowered by practitioners who see the patient as an expert in his or her own life.

Saleebey (1996) suggests that it is not normal in a caring service to pursue practice based on ideas of resilience, strength, and the possibility of transformation. There is often an assumption that people are more dependent than they are. Thompson (2003) suggests that the assumption that disabled people should be dependent leads to a self-fulfilling prophecy in which disabled people become more dependent than they need to be. An approach which aims to build upon strengths requires a different starting point for health care practitioners. Instead of starting with 'what is wrong' a strength-based approach starts with 'what is going right', 'what might be achieved', and 'what are the possibilities'.

Healy (2005) suggests that a strengths approach to listening requires us to pay attention for signs of capacity and resourcefulness rather than to problems and deficits in patients' lives. In other words, refocusing on working in partnership and prioritising time to actively listen and build on strengths can in itself lead to positive change and greater resilience. Developing these core skills will enable health care professionals to have some understanding of what the vulnerable person wants to achieve, and in turn the health care professional can be clear about what they are trying to achieve with the vulnerable person.

Critical reflection, introspection, and self-awareness

It has been stated earlier (Chapters 1, 2, 3, and 5) that all of us are capable of increasing the vulnerability of others through oppression and discrimination, but not always in an intentional or conscious way. Each of us is an individual with our own unique collection of values, beliefs, prejudices, assumptions, and stereotypes, all of which can influence our practice in unthinking ways and thus may play a part in the vulnerability of the people we seek to care for. Therefore, one of the most frequent strategies put forward by various writers on this topic is the skill of reflection and the development of enhanced self-awareness (Healy 2005, Dalrymple and Burke 2006, Clifford and Burke 2009, Nzira and Williams 2009, Okitikpi and Aymer 2010, Thompson 2011). Various terms are used, e.g. reflexivity, reflectivity, and reflection, to refer to similar and overlapping processes; however, for simplicity, this chapter will employ the term 'critical reflection' whilst acknowledging the nuances and variability in term usage (D'Cruz *et al.* 2007).

Critical reflection can take several forms and has different dimensions which require consideration. At one level, critical reflection refers to a process of *introspection*, inspecting and examining the 'self' of the practitioner and the part that he or she plays in the vulnerability or potential vulnerability of clients. However, it can also refer to a deep consideration of the actions of others within situations. Thus, the focus of critical reflection can range from the self as an individual, through others, peers, or colleagues, to individual situations. In all events, the self will always be a component of any reflection, since it is argued here that the self of the practitioner is always involved even if not directly participating. Reflection upon *in*-action or *re*-action is as much a focus for reflection as direct action is.

When focusing upon the self, critical reflection requires a multi-layered depth of consideration. It requires us to examine every potential influence upon our interactions with others (see Box 9.5).

This list (Box 9.5) is not exhaustive but clearly shows the wide and diverse range of factors which full reflection needs to focus upon as an anti-oppressive strategy. Consideration of your potential influence upon a situation is required, even taking account of factors which are unchangeable, e.g. gender, class, ethnicity, style of speaking, style of dress.

> taking account of your own social location, powers, values and perspectives, and your membership of the social divisions, in relation to specific others, recognising the inequalities and diversities of particular social situations in all your interactions with others. (Clifford and Burke 2009: 38)

Box 9.5 Factors to reflect upon (drawn from Dalrymple and Burke 2006, D'Cruz *et al.* 2007, Clifford and Burke 2009, Okitikpi and Aymer 2010)

Language used
Thoughts
Feelings
Impressions
Values
Prejudices and biases
Assumptions made
Judgements made
Behaviours and actions
Motives and motivating factors
Personal power
Personal biography
Prior experiences
Social position
Social identity
Knowledge and theory used
Knowledge and theory discarded and ignored

The process requires an honest assessment of the factors and a real openness to the full range of issues which could lead to vulnerability. Clifford and Burke even refer to the process as an 'interrogation' (2009: 36) suggesting the level of rigour required and the commitment to the goals of reducing vulnerability. Without this commitment, 'real' and 'genuine' critical reflection is unlikely to occur.

A further level of critical reflection moves beyond introspection or mere reflection and self-discovery to include the questioning or challenging of situations, practices, or beliefs; this involves a desire to move beyond face value and the status quo to challenge the 'taken for granted' (Dalrymple and Burke 2006: 48). As such, critical reflection can include the challenging of dominant discourses (D'Cruz *et al.* 2007: 86), allowing more marginal discourses to be heard and considered. This added element of critical reflection is vital for reducing vulnerability, since it requires all individuals to be prepared to follow-up on their initial reflections and not be content to continue with ritualistic, routine, or taken-for-granted practices. Here, again Thompson's exhortation to be part of the solution or else accept that you are part of the problem is ringing in the ears (Thompson 2011).

Okitikpi and Aymer (2010: 109) have characterised critical reflection in terms of four key questions:

- What are you doing?
- Why are you doing it?
- What is influencing what you are doing?
- What else could you do?

This suggests not just bringing your thoughts, feelings, values, and behaviours under scrutiny and into consciousness, but also encompasses the need to follow-up with action to question, challenge, or change situations, practices, or beliefs. Critical reflection is the cornerstone to reducing vulnerability as a result of unthinking or unintentional oppression by allowing you as the practitioner to step back and review current practice with a view to moving towards practice which is anti-oppressive.

Elegant challenging

Take a few minutes to address the questions in Box 9.6. Challenging the practice of others is something that many will recoil from, feeling it is fraught with difficulty and tension. However, challenge is a necessary element of reducing vulnerability and is a key aspect of critical reflection and anti-oppressive practice, as we have seen. Thompson introduced the term 'elegant challenge' (Thompson 2011), and the phrase clearly softens the sense of tension and confrontation that many associate with challenge. This is important as the process of challenge should not be aggressively confrontational; indeed, such an approach would reduce the chances of a successful challenge and be a waste of time and energy. Goleman (1996) suggests that emotionally intelligent individuals manage relationships effectively through interactions that are constructive and have a positive outcome. To challenge strongly or aggressively is unlikely to achieve this and might be deemed emotionally unintelligent. Thompson (2006, 2011) suggests that poor or unskilled challenge may be damaging to the other person and ultimately counterproductive, creating resistance and barriers to change.

Elegant challenging is one means of tactfully yet effectively challenging oppressive practice in others. It is a form of sensitive challenge which is firm, yet diplomatic. Heron's conception of a 'confronting intervention' seems to capture the sense of the elegant challenge as an intervention which:

> … unequivocally tells an uncomfortable truth, but does so with love, in order that the one concerned may see it and fully acknowledge it. (Heron 2001: 59)

Thompson (2006, 2011) offers some guidance on how to conduct an 'elegant challenge' which we have included here, together with further details drawn from Heron's guidance on 'confronting interventions' (2001):

• Be tactful and constructive, offering advice on what was a problem and how practice could be different and non-oppressive. The challenge should focus on the oppressive action that needs to be amended, rather than conducting a personal attack on the other person. Heron (2001) adds that the challenge should be 'on target in content' (60),

---

Box 9.6   Time for reflection

• How easy or difficult do you find it to express your opinions, particularly if they differ from the people you are talking to?
• What feelings do you experience when you think of challenging another person?
• What does the word 'challenge' suggest for you?
• Does adding the word 'elegant' make it better?

suggesting that the challenge needs to be accurate, relevant, and 'to the point'. It should not get caught up in unnecessary detail but equally should offer sufficient information so that the listener understands the issue clearly and recognises the points being made. Using observed evidence can help to achieve this.

- The challenge should avoid leaving the person feeling 'cornered' and humiliated.
- It is important to choose right time and place. There is no easy answer to this, but a thoughtfully chosen moment to challenge someone's behaviour may be more effective than an impetuously chosen one. Appropriate timing would be near to the event, not too long after, but also at a time when the situation is not too emotionally charged. Heron (2001) adds that the individual should be ready and willing to listen to what is said; they may be unaware of the issue, but they should be in a state of readiness to listen to what is said.
- We should avoid being punitive, thus reducing the potential for a hostile outcome. Heron further distinguishes that the intervention should be poised somewhere between the extremes of a 'sledgehammer' and 'pussyfoot' approach (Heron 2001: 61). Thus, the challenge should avoid 'clobbering' the person in a destructive and punitive way, but equally should not skirt around the issues, 'going round the mulberry bush' or avoid the challenge.
- The challenge should recognise in some way our own vulnerabilities to less than good practice, in that we are all capable of thoughtless or unskilled comments and behaviours, and that we are all attempting to do the best we can in sometimes difficult circumstances. This emphasises a more collaborative shared approach to development which avoids taking the moral high ground but should resist offering excuses for oppressive actions.
- Challenge should be offered with a real sense of concern and consideration for the individual and not just point scoring. Heron adds that the intervention should be 'deeply affirming of the worth' of the individual (Heron 2001: 59) and supportive in its manner. This would suggest that an elegant challenge is delivered whilst using the key communication and relationship skills referred to earlier such as empathy, unconditional positive regard, and congruence or genuineness.
- Challenge with humility and modesty rather than a bullying or overzealous approach. Educating and convincing need to be the focus rather than bullying and lecturing.

Readers are recommended to read Heron's work for further detail on how to construct the intervention, what to say and what not to say, and how to avoid the pitfalls that occur (2001). It should be noted that elegant challenge and confrontation are just a few of a vast range of communication skills involved in reducing vulnerability; others include negotiation, advocacy, and facilitation (Dalrymple and Burke 2006), whilst Heron's work refers to informative or cathartic interventions which are useful in this context (2001). Advocacy and empowerment have been explored within Chapter 5 and readers are urged to explore these skills through further reading – space does not permit further consideration here.

Minimal intervention

The concept of minimal intervention has been put forward as a core principle underpinning anti-oppressive practice (Healy 2005) and has largely appeared within

---

Box 9.7 Activity

1 Refer back to Sanjay's story in 4? (Chapter 4, Box 4.14) and the discussion of welfarism (Chapter 4, page 81).
   ○ Did the nurses' recommendation for going into a care home meet the criterion of minimal intervention?
   ○ Where would you place the 'fine line' for Sanjay in terms of 'minimal intervention'?
2 Reflect upon your experiences of practice.
   ○ Can you think of situations where the intervention by health carers has been intrusive, excessive, and perhaps disabling or disempowering?

---

the context of social work practice (Healy 2005, Dalrymple and Burke 2006). However, there is a value in mentioning it here as a personal level strategy for health care practitioners. Minimal intervention urges practitioners to 'try to intervene in people's lives with as little intrusion as possible …' (Dalrymple and Burke 2006: 151). Immediately this casts a fine line in judging vulnerability; too much intrusion is seen as disempowering and disabling for clients, whilst too little intervention risks leaving clients at greater risk of vulnerability. However, it is our argument here that critical reflection upon this fine line with each client is of crucial importance in reducing vulnerability. In order to examine this further, please undertake the activity in Box 9.7.

Clearly minimal intervention is a complex issue which has no simple answers. In relation to Sanjay, it is easy to see the two sides of the fine line: an over-intrusion into his life and his autonomy could result from admission to a care home, thus increasing his emotional vulnerability, whilst allowing him to be at risk of choking alone is equally increasing his physical vulnerability. The answer lies in careful consideration, negotiation, advocacy, and respect for Sanjay's autonomy in the process. Equally, it lies in critical reflection upon the degree to which interventions are 'minimal' and non-intrusive or where they go beyond this.

Welfarism as discussed in Chapter 4 is clearly a risk for intrusion in the lives of some beyond that which is required, thus creating dependency. Additionally, you may have identified some instances where the functional ability of clients has decreased whilst receiving care. Lafont *et al.* (2011) have labelled this as 'iatrogenic disability' where avoidable dependence occurs during the course of care for some clients. You may have seen instances where health carers undertake activities which the client is capable of doing for themselves but which 'saves time' for the health carers or where a client is able to mobilise, but where health carers 'wheel' them around without encouraging mobilisation, again perhaps because it saves time. You may have noticed that for some clients this process leads them to lose their ability to mobilise or carry out activities they were previously able to undertake. These would be instances of 'iatrogenic disability', where minimal intervention would have reduced the vulnerability of the client. In these instances, minimal intervention would be to offer only the assistance that the client needs to fulfil activities they are unable to complete themselves, therefore only meeting the actual needs of the client, rather than the health carers' needs.

Having a clear and explicit theory base

Above all, a key personal level intervention as described by many (Dominelli 2002; Thompson 2011, 2012) is to have a clear and explicit theory base. This should be used to understand the impact of vulnerability or oppression, to understand its causes, and to understand and gain the skills in order to address vulnerability and oppression. Much of this book has been devoted to exploring a knowledge base which can help the health and social care practitioner develop an awareness of where vulnerability and oppression exists, how it can affect people, and, most importantly, its causes and what can be done to reduce vulnerability and oppression when it is possible to do so. A key aim of this book is to equip practitioners with the knowledge base to work in an anti-oppressive manner and to reduce vulnerability for the individuals they work with.

Having a clear and explicit theory base to underpin practice is vital to avoid 'drift' where people can lose sight of what should be the aims of practice in the day-to-day chaos and busyness of contemporary health and social care (Thompson 2011: 165). Thompson also argues that having this clear and explicit theory base can also help us avoid resorting to poorly thought through 'common sense' approaches which might be based on 'taken-for-granted' sexist, racist, or other discriminatory assumptions in the absence of a clearly thought out theory base (Thompson 2012: 191–192).

Cultural level strategies

This section will explore:

* Anti-oppressive practice as a core central value
* Developing a shared team culture
* Small acts of resistance
* Working collectively
* Personal research on oppression and anti-oppression
* Language and terminology
* Openness, transparency, and demystification

Anti-oppressive practice as a core central value

Reducing vulnerability and anti-oppressive practice are clearly passionately held commitments and goals for all of the authors in this book. This commitment is underpinned by a shared set of values and beliefs; central amongst these is the valuing of equality, diversity, respect, and anti-oppression. We are passionate about sharing these values hence we have committed to writing this book. Equally, the professional bodies, such as the Nursing and Midwifery Council, have embedded such values within their codes of practice (NMC 2008) as evidence of their commitment to such values and goals. The question for you the reader is:

> Are *you* passionate about these values and are you committed to the goals of reducing vulnerability and anti-oppressive practice?

Because unless you are, there will be minimal change in your ability to reduce the vulnerability of clients you work with. This is a stark and rather brutal way of saying that reducing vulnerability is not simply about learning a list of terms and knowledge, it is much more than this. Anti-oppressive practice needs to be a commitment rather than just a technique. It requires an emotional commitment, a passion and desire to keep trying, to keep knocking on doors, to keep vigilant to the harm (both actual and potential) being caused to clients.

Thompson (2006, 2011) comments on the dangers of 'tokenism' and 'superficiality' in addressing anti-oppressive practice; here he refers to the practice of just 'saying the right things' or 'going through the motions' of anti-oppressive practice, but without any real and genuine commitment to its principles and values. As a result, the status quo remains; there is little progress or reduction in vulnerability. Hence our exhortation to you to question and review your own level of commitment.

Anti-oppressive practice is not just an add-on part to your practice, something you choose to do or not do, it must be a central and core element of your practice if real protection against vulnerability is to be achieved. Nzira and Williams have stated:

> The duty of care accepted by all who choose a career in health and social care .... places a responsibility upon these professionals to challenge discrimination. It is also morally right and just to do so. (Nzira and Williams 2009: 75)

They are quite clear that anti-oppressive practice is both a professional and moral responsibility and duty, and as health carers we are beholden to challenge discrimination and to reduce vulnerability. This is a core and central aspect of our practice, not an optional added extra.

But what of Thompson's 'tokenistic' carers, those that give the appearance of being anti-oppressive but who do not commit to its values and principles? They may be governed by the same code of practice, have studied on the same courses, read the same books urging anti-oppressive practice, and yet somehow it is not enough. This emphasises the personal nature of this commitment and about the nature of your own personal value base. Yes, we all answer to our governing bodies, but they alone cannot prevent all instances of vulnerability as evidenced by the many reports mentioned in the introduction. For vulnerability to be reduced, there is a need for health carers to support and complement the structural level of governing bodies by working to enhance the cultures we work in, endeavouring to provide cultures which are anti-oppressive and which reduce vulnerability. A key element of this relies on our underpinning passion and commitment to anti-oppressive practice and our own moral code and conscience.

Developing a shared team culture

Whilst individual moral codes are important, the efforts to reduce vulnerability can be significantly eased by developing a shared culture where team members have anti-oppressive practice as a shared core value and where mutual yet respectful challenge is accepted and valued. A team where there is openness to offering constructive and respectful challenge or to receive it openly with appreciation. Benjamin (2007: 201) and

Thompson (2011: 222–223) emphasise the need to develop the right work place culture and spirit so that all team members can feel supported to engage in anti-oppressive practice, which can include occasional difficult requirement to challenge others. They emphasise the importance of mutual care and support within the team or professional network which can both offer psychological and emotional support and also ensure that no one member of the team feels victimised or labelled as a troublemaker.

Small acts of resistance

When anti-oppressive values are core and 'non-negotiable' within your own belief system or within the team culture then this will drive the passion and commitment to reducing vulnerability. These qualities are vital at times in the face of opposition or threats. Cooper (2004) suggested that challenging accepted yet oppressive norms, policies, and practice could be viewed as 'being a nuisance'. However, she argues that if challenging oppression or opposing oppressive processes means being a nuisance or causing irritation to managers or others, 'so be it'. In her view, this is better than colluding or going along with oppressive practice, and she points to the success of awkward protest movements in achieving significant advances such as the women's movement or the disability movement, who have used direct action and constant critical challenge in order to advance their cause. An underpinning passion, commitment, and strong value base are crucial for such achievements. In your setting, the changing of a routine or ritual or the offering of choice to clients might be your achievement, but the passion and commitment required are no less.

Baines argues that 'micro-resistance' can foster more resistance and can overcome feelings of futility and pointlessness and can help to 'keep hope alive', to encourage others to choose resistance over compliance with oppressive exploitative systems (Baines 2007: 61). De Certeau (1988) also refuses to see us as passive victims of an oppressive society. He argued that we can all employ all sort of techniques and minor acts of resistance and disobedience, which can create a challenge to oppressive processes and systems. The political philosopher Herbert Marcuse constantly advocated the 'Great Refusal' (Marcuse 1969, 2002) as the proper political response to any form of irrational repression or oppression. He argued we should all join in challenging and opposing all forms of oppression and domination and use relentless criticism of all policies that impact negatively on others. He criticised the era of 'positive thinking,' conformity, and the drive for self-interested promotion before any moral and ethical principles. Marcuse's emphasis on critical thinking, refusal, and opposition to the oppression and domination of others provides a philosophical underpinning for anti-oppressive practice and reducing vulnerability.

Baines (2007) recognises that micro-resistance alone may only slow down or temporarily sidetrack oppressive agendas and will do little to fundamentally change them. However, De Certeau (1988) suggests, we may not be able to change the whole world, but we may be able to make small changes that may lead to larger and longer term changes.

Baines offers six principles that can help to create a more anti-oppressive culture and a more effective anti-oppressive practitioner (Figure 9.1).

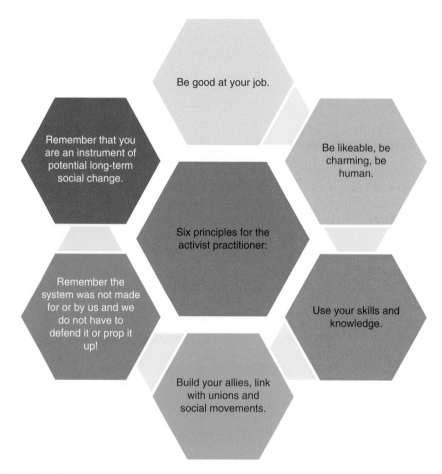

Figure 9.1   Six principles for the activist practitioner (adapted from Baines 2007: 61).

Working collectively

Cooper (2004), Baines (2007), and Thompson (2011) have suggested that for anti-oppressive activism and challenge to be effective and not end up with the anti-oppressive practitioner being overwhelmed, 'burnt out', and experiencing vulnerability of their own, collaborative and collective action is advisable and more effective, so that group lobbying and campaigning is both safer and more effective than individuals acting alone. Benjamin (2007: 201) and Thompson (2011: 222–223) emphasise that collective whole team approaches may be more effective and influential than the isolated efforts or actions of a single practitioner working alone. Working collaboratively as a staff group also means that members of the team can learn from each other about how to tackle difficulties and barriers to anti-oppressive practice. Although Thompson (2011) does recognise that there is the small risk that this collective action could be used to overwhelm individuals so they may succumb publicly, yet still hold oppressive beliefs privately.

Personal research on oppression and anti-oppression

Carrying out reading and research into the first-hand, lived experience of oppression and vulnerability experienced by others can be a powerful tool at the cultural level of anti-oppressive practice (Hood *et al.* 1999, Nzira and Williams 2009). Anti-oppressive social research can include the collecting, cataloguing, and recording of the oppression and discrimination experienced first hand by various individuals and groups. This can be supplemented by more objective research evidence to demonstrate the extent of such vulnerability and oppression. For example, the Care and Compassion report (Parliamentary and Health Service Ombudsman 2011) showed that the experience of vulnerability and degradation was shared by the ten different individuals and families on which the report focuses. This book has so far been based on the inclusion of both first-hand personal evidence as well as more third-hand research evidence that people have experienced vulnerability and oppression even in very recent times and may still continue to do so.

Nzira and Williams (2009: 1–8) give three examples to illustrate the value and use of such an approach. By identifying the experiences of women, experience of racism by people throughout history, or the lived experience of disabled people, it may be possible to get a greater understanding of how oppression occurs, the impacts of that oppression, and insight into what can be done to challenge that oppression. When collected together, this evidence can be used to demonstrate approaches that may be oppressive and those that are anti-oppressive. For example, one of the contributing factors in the oppression of the individuals and groups described is that there was an ideology prevalent in earlier ages that these groups were socially or biologically 'inferior'. This belief was used to justify discriminatory and even oppressive treatment and represents a process of stigmatisation, depersonalisation, and dehumanisation (see Chapter 4). Such insights are valuable in reducing vulnerability, and there is a need to collect together much more recent and contemporary examples of where people have experienced depersonalisation and dehumanisation. Thus, the researcher takes on a journalistic role similar to that of Charles Dickens or Friderich Engels when they recorded the miserable conditions experienced by the poor, working class in Victorian Britain (Hood *et al.* 1999).

Nzira and Williams (2009) and Thompson (2011) highlight some possible benefits for taking such an approach. By researching and collecting evidence together of the achievements and experiences of vulnerable and oppressed groups throughout the past and up to the present, it is possible to see vulnerable and oppressed individuals and groups not as passive victims, there to be rescued by people from more dominant groups, but we can see their experiences often as stories of survival and 'self-contribution' where many of the individuals and groups have been instrumental in advancing their own rights and interests. Collecting together the experiences and views of people from these traditionally oppressed or marginalised groups can help us as they often have a more positive experience of their own identity that we can learn from (Nzira and Williams 2009: 17).

This creates a slightly different cultural perception of vulnerability and oppression which changes it from the story of victims and oppressors to one where we are all seeking mutual respect and emancipation. The story of the disabled persons or feminist movement through their own protest and campaigning creates a more positive image about oppressed groups and their own ability to achieve change in partnership with others from more 'dominant' groups. Two examples of a memoir written by authors writing about their experience of disability are Nolan (1999) and Mukhopadhyay (2003). One rich example is the poem *Crabbitt Old Woman* (Chapter 4, Box 4.5) which shows the experience of an older patient in a hospital and what it is like to be disregarded and discounted by nurses. There are numerous other examples of the first-hand experience of many other people with many other experiences to tell (revisit Box 4.2).

Keeping newspaper, web-based, or material in other formats in personal scrapbooks, diaries, or saving files electronically can help you gather up a substantial database as evidence that vulnerability, discrimination, and oppression are still an all too common experience for too many people. Why not record incidents or reflect on situations where oppression may have occurred or where someone may have experienced it, and record what happened and reflect on possible reasons for it and the possible impact of that experience of oppression for the individual. These reflections could be included in your personal work diary or Portfolio, and the themes that emerge could be used as part of a staff team discussion or training workshop on how to reduce or otherwise address vulnerability and oppression within the care setting.

The power of people's own personal stories and accounts of their own oppression and vulnerability, collected together through this type of research, can be insightful and useful in the effort to reduce vulnerability and as a minimum is useful in increasing levels of empathy and understanding. This shows the value of this research approach.

Language and terminology

Another cultural level intervention which may be important is paying due attention to the language, labels, and terminology used in health care setting which can either contribute to people's vulnerability and oppression or serve to reduce it. The potential of language, labels, and terminology to oppress, marginalise, or make people feel vulnerable has been explored throughout much of this book (see, for example, Chapters 4 and 6). The language and terminology we use both with service users and with colleagues can reinforce stereotypical and stigmatising perceptions held by others and needs constant self-awareness and self-monitoring (Thompson 2011, 2012).

Clements and Spinks (2009) suggest that sensitivity and insensitivity to the oppressive use of language and labels could be conscious or unconscious – see Figure 9.2. For example, at one level, you might really offend someone by what you say, but have no awareness or idea that you are doing it; this could be described as unintentional and unconscious offence. To deliberately and knowingly offend, would obviously be at the other end of that level. However, both examples, the knowing or unknowing use of discriminatory language, can still cause offence.

However, many authors such as Nzira and Williams (2009) and Thompson (2012) recognise that a rigid, inflexible, and dogmatic attention to language and labels can create hostility and a backlash against so-called political correctness (see the discussion of 'Trivialisation' in Chapter 4). Sensitivity to the impact of language and labels is recommended, recognising why they may be offensive or difficult for others and being

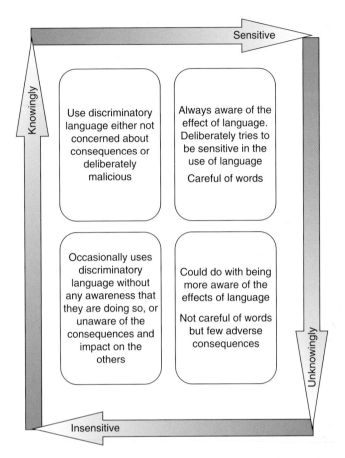

Figure 9.2   How sensitive and insensitive language can be conscious or unconscious (adaptation based upon data from Clements and Spinks 2009: 26).

willing to negotiate and consult about preferred terminology with people with whom we work. One approach to the difficult issue of language and labels is to find out the preferred terms of language of the individual or group with whom we are working and to use that advice and guidance about the language which is appropriate in that context.

To illustrate, according to Modood (1994, cited in Macionis and Plummer 2012: 350), the all-encompassing term 'black' person or 'black Briton' is problematic. This is because the term 'black' does not adequately address the separate and distinct identity of Asians and Chinese, especially given that the term 'black' is also used to specifically mean African and African Caribbean people in other contexts. People of African descent may not accept the term 'black' and may prefer alternatives such as person of colour, which again might not be acceptable to all. Modood suggests we should continually explore alternative terms for black, 'Asian', or 'Oriental' identity with the respective communities to find acceptable alternative concepts to the all-encompassing term 'black' if preferred.

> **Box 9.8** Openness and demystification: Creating an open and inclusive communication culture (Thompson 2011: 227)
>
> • Interactions between staff and service users should be based on openness and honesty, with no collusion, hidden agendas, deceptions, or the withholding of information.
> • All forms of communication, both written and verbal, should use language which is 'user friendly' or easy to read where appropriate, with no jargon or complex terminology used to mystify.
> • Interpreters should be used for people who may not be fluent in spoken or written English. This might include people who may have dyslexia and cannot access written language in the same way as other people can use written language.
> • Service users should always be involved fully within decision making processes or where this is not possible; a full and appropriate explanation should be given to them, as well as information about the complaints and appeals procedures. Here the links to power with and power within (Chapter 3) are clear.

A sense of modesty and humility is needed in order to avoid arrogance and complacency and to remain open and critical about our use of language, avoiding critical and punitive approaches to others in their use of language (Nzira and Williams 2009; Thompson 2011, 2012).

Openness, transparency, and demystification

Another facet of creating an inclusive non-oppressive culture is being open and transparent, demystifying language and labels used, and the care and the decision-making process. The intention being to ensure that vulnerability is not created through lack of information or understanding. The goal should be for full and equal participation for all clients/service users in their care. This is restricted if individuals do not understand situations, processes, or decisions involving them. For example, the use of abbreviations, professional jargon, or academic language such as #NOF, MI, dementia, acopia, Parkinson's can shroud the communication in mystery and misunderstanding. Additionally, the provision of appropriate interpreters rather than relying inappropriately on family members to translate and the provision of multilingual, easy read, and accessible printed information is important in creating a culture and climate of inclusiveness and avoids excluding or marginalising people who may be using our service.

Where machinations or any decision takes place behind closed doors and decisions and events are shrouded in mystery, the scope for the inequality and the abuse of power to flourish is greatly increased, Thompson (2011). Thompson adds that to be open, inclusive, and free of mystification, a number of principles may help (see Box 9.8).

Structural level strategies

This section will explore:

• Politicisation and conscientisation
• Using the law
• Participation in the democratic process

The third level of structural interventions is possibly the most difficult, the reason being that personal level and cultural level interventions are part and parcel of the practitioners' everyday practice within the work setting. Addressing structural level factors means directing one's attention to factors outside of the immediate workplace and may involve activity outside of work such as engagement with the political and democratic process in order to influence changes in policy and practice or even legislation and wider levels.

However, structural level interventions are as important as any other levels of intervention in that it goes to the heart of definitions of what an anti-oppressive practitioner should be. If we accept the definitions of anti-oppressive practice given at the beginning of the chapter, that it seeks to 'reduce, undermine, challenge and eliminate discrimination and oppression, and to promote equality' (adapted from Thompson 2006, 2011), then personal level intervention alone is insufficient and incomplete practice. Just like fire fighters, the anti-oppressive practitioner needs to put out fires where they occur and save or protect individuals; however, firefighting would be ineffective without good quality fire prevention addressing the possible causes of fires, providing people with information and advice on how to be safe. In the context of anti-oppressive practice, practice which does not take account of addressing the structural causes or factors which create oppression and vulnerability for service users could be said to be poor practice (Dominelli 2002, Thompson 2011, Thompson 2012). Within the context of the PCS model, Thompson (2011: 182) describes practice which focuses exclusively or primarily on P level interventions, with little or no attention to cultural or structural level factors, as a 'Polo Mint' approach where the centre has been taken out of the whole approach. He is equally critical of practice which may just focus on cultural or structural level intervention.

A number of different structural level interventions are described here for your consideration in order to determine whether any of these may have potential value in addressing discrimination and oppression and dealing with some of the wider social and structural factors that may contribute to people feeling vulnerable and powerless.

Politicisation and conscientisation

The first challenge of structural level intervention is raising awareness and consciousness, the process described by the Brazilian educationalist Paulo Freire as conscientisation (1970). This is described as 'becoming aware of how oppression works and is reproduced through daily interactions' (Essed 1991, cited in Dominelli 2002: 13).

Freire explained conscientisation as:

> In order for the oppressed to be able to wage the struggle for their liberation they must perceive the reality of oppression, not as a closed world from which there is no exit, but as a limited situation which they can transform … this perception must become the motivating force for liberating action (Freire 1970: 31).

For Thompson, this raising of awareness is also political and can then lead onto political or structural action to address the factors that are contributing to oppression that become apparent through raised awareness.

Conscientisation can be seen as the process of helping to make people aware of the broader context of the situations they face: politicisation is the process of seeking to address problems at the broader socio-political level (Thompson 2011: 221).

For Thompson, this is about helping people understand and become aware of the extent to which their situations or predicaments are influenced by wider cultural or social processes. Dominelli (2002: 147) highlights the value of consciousness raising in terms of mobilising differing groups such as women, black activists, and in the disability movement to define their own experience and goals and then to achieve personal and structural improvements in their situation through their own efforts or actions. Therefore, in order to address racism or gender oppression, the practitioner or the community at large may need to address the social and structural causes of that racism or gender oppression, whether it be through the perpetuation of stereotypes in the media, dominant discriminatory discourses surrounding certain marginalised groups, or to do with the lack of protection or the lack of positive action to promote better life chances for those who historically belong to marginalised groups.

According to Dalrymple and Burke (2006: 283), becoming aware of the reality of oppression and injustice and having the core aims of social justice and social equality can help us maintain a 'sense of outrage' that can energise us to do something about it. This is in the spirit of Freire's idea that conscientisation and growing political awareness of the cause and effect of oppression can be the engine of anti-oppression (Nzira and Williams 2009: 26).

As well as being about raising personal level awareness and consciousness of discriminatory and vulnerability and using factors, conscientisation could also include raising societal level awareness through education and providing information for communities as to what might actually be happening (Dominelli 2002: 34). This contributes to the empowerment of individuals and communities to address those factors politically and structurally through the political process. This raised awareness of oppression and its causes could lead to recognition that, because these are often created through structural and social processes, these need to be changed or challenged in order to prevent future oppression or address factors that contribute to vulnerability. A few differing methods of achieving anti-oppression through political activity or seeking structural change are described hereafter but it starts with this raised awareness.

Using the law

One structural approach that can come through raised awareness is to 'use the law' (Dalrymple and Burke 2006, Nzira and Williams 2009, Thompson 2011). Dalrymple and Burke (2006: 171) argue that although the existing legal structures may have helped reinforce discrimination, oppression, and social control, it also has the potential for anti-discriminatory and anti-oppressive change. Firstly, the law clearly stipulates a legal requirement to address discrimination, oppression, and factors that might be adding to the vulnerability of patients and service users. Two very relevant piece of legislation which outlines the practitioners' legal duty to practice in an anti-discriminatory and anti-oppressive fashion are the Human Rights Act (1998a, 1998b) and the Equality Act 2010.

The UK government was an early signatory of the 1950 European Convention on Human Rights (ECHR) after the abuse of human rights and genocides evident before and during World War II. The ECHR was a binding international agreement that the UK helped draft and has sought to comply with for over half a century (Department of Constitutional Affairs 2006).

In order to strengthen the legal basis of these rights outlined in the ECHR for UK citizens, the UK government enshrined these key human rights in UK law when they passed the Human Rights Act (HRA) 1998 into law. The HRA protects and upholds certain human rights and it would be an offence to knowingly abuse these rights of other individuals. Therefore, health and social care practitioners should make themselves aware of these rights and what they entail so that they do nothing to infringe or breach the rights of others and work to protect the rights of those with whom they work. This is especially important when someone through illness, disability, or other incapacity is vulnerable and therefore unable to defend or protect their own human rights. That is why advocating for the interests and rights of others is such an important part of the professional codes, i.e. NMC 2008 (HCPC 2012a). Please read the summary of the Human Rights Act provided and complete the reflective exercises (Box 9.9).

Clearly, there are potentially many instances where the rights of service users or patients in your care could be violated or undermined. The Equality and Human Rights Commission (EHRC, undated b), a body set up through the Equality Act 2010 to monitor equality and human rights in the UK, has given a number of examples, including where people have been judged to have had Human Right no 2, 'Freedom from torture and degrading treatment', undermined (Box 9.10).

Box 9.9   Time for reflection

Summary of human rights outlined in Human Rights Act 1998 (Source: Equality and Human Rights Commission, undated a)

- Right to life
- Freedom from torture and inhuman or degrading treatment
- Right to liberty and security
- Freedom from slavery and forced labour
- Right to a fair trial
- No punishment without law
- Respect for your private and family life, home and correspondence
- Freedom of thought, belief, and religion
- Freedom of expression
- Freedom of assembly and association
- Right to marry and start a family
- Protection from discrimination in respect of these rights and freedoms
- Right to peaceful enjoyment of your property
- Right to education
- Right to participate in free elections

Which of these rights do you think could be intentionally or unintentionally violated in a health care situation? List any potential examples you can think of.

Box 9.10   Protection from torture and mistreatment – examples of human rights breach (Equality and Human Rights Commission, undated b)

Example 1: A young man with mental health problems was placed in residential care. During a visit, his parents noticed unexplained bruising on his body. They raised the issue with managers at the home, but their concerns were dismissed. They were also told that they were no longer allowed to visit their son. The parents approached the home and raised their son's right not to be treated in an inhuman and degrading way and their right to respect for family life. As a result, the ban on their visits was revoked and an investigation carried out into the bruising on the son's body. *(Taken from The Human Rights Act: Changing Lives, British Institute of Human Rights 2006, cited EHRC undated b).*

Example 2: *McGlinchey and others v United Kingdom* (2003)
A woman who had a heroin addiction and suffered from asthma was sentenced to four months in prison. While there, she suffered severe heroin withdrawal symptoms, including vomiting and weight loss. A doctor who visited her when she arrived advised the nursing staff to monitor her symptoms. Her condition deteriorated over a weekend, but the nursing staff did not call a doctor, nor did they transfer her to a hospital. On Monday morning, she collapsed and was immediately admitted to hospital, where she died. The European Court of Human Rights held that the Prison Service had not protected the woman from inhuman treatment, because it had failed to take appropriate steps to treat the prisoner's condition and relieve her suffering and had failed to act sufficiently quickly to prevent the worsening of her condition.

(Case summary taken from Human Rights, Human Lives, Department for Constitutional Affairs 2006, cited by EHRC undated).

Another key piece of legislation concerned with protecting the rights of others and avoiding and even challenging discrimination and oppression aimed at others is the Equality Act 2010. Since the mid-1960s, successive UK governments have attempted to challenge discrimination and inequality through legislation with varying success (Box 9.11). The Equality Act 2010 harmonises previous anti-discriminatory legislation under the umbrella of this single act, i.e. incorporates provisions from earlier Race Relations Acts, Disability Discrimination Acts, and so on (Home Office undated; Equality Act 2010).

The Equality Act covers discrimination and inequalities against people from all 'protected characteristics': gender, race and ethnicity, religion, sexual orientation, age, and disability. It provides protection for individuals, especially for those with 'protected characteristics', against direct and indirect discrimination, harassment, and victimisation. It provides protection in services and public functions, premises, work, education, associations, and transport. This clearly covers anyone receiving health and social care in whatever context or setting, whether through statutory health or social services settings or through private or 'not for profit' sector services. The Act also provides protection for people discriminated against because they are perceived to have or are associated with someone who has a protected characteristic, so providing new protection for people like carers from discrimination or unfair treatment.

The Act places a statutory requirement on all public bodies to have provision in place to make adjustments for people with *protected characteristics* (a *general* equality duty) and meet *specific* additional duties, i.e. a specific race equality duty, disability equality

---

Box 9.11   Examples of anti-discriminatory legislation since the 1960s

- Race Relations Act 1965
- Equal Pay Act 1970
- Chronically Sick and Disabled Persons Act 1970
- Sex Discrimination Act 1975
- Race Relations Act 1976
- Mental Health Act 1983
- Disability Discrimination Act 1995
- Human Rights Act 1998
- Race Relations Amendment Act 2000
- Disability Discrimination Act 2005
- Mental Capacity Act 2005, Deprivation of Liberty Safeguards 2007
- Equality Act 2006
- Equality Act 2010

---

duty. Public bodies need to carry out equality impact assessments on their policy and practice and how any change in policy and practice will impact on people with protected characteristics. This means that whether you are an unqualified member of staff or a qualified health or social care professional, or even a student in training on placement, any agency in which you work should have policies in place on how the organisation will meet these statutory *general* and *specific* equality duties, with appropriate training available for all staff in how to meet the requirements of these duties. The requirement of all staff working in an organisation to meet these equality act duties and responsibilities is likely to be reflected in their employment contract, job description, and employer policies that apply to all staff. Therefore, employees whose practice is discriminatory or oppressive or does not take account of equality duties may face disciplinary action by their employers, in addition to being accountable to their professional body possibly through litigation (see activity in Box 9.12).

Whilst there have been many legislative attempts to prevent or address discrimination through legislative approaches, there are limitations on what this has or could achieve (Dalrymple and Burke 2006). For example, the numerous pieces of race relations legislation introduced into UK law since 1960s has done little to completely remove racism from the UK. All it can do is to make it illegal to express racist views or behave in an overtly racist way, but it may just drive people's racist beliefs or actions underground. Having an Equality Act on its own can do little to provide the material resources and opportunities that people need to make equality a reality. As explored throughout this book, poverty and social class can affect someone's ability to fully enjoy their rights of citizenship (Dominelli 2002, Baines 2007, Thompson 2011). Thompson (2012: 15) uses the example of poverty and social exclusion in relation to people with disabilities in that poverty and social exclusion interlink with the discrimination faced by disabled people. Unless we challenge disability discrimination such as in the employment market, disabled people may go on to experience further social exclusion and poverty which undermines their rights. However, tackling poverty and social exclusion can also help disabled people enjoy the rights which are enshrined in equality and anti-discrimination legislation.

Box 9.12   Activity

Read the Home Office Equalities Dept Guidance (2011) *Equality Act* 2010: *Public Sector Equality Duty What Do I Need To Know? A Quick Start Guide For Public Sector Organisations* (*) http://www.homeoffice.gov.uk/publications/equalities/equality-act-publications/equality-act-guidance/equality-duty?view=Binary

- What does the Equality Act 2010 say about the general equality duty of public sector organisations such as a hospital or NHS Trust? List or make notes of what these requirements are.

The Equality Act places further specific equality duties on these organisations too; see Home Office Equalities Dept guidance on these specific duties, Equality Act 2010: Specific Duties To Support The Equality Duty What Do I Need To Know? A Quick Start Guide For Public Sector Organisations (*) http://www.homeoffice.gov.uk/publications/equalities/equality-act-publications/equality-act-guidance/specific-duties?view=Binary

- What specific actions should public sector organisations carry out to meet the specific equality duties outlined in the Equality Act?
- Find out what policies your organisation has in place to meet the general and specific equality duties as required by the Act and familiarise yourself with them and what your own responsibilities are.
- Find a copy of your employment contract or job description. What does it say about your responsibility to act in an anti-discriminatory or anti-oppressive way?

(*) nb: slightly different guidance applies to voluntary or 'not for profit' organisations – please refer to Home Office Equality Act guidance if working in non-statutory services: http://www.homeoffice.gov.uk/publications/equalities/equality-act-publications/equality-act-guidance/

For Dominelli (2002: 90), the failure of legalistic approaches is not just in the limitations of the anti-discrimination legislation itself, but in the way that it is operated or implemented by the various agencies of the state. She gives the example of the failure of the police, probation officers, and the criminal justice system to cater to the needs of abused women or rape victims which tends to add to abuse and disregard that they may have already suffered. Dalrymple and Burke (2006) caution against the overreliance on a legalistic approach, suggesting there are many situations where the direct application of law may be of limited value in addressing discrimination and vulnerability experienced by the people you work with. Anti-discrimination legislation does not and could not ever cover every situation which the anti-oppressive practitioner may encounter. Therefore, much more proactive and challenging approaches are needed to identify and address the other factors such as prejudicial attitudes or dominant and oppressive discourses, imagery, and language at the cultural level which may reinforce people's prejudicial attitudes and behaviours as an example where the existence of relevant legislation alone is insufficient (Thompson 2011).

Another possible anti-oppressive dimension in 'using the law' is that it can provide us with the means to both influence and persuade others to improve or change policy or practice, or request statutory interventions (Dalrymple and Burke 2006, Thompson 2011). This could be described as the proactive use of law. They argue that legislation can be used as a persuasive justification for anti-discriminatory or anti-oppressive policy and action.

As a last resort, legislation opens up the possibility of using legal powers to address oppressive or discriminatory situations or processes (Dalrymple and Burke 2006, Thompson 2011). Dalrymple and Burke argue that a detailed knowledge and understanding of the provisions of different equality or anti-discrimination legislation is needed to identify when legal requirements and obligations are being breached or to know what people's entitlements and rights are. For example, legislation such as the Mental Health Act 1983 involves having a good understanding of what protections and safeguards exist to protect the rights of any individual detained or compulsorily treated.

Caution is needed though, as persuasion may be better and more productive than legalistic threats, so that using legal powers to challenge the practice of others may not be a first-resort action (Dalrymple and Burke 2006). Also, as noted earlier, overreliance on legal powers and legal rights can ignore the material and other factors that create or contribute to vulnerability and oppression in the first place.

This leaves the anti-oppressive practitioner with a further challenge: how are any structural level changes to come about? For example, if a piece of legislation, policy, wider social process, or structural institution requires change or improvement, then how could the practitioner achieve this, individually or collectively with others. Some authors (Nzira and Williams 2009; Thompson 2011, 2012) discuss the need for social, structural, and political change but sadly devote little space to detailed discussion as to how this could be achieved. Thompson himself demonstrates 'the Polo Mint effect' (2011: 182) in the rather brief discussion of strategies for promoting equality at the end of his work.

Participation in the democratic process

On the most immediate and basic level, UK citizens have the right to vote every four or five years in local, national, and even European elections (Heywood 2007). Voting for a political party that is more likely to represent a fairer or less discriminatory approach, a change of policy which you think will address some of your concerns about health and social care, or the factors that can lead to discrimination and oppression might influence your decision on who to cast your vote for. Making a personal commitment and encouraging others to vote in the first place could be seen as an important first step to achieve change given historically low turnouts in general elections (Box 9.13).

Nzira and Williams (2009: 196) describe anti-oppression as a political stance, but one which means gaining more influence and rights for people at risk of discrimination and oppression. This could be achieved through discussing the various policies and manifestoes of political parties at election time with colleagues or at meetings either through your union or professional association (Hart 2004). A relevant point is exploring whether the

---

Box 9.13   Turnout of registered voters in recent UK general elections (Electoral Commission 2010)

- 7 June 2001 general election: 59.54%
- 5 May 2005 general election: 61.4%
- 6 May 2010 general election: 65.1%

analysis and debate of relevant health and care policy have a place in team meetings given the political nature of care work and given that it is impossible to be apolitical anyway (Goodwin 2007, Thompson 2011, Heywood 2012). It might also involve speaking out publicly whether within a team meeting, through the media, or more publicly through joining a legal march or demonstration or even joining a protest movement such as Amnesty International or another campaigning group or even political party in order to achieve equality or anti-discrimination or anti-oppression.

Such participation in the political process could also involve 'lobbying', which seeks to influence the attitudes, behaviour, or policy of local or national politicians and government (Giddens 2009). This might involve attempts to influence politicians or others on oppressive and discriminatory policy in order to secure support; challenging prevailing social attitudes and discourses spread by journalists; and writing to the letters page in newspapers and contacting TV producers and broadcasters about TV programming (both good and oppressive programmes). Many authors (Heywood 2007, Goodwin 2007, Giddens 2009) suggest that there has been a change from representative politics, which lobbies politicians, to a more participatory approach where people are joining campaigns or even protest groups rather than putting faith in politicians.

On the most immediate level, with the advent of the Internet and e-mail, it has never been easier to directly contact your local or national elected political representative. Websites such as 'They work for you' and 'Write to them' provide direct e-mail links to your own elected representative via the searchable websites. It is also possible to search through the voting record and major interests and speech history of your local elected politicians. It is also possible to contact your politicians through the Parliament website (Box 9.14).

If seeking to influence the views or actions of newspaper journalists or TV producers and broadcasters, postal or e-mail addresses of these organisations in order to make a

---

Box 9.14   Contacting your member of Parliament or local councillor

Via Parliament website: http://www.parliament.uk/about/contacting/mp.cfm

'Write to Them': http://www.writetothem.com/

'They Work For You' http://www.theyworkforyou.com/

No 10 Downing Street e-petition website: http://www.number10.gov.uk/take-part/public-engagement/petitions/

Box 9.15   Activity

If in the future you see a derogatory or potentially oppressive portrayal of an issue, individual, or group in the media, why not contact that broadcaster or journalist in order to challenge that representation and suggest less oppressive ways of addressing or covering that issue or group.

   Consider why this might be productive and helpful to prevent future reinforcement of oppressive or discriminatory messages in the media.

complaint or offer suggestions will be available on their websites (see activity in Box 9.15). Wingfield (2008) offers practical suggestions and advice on lobbying. Joining a union, campaign group, or professional association such as the RCN can help in practical support, advice, and guidance on more effective lobbying. There is also a good resource for nurses wanting to get political at Nurse Activism Website (http://nurse-activism. com); although a US site, it has some useful resources on effective lobbying and campaigning.

It is recognised that lobbying and engagement in this process can be time-consuming, especially in a busy working life. However, anyone serious about tackling the root causes of oppression and discrimination may consider some level of action at this level is justifiable. However, as Baines (2007) and Thompson (2011) suggest, doing this collectively as a group may be more powerful and persuasive, i.e. if a politician or a broadcaster was either to receive a petition or 100 letters rather than just one.

Whatever the level of structural or political action, some might question whether health and social care professionals should be political anyway? Goodwin (2007), Thompson (2006, 2011), and Heywood (2012) all argue that to 'not be political' and sit on the fence is being political itself as it suggests acceptance or support for the status quo and the perpetuation of the current state of affairs. As Thompson says:

> …if you're not part of the solution, you must be part of the problem (Thompson 1992, cited in Thompson 2012: 9)

Conclusion

This chapter has explored a range of strategies, interventions, and actions that can be used at the personal, cultural, or structural level in order to address some of the factors and processes that contribute to someone feeling vulnerable or oppressed. It must be acknowledged that this chapter is merely an introduction to some of these strategies and that more detailed discussion of each of these intervention strategies might take up a whole book. However, the chapter authors hope that they have signposted some of the possible strategies and signposted a few practical tips and resources for further consideration of these strategies.

A key issue, as reinforced by Thompson himself (2011, 2012) and also others such as Nzira and Williams (2009), is that it may be ineffective and inappropriate to work at one level of intervention whilst excluding the other levels. If we recognise that cultural and structural level factors can influence personal actions, or conversely that personal actions can influence and alter organisations and wider culture, then it is desirable to consider working at all three levels simultaneously or in parallel. To illustrate, if everyone bought in to the value of being anti-oppressive, this would have far reaching consequences on people's individual actions, the values which the next generation might be socialised into, media portrayals, as well as the policy decisions and actions of politicians. However, that might be a bit idealistic in the short term but is something to work towards in the long term so that social justice and reduction and prevention of oppression could be a long-term social aim for all of us.

Links to other chapters

- Chapter 3 identifies the concepts of 'power with' and 'power within' which are two forms of power that underpin empowerment.
- The 'Processes of Oppression' whereby people can be oppressed and made to feel vulnerable are explored in Chapter 4. These include some accounts of everyday real experiences of vulnerability and the role of language in vulnerability.
- Chapter 5 explores the values identified by the professional bodies. It also discusses the strategy of 'advocacy' and 'empowerment'.
- Chapter 6 explores the power of discourse and language to construct the experience of vulnerability and oppression.
- Chapter 8 explores the processes of conformity and compliance and how these group pressures might prevent an individual taking action against observed vulnerability.

References

Baines, D. (2007) Bridging the practice activism divide in mainstream social work. In: *Doing Anti Oppressive Practice: Building Transformative Politicised Social Work* (Baines, D. ed.), pp. 50–66. Fernwood, Halifax.

Benjamin, K. (2007) Doing anti-oppressive social work: The importance of resistance, history and strategy, afterword. In: *Doing Anti Oppressive Practice: Building Transformative Politicised Social Work* (Baines, D. ed.), pp. 196–201. Fernwood, Halifax.

Burton, G. and Dimbleby, R. (1995) *Between Ourselves – An Introduction to Interpersonal Communication*. 2nd ed., Arnold, London.

Clements, P. and Spinks, T. (2009) *The Equal Opportunities Handbook: How to Recognise Diversity, Encourage Fairness and Promote Anti-Discriminatory Practice*. Kogan Page, London.

Clifford, D. and Burke, B. (2009) *Anti-Oppressive Ethics and Values in Social Work*. Palgrave Macmillan, Basingstoke.

Condon, W.S. (1980) The relation of interactional synchrony to cognitive and emotional process. In: *The Relationship of Verbal and Non-Verbal Communication* (Key, M.R. ed.), pp. 49–65. The Hague, Mouton.

Cooper, D. (2004) *Challenging Diversity: Rethinking Equality and the Value of Difference*. Cambridge University Press, Cambridge.

D'Cruz, H., Gillingham, P. and Melendez, S. (2007) Reflexivity, its meanings and relevance for social work: A critical review of the literature. *British Journal of Social Work*, January 37 (1), 73–90.

Dalrymple, J. and Burke, B. (2006) *Anti-Oppressive Practice – Social Care and the Law*. 2nd ed., Open University Press, Maidenhead.

De Certeau, M. (1988) *The Practice of Everyday Life*. (trans. Rendall, S.) University of California Press, Berkeley.

Department of Constitutional Affairs (2006) *A Guide to the Human Rights Act 1998*: 3rd ed. Available from http://www.justice.gov.uk/downloads/human-rights/act-studyguide.pdf [accessed on 5 October 2012].

Devito, J.A. (2008) *The Interpersonal Communication Book*. 12th ed., Pearson Education, Boston.

Dominelli, L. (2002) *Anti-Oppressive Social Work Theory and Practice*. Palgrave Macmillan, Basingstoke.

Electoral Commission (2010) *The 2010 Turnout Factsheet*. Available from http://www.electoralcommission.org.uk/__data/assets/electoral_commission_pdf_file/0003/13278/Turnout.pdf [accessed on 8 October 2012].

Equality and Human Rights Commission (undated a) *The Human Rights Act*. Available from http://www.equalityhumanrights.com/human-rights/what-are-human-rights/the-human-rights-act/ [accessed on 19 October 2012].

Equality Act (2010) *The National Archives at Legisltation.gov.uk*. Available from http://www.legislation.gov.uk/ukpga/2010/15/contents [accessed on 5 October 2012].

Equality and Human Rights Commission, (undated b). *Protection from Torture and Mistreatment*. Available from http://www.equalityhumanrights.com/human-rights/what-are-human-rights/the-human-rights-act/protection-from-torture-and-mistreatment/ [accessed on 5 October 2012].

Freire, P. (1970) *Pedagogy of the Oppressed*. Penguin, Harmondsworth.

General Medical Council. (2012) *Raising and Acting on Concerns About Patient Safety*. Available from http://www.gmc-uk.org/guidance/ethical_guidance/raising_concerns.asp [accessed on 5 October 2012].

Giddens, A. (2009) *Sociology*. 6th ed., Polity Press, Cambridge.

Goleman, D. (1996) *Emotional Intelligence*. Bloomsbury, London.

Goodwin, B. (2007) *Using Political Ideas*. 5th ed., John Wiley and Sons, Chichester.

Hargie, O. and Dickson, D. (2004) *Skilled Interpersonal Communication – Research, Theory and Practice*. 4th ed., Routledge, London.

Hart, C. (2004) *Nurses and Politics: The Impact of Power and Practice*. Palgrave Macmillan, Basingstoke.

Health and Care Professions Council (HCPC) (2012a) *Standards of Conduct, Performance and Ethics*. Available from http://www.hpc-uk.org/aboutregistration/standards/standardsofconduct-performanceandethics/ [accessed on 5 October 2012].

HCPC (2012b) *Guidance on Conduct and Ethics for Students*. Available from http://www.hpc-uk.org/assets/documents/10002C16Guidanceonconductandethicsforstudents.pdf [accessed on 5 October 2012].

HCPC (2012c) *Raising and Escalating Concerns in the Workplace*. Available from http://www.hpc-uk.org/registrants/raisingconcerns/ [accessed on 28 February 2013].

Healy, K. (2005) *Social Work Theories in Context: Creating Frameworks for Practice*. Palgrave Macmillan, Basingstoke.

Heron, J. (2001) *Helping the Client – A Creative, Practical Guide*. 5th ed., Sage, London.

Heywood, A. (2007) *Politics*. 3rd ed., Palgrave Macmillan, Basingstoke.

Heywood, A. (2012) *Political Ideologies: An Introduction*. 5th ed., Palgrave Macmillan, Basingstoke.

Home Office (undated) *Guide to the Equalities Act 2010*. Available from http://www.homeoffice.gov.uk/equalities/equality-act/ [accessed on 5 October 2012].

Hood, S., Mayall, B. and Oliver, S. (eds) (1999) *Critical Issues in Social Research: Power and Prejudice*. Open University, Buckingham.

Human Rights Act (HRA) (1998a) *Summary. Directgov 2012*. Available from http://www.direct.gov.uk/en/governmentcitizensandrights/yourrightsandresponsibilities/dg_4002951 [accessed on 5 October 2012].

Human Rights Act (1998b) *The National Archive at Legislation.co.uk*. Available from http://www.legislation.gov.uk/ukpga/1998/42/contents [accessed on 5 October 2012].

Itzhaky, H. and Bustin, E. (2002) Strengths and pathological perspectives in community social work. *Journal of Community Practice*, 10 (3), 61–73.

Kirschenbaum, H. and Henderson, V.L. (eds) (1990) *The Carl Rogers Reader*. Constable, London.

Lafont, C., Gérard, S., Voisin, T., Pahor, M. and Vellas, B. (2011) Reducing iatrogenic disability in the hospitalized frail elderly. *The Journal of Nutrition, Health & Aging*, 15 (8), 645–660.

Macionis, J. and Plummer, K. (2012) *Sociology: A Global Introduction.* 5th ed., Pearson/Prentice Hall, Harlow.

Marcuse, H. (1969) *An Essay on Liberation.* Beacon Press, Boston.

Marcuse, H. (2002) *One-Dimensional Man: Studies in the Ideology of Advanced Industrial Society (Routledge Classics).* Routledge, London.

Mukhopadhyay, T. (2003) *The Mind Tree: A Miraculous Child Breaks the Silence of Autism.* Arcade, New York.

Nolan, C. (1999) *Under the Eye of the Clock: A Memoir.* Phoenix, London.

Nurse Activism Website. Available from http://nurse-activism.com/index.html [accessed on 5 October 2012].

Nursing and Midwifery Council (NMC) (2008) *The Code: Standards of Conduct, Performance and Ethics for Nurses and Midwives.* Available from http://www.nmc-uk.org/Documents/Standards/The-code-A4–20100406.pdf [accessed on 5 October 2012].

NMC (2010) *Raising and Escalating Concerns: Guidance for Nurses and Midwives.* Available from http://www.nmc-uk.org/Documents/NMC-Publications/NMC-Raising-and-escalating-concerns.pdf [accessed on 5 October 2012].

NMC (2011) *Guidance on Professional Conduct for Nursing and Midwifery Students.* 3rd ed. Available from http://www.nmc-uk.org/Documents/NMC-Publications/NMC-Guidance-on-professional-conduct.pdf [accessed on 28 February 2013].

Nzira, V. and Williams, P. (2009) *Anti-Oppressive Practice in Health and Social Care.* Sage, London.

Okitikpi, T. and Aymer, C. (2010) *Key Concepts in Anti-Discriminatory Social Work.* Sage, London.

Parliamentary and Health Service Ombudsmen (2011) *Care and Compassion?: Report of the Health Service Ombudsman on Ten Investigations into NHS Care of Older People.* Available from http://www.ombudsman.org.uk/__data/assets/pdf_file/0016/7216/Care-and-Compassion-PHSO-0114web.pdf [accessed on 5 October 2012].

Rogers, C.R. (1957) The necessary and sufficient conditions of therapeutic personality change. In: *The Carl Rogers Reader* (Kirschenbaum, H. and Henderson, V. eds), pp. 219–235. Constable, London.

Rogers, C.R. (1980) *A Way of Being.* Houghton Mifflin Co, Boston.

Rogers, C.R. (2003) *Client-Centered Therapy: Its Current Practice, Implications and Theory.* Constable, London.

Saleebey, D. (1996) The strengths perspective in social work practice: Extensions and cautions. *Social Work*, 41 (3), 296–305.

Spiers, J.A. (2005) A concept analysis of vulnerability. In: *The Essential Concepts of Nursing* (Cutcliffe, J.R. and McKenna, H.P. eds), pp. 331–348. Elsevier Churchill Livingstone, Oxford.

Thompson, N. (2003) *Promoting Equality: Challenging Discrimination and Oppression.* Palgrave Macmillan, Basingstoke.

Thompson, N. (2006) *Anti-Discriminatory Practice.* 4th ed., Palgrave Macmillan, Basingstoke.

Thompson, N. (2011) *Promoting Equality: Working with Diversity and Difference.* 3rd ed., Palgrave Macmillan, Basingstoke.

Thompson, N. (2012) *Anti Discriminatory Practice: Equality, Diversity and Social Justice.* 5th ed., Palgrave Macmillan, Basingstoke.

Wingfield, K. (2008) Strategic thinkers in the making. *Cancer Nursing Practice*, 7 (8), 10.

Chapter 10

Conclusion

Julie Ryden and Vanessa Heaslip

Vulnerability is an experience that most, if not all of us will encounter at some stage in our lives as was discussed in Chapter 2. For some vulnerability will be an everyday experience whilst for others it may occur less frequently. There are occasions where it can be a positive life experience, but more usually the impact will be harmful and destructive. This text has sought to explore vulnerability within the context of healthcare settings, a context which clearly increases the risk of vulnerability, and which exposes clients and service users to a greater susceptibility for harm (NMC 2002).

It has been a key contention of the book that vulnerability is an experience which can result from oppression, discrimination, and ultimately the use, abuse, or misuse of power. These concepts are core to the socially constructed experience of vulnerability, showing that vulnerability does not emerge just because someone has a disability, or they have a mental health condition, or that they have been admitted to hospital. These issues on their own are not the major cause of vulnerability, rather it is the relationship between the individual and the world around them which is the major determinant – whether that be the direct or indirect action of health carers; the cultural norms of the care team or society; the policies of the setting; or our experience of the social structures of that world (such as our experience of gender, social class, age). So for example, reaching an age over 65 may introduce the *potential* for *some* vulnerability in *some* people, but it is the attitudes of others around the person which is likely to amplify and solidify vulnerability as the experience for someone over 65. There is no inevitability in the creation of vulnerability as the 'etic' approach (Spiers 2000) would lead us to believe (see Chapter 2), and even for those who may become limited in some aspects of daily living, we should question whether this should inevitably expose an individual to the harm of vulnerability. Our contention is that this risk of harm only occurs in a world where older people are devalued, discarded, and considered to be a burden. In cultures where older people with limited abilities are revered, valued, respected, and celebrated, it is less likely that their risk or susceptibility to harm would be raised. This is the nub of this book and its emphasis on the socially constructed and created nature of vulnerability.

Throughout the text we have emphasised that much vulnerability is unintentionally caused, and that the vast majority of practitioners are conscientious and morally responsible people. By choosing to read this book you have clearly shown such qualities. However, all of us are subject to the pushes and pulls of cultural and structural factors of which we may be unaware. Discourses (Chapters 3, 4, and 6), rituals, and routines (Chapter 5), peer culture (Chapter 5), media culture (Chapter 4), compliance and conformity (Chapter 8), and attribution processes (Chapter 7) are just some of the processes explored within the book which may lead us into being unaware of the impact of our actions. The aim of this book has been to enable practitioners to reflect upon and consider ways that their own practice may unintentionally be creating or contributing to vulnerability. It aims to raise awareness and to bring into the consciousness of its readers the many ways by which we may be causing vulnerability. As such the text provides practitioners with the theoretical and practical base for reviewing their own practice and that of others around them.

We want to emphasise, readers should not feel guilty or ashamed of their reflections upon practice; all of us have at times unintentionally caused vulnerability. Recognition of past actions is a necessary and commendable first step; however, it does then oblige readers to go a step further and explore alternative practises and alternative strategies. To avoid addressing our own practice, would make the reader vulnerable to being 'part of the problem rather than the solution' (Thompson 1992, cited in Thompson 2012: 9), and to be guilty of a degree of conscious negligence. Apologies for the harsh language, but it is a reflection of the seriousness of the issue, and the clear line between being anti-oppressive and being oppressive. There is, as Thompson suggests, *no* 'middle road' (2012: 190). It is not enough to just 'understand' the situation and to recognise where vulnerability is caused; there is a duty for all of us to take some action to address it. These actions need not and may not change the world, they may not be earth shattering, they may only be small and subtle actions, but action must surely follow from the recognition of vulnerability.

> In the end, we will remember not the words of our enemies, but the silence of our friends.
> (Martin Luther King Jr. 'The Trumpet of Conscience' Steeler Lecture, November 1967, cited in Boothe 2011)

This quote from Martin Luther King Jr. is a spur to action rather than silence. It suggests that the vulnerable client will expect evil and harm from an enemy or a bully but a friend who does not challenge the harm being caused will ultimately cause greater hurt and harm. Surely health carers would expect clients to view them, maybe not as friends, but certainly as friendly people who are on the side of the person receiving care. Thus if we do nothing, we may be causing greater harm and vulnerability to the client by our silence and inaction.

This lays down a challenge for all aspiring anti-oppressive practitioners and goes to the heart of what the Health and Care Professions Council (HCPC), the Nursing and Midwifery Council (NMC), and other professional bodies regard as a 'professional'. They require all professionals, including those students who aim to be professionals, 'to always act in the best interests of service users' (HCPC 2012) and 'to make the care of people their first concern' (NMC 2008). It is inconceivable that allowing vulnerability, which after all is a 'susceptibility to harm', to occur and remain unchallenged could fit within either code of practice and thus does clearly direct the practitioner to action. This however does not mean the process is easy and we recognise the difficult path this places us all on, but it is a necessary path if we are to maintain professional integrity and to prevent the harm that results from vulnerability for those in our care.

Let us consider the actions available to all of us; firstly there are *personal* level actions such as communication skills, advocacy, and empowerment. Some of the actions at this level might be deemed easier to implement for the anti-oppressive practitioner and may not prove so daunting for practitioners, others such as 'elegant challenge' may raise greater anxiety. Actions at the *cultural level* such as holding anti-oppressive practice as a core central value, sensitive use of language, and terminology or personal research on oppression and anti-oppression may again be less daunting. Others may be more difficult such as developing a shared team culture or small acts of resistance against oppressive practices and routines. Equally the *structural* level actions may also be challenging for many. Unfortunately, to be effective in reducing vulnerability, may require you being prepared to use many of the strategies, some easy, some not so.

It is at this point that some healthcare practitioners may hold back, afraid of the impact, or concerned that they cannot achieve anything, or preferring 'not to rock the boat' (as explored in Chapters 5, 7 and 9). However, the standards of practice required for health carers are clear that protection for those service users 'at risk' is an essential element, regardless of the level of action. This action may be undertaken alone or undertaken collaboratively, by drawing on the support of colleagues, managers, union representatives, or wider support services. Apart from anything else the research advocated in Chapter 9 on the experiences of people who are vulnerable, together with our own personal knowledge of the harm and distress that comes with vulnerability, will surely convince anyone that action is required regardless of the inconvenience or time needed to do so.

This returns to the issue raised in Chapter 9, that unless anti-oppressive practice and the service user are at the centre of our value system then we will be more easily persuaded out of action. We need to passionately believe in the importance of reducing vulnerability and anti-oppressive practice. Lago and Smith (2010: 1) urge the practitioner to:

> … dare to really feel the consequences of assuming this deeply philosophic stance in their personal and professional transactions with others.

This suggests that anti-oppressive practice is a philosophical position, centred around values and beliefs, but that there is a degree of courage required in the practitioner who chooses to adopt this position and to be true to their core beliefs and values. You will need to 'dare' to be an anti-oppressive practitioner … are you up to it?

Christopher Hitchens recounted the words of his grandmother, 'Thou shalt not follow a multitude to do evil' (Hitchens 2001, cited in Lago and Smith 2010: 2). Following the crowd may feel comfortable and may feel personally safer; however, it does mean that you lose control of the direction. It means that you are then held accountable for the actions of the crowd, regardless of how high your personal values. Again we pose the challenge – can you 'dare to be different' and stand up for what you believe to be right?

Having the courage to question practice which is not compassionate or caring is part of the draft vision proposed by Cummings and Bennett (2012). Entitled 'Developing the culture of compassionate care', Jane Cummings (Chief Nursing Officer for England) and Viv Bennett

(Director of Nursing for the Department of Health) recognise people can and do find themselves in vulnerable circumstances in healthcare, and that health carers play a pivotal role in their experience. However, they are concerned at the recent reports which undermine the high-public regard that they have so often attracted. This consultation document is then a response to this situation and draws out the six core values that thread through and underpin the roles of nurses, midwives, and caregivers – these are referred to as 'the 6 C's':

• Care, delivering high-quality care
• Compassion, how the care is delivered and relationships are developed
• Competence, knowledge and skills to do the job
• Communication, better listening and shared decision making
• Courage, to do the right thing for the people we care for; to speak up when things go wrong
• Commitment, to take action to achieve this vision

These values have been loud and clear throughout this book. Of particular note here are the values of 'courage' and 'commitment'. Courage and boldness is urged in the pursuit of high quality care. In the view of these authors, it is our 'duty', regardless of whether we are on a register or not, to challenge poor quality care. They are unequivocal that the interests of patients, clients, and service users should be at the forefront:

> We must not place our own personal interests or those of our organisation before the interest of the people we care for. We have a collective commitment to make care better. (Cummings and Bennett 2012: 12)

Personal or organisational interests should not be allowed to render us silent or passive; we are therefore urged to be bold and to be committed to delivering compassionate care which reduces the vulnerability of clients. Box 10.1 relays a tale which can be of help in driving

---

Box 10.1   The starfish

One day a man was walking down the beach just before dawn. In the distance, he saw a younger man picking up stranded starfish and throwing them back into the sea. As he approached the younger man, he said: 'Good morning! What are you doing'?
    The young man paused, looked up and replied, 'Throwing starfish into the ocean'.

'I can see that, but WHY'?
'The sun is up and the tide is going out. If I don't throw them in they'll die'.

The boy stated this so matter-of-factly that the old man was taken aback at first, wondering if there was some logic he was missing. He said quietly, 'young man, don't you realize that there are miles and miles of beach and thousands of starfish all along it? You can't possibly make a difference'!
    The young man listened politely then bent down, picked up another starfish and threw it into the sea, past the breaking waves. He turned to the old man with a smile and said,

'it made a difference for that one'.

Based on *The Star Thrower* by Loren Eiseley (1979)

us forward when personal interests, such as fear, anxiety and the need to 'fit in', or organisational interests such as cost efficiency and staff shortages are persuading us out of action.

The anti-oppressive practitioner is driven by the desire to 'make a difference' to the vulnerability of service users, and as such will be as concerned with each small step on the journey as they are with changing the world. Even changing the experience for one service user is a major and commendable achievement, and it is something that we as health carers have the 'power to' achieve (see Chapter 3 for further detail on this concept). It is in our power as practitioners to make a difference, regardless of how big the impact.

At this point we should offer some cautionary advice and support for you as an individual. Challenging the practice of others is certainly a daunting and potentially frightening role, it can be a 'painful, confusing and isolating quest' (Lago and Smith 2010: 1). So while we, together with the professional bodies, strongly advocate this quest; we also acknowledge that on occasions it may be difficult. We therefore would urge the advice offered within Chapter 9, wherever possible try to *work collectively*. This may be with colleagues in your practice area, or it might mean drawing upon the knowledge, skills, and support of wider resources. This could include:

- Your mentor or clinical supervisor
- Your peers
- Other members of the inter professional team
- Your manager
- Your employer
- Colleagues working in the voluntary sector
- Advocacy and service user representative groups
- Your lecturers or past lecturers
- The Human Resources department for your organisation
- Your professional body or association
- Your union
- Public Concern at Work (a confidential whistleblowing support charity)
- NHS Whistleblowing Helpline
- The Patients Association
- Care Quality Commission
- Your MP

Our recommendation would be to find someone, anyone that you feel safe talking to in order to help you explore and tease out the concerns. Alternatively, you might spend time reading the advice on whistleblowing offered by any of the professional bodies (see Activity in Box 9.1) or use the support and guidance offered by any of the support agencies (a list of resources is given at the end of the chapter). This process gives time for reflection, consideration of the most appropriate way forward, and more importantly the opportunity to share the burden. It is equally important that you use the wider support in order to protect yourself from vulnerability. Caring for yourself enables you to go on caring for others and making a bigger difference to the potential vulnerability of those you work with.

Final thought

This book has explored the issue of vulnerability within health social care contexts from a range of perspectives and whilst raising your awareness of issues, it may also have taken you out of your comfort zone; it may have made you aware of challenges you may need to face. Hopefully at the same time we have provided some useful advice and resources which can be used to aid you on the next steps of your journey. There is plenty of support and guidance available and with the knowledge that we do not always get it right the first time, we hope you might be tempted to further improve the lives of clients you work with and to reduce their experiences of feeling vulnerable. Caring for others is a privilege as stated at the outset of this journey (Chapter 1), but we need to earn the right to enjoy that privilege and to challenge others who abuse or misuse that privilege.

Where can I get further help or advice?

Public Concern at Work (a confidential whistleblowing support charity)
020 7404 6609
helpline@pcaw.co.uk
www.pcaw.co.uk

NHS and Social Care Whistleblowing Helpline
08000 724 725
http://wbhelpline.org.uk/
NHS Speaking Up Charter - http://www.nhsemployers.org/EmploymentPolicyAndPractice/
UKEmploymentPractice/RaisingConcerns/SpeakingUpCharter/Pages/SpeakingUp
Charter.aspx

The Patients Association
020 8423 9111
Helpline 0845 608 4455
helpline@patients-association.com

Equality and Human Rights Commission – Advice and Guidance http://www.equalityhu
manrights.com/advice-and-guidance/
Equality Advisory Support Service
0800 444 205
Textphone: 0800 444 206
http://www.equalityadvisoryservice.com/

British Institute of Human Rights – Rights in Healthcare http://www.bihr.org.uk/projects/
human-rights-in-healthcare-public-sector
Liberty – Protecting Civil Liberties, Promoting Human Rights
http://www.liberty-human-rights.org.uk/index.php

Stop Hate UK – Supporting Victims of Hate Crime
0800 138 1625
http://www.stophateuk.org/

Healthcare professional regulators

Nursing and Midwifery Council
020 7637 7181
http://www.nmc-uk.org/
Raising and Escalating Concerns http://www.nmc-uk.org/Nurses-and-midwives/Regulation-in-practice/Safeguarding-New/Raising-and-escalating-concerns/

Health and Care Professions Council
Regulator for the allied health professions
020 7582 0966
www.hpc-uk.org
Raising and Escalating Concerns http://www.hpc-uk.org/registrants/raisingconcerns/

General Medical Council
Regulator for medical doctors throughout the UK in all healthcare sectors
0161 923 660215
www.gmc-uk.org
Raising concerns about patient safety http://www.gmcuk.org/guidance/ethical_guidance/raising_concerns.asp

Regulators of health and social care services

Care Quality Commission (UK)
03000 616161
www.cqc.org.uk
Care Quality Commission – Whistleblowing information and guidance – http://www.cqc.org.uk/contact-us#tab-2
Care and social Services Inspectorate Wales (for social services and care homes)
http://wales.gov.uk/cssiwsubsite/newcssiw/?lang=en01443 848450

Health Inspectorate Wales (for all NHS funded care including independent hospitals)
Health Inspectorate Wales
029 2092 8850

Care Inspectorate (Social Care and Social Work in Scotland)
http://www.scswis.com/index.php
0845 600 9527

Healthcare Improvement Scotland
http://www.healthcareimprovementscotland.org/about_us.aspx 0131 623 4300

Regulation and Quality Improvement Authority Northern Ireland
http://www.rqia.org.uk/home/index.cfm
028 9051 7500

Council for Healthcare Regulatory Excellence (soon to become the Professional Standards
Authority for Health and Social Care)
020 7389 8030
https://www.chre.org.uk/

Monitor – NHS Foundation Trust regulator
020 7340 2400
http://www.monitor-nhsft.gov.uk/

Trade Unions
Royal College of Nursing (RCN)
0345 772 6300 (Whistleblowing hotline)
www.rcn.org.uk/raisingconcerns

Royal College of Midwives (RCM)
020 7312 3535
www.rcm.org.uk

UNISON
0845 355 0845
www.unison.org.uk
Whistleblowing FAQ's http://www.unison.org.uk/healthcare/thinkclean/faqwhistle
blowing.asp

CPHVA/Unite
020 7611 2500
www.unite-cphva.org

Medical Defence Union
Freephone 24-hour advisory helpline 0800 716 646
www.the-mdu.com

Advocacy and service user representative groups

There are many of these organisations, unfortunately too many to mention, however a
very small selection are offered next to give an idea of the support available

Age UK
0800 169 6565
http://www.ageuk.org.uk/

Mencap
0808 808 1111 (Mencap Direct)
http://www.mencap.org.uk/
People First – National Self Advocacy Group
0208 874 1377
http://peoplefirstltd.com/

Mind
0300 123 3393 (Mind Infoline)
http://www.mind.org.uk/

Refugee Council
020 7346 6700
http://www.refugeecouncil.org.uk/

Friends, Families and Travellers
01273 234 777
http://www.gypsy-traveller.org/

Gypsy Council
07963 56 59 52
http://www.gypsy-association.co.uk/

References

Boothe, I. (2011) *Martin Luther King Jr. in his Own Words: Radical, Revolutionary, and Opposed to War*. Available from http://forusa.org/blogs/ivan-boothe/martin-luther-king-jr-his-own-words-radical-revolutionary-opposed-war/8435 [accessed on 24 October 2012].

Cummings, J. and Bennett, V. (2012) *Developing the Culture of Compassionate Care – Creating a New Vision for Nurses, Midwives and Caregivers*. NHS Commissioning Board. Available from https://www.wp.dh.gov.uk/commissioningboard/files/2012/10/nursing-vision.pdf [accessed on 29 October 2012].

Eisely, L. (1979) *The Star Thrower*. Mariner Books, Orlando.

Health and Care Professions Council (HCPC) (2012) *Standards of Conduct, Performance and Ethics* (revised 2012). Available from http://www.hpc-uk.org/aboutregistration/standards/standardsofconductperformanceandethics/ [accessed on 5 October 2012].

Lago, C. and Smith, B. (2010) *Anti-Discriminatory Practice in Counselling & Psychotherapy*. 2nd ed., Sage, London.

Nursing Midwifery Council (NMC) (2002) *Practitioner – Client Relationships and the Prevention of Abuse*. London: Nursing Midwifery Council.

NMC (2008) *The Code: Standards of Conduct, Performance and Ethics for Nurses and Midwives*. Available from http://www.nmc-uk.org/Documents/Standards/The-code-A4-20100406.pdf [accessed on 5 October 2012].

Spiers, J. (2000) New perspectives on vulnerability using emic and etic approaches. *Journal of Advanced Nursing*, 31 (3), 715–721.

Thompson, N. (2012) *Anti-Discriminatory Practice*. 5th ed., Palgrave Macmillan, Basingstoke.

Index

Note: Page numbers in *italics* refer to Figures; those in **bold** to Tables.

abuse of power
  categories, 42
  definition, 42
  prevention, 43–5
  risk factors, vulnerability, 42, 43
activity infantilisation, 78
'anti-oppressive practice'
  description, 177
  as emotional commitment, 190
  guidance and support, councils, 179
  moral duty of care, 178–9
  principles, activist practitioner, 191–2, *192*
  standard and quality, care, 178
  Thompson's PCS model *see* Thompson's
    PCS model
attribution
  cognitive bias, 140–141
  external/situational attribution, 139
  fundamental attribution error, 139–40
  internal/dispositional attribution, 138–9
  rudeness, 140
  theory, 138
authority form of power, 40

behaviour infantilisation, 77–8
biomedical discourse, 114, 127, 162
Black and Minority ethnic (BME) societies,
  112, 121

capitalism, exploitative nature
  fixed structural inequalities, 158
  'hidden curriculum', school, 159
  religion, 158
  welfare state, 159
care work as stressful work, 167–8

Carl Roger's core conditions, therapeutic
  relationship, 182–3
chronic fatigue syndrome *see* myalgic
  encephalomyelitis (ME)
'civilised oppression', 30
coercion, Weber's notion of, 40–41
coercive power, 46–7
cognitive bias
  confirmation bias, 141
  description, 140
  'in-group' bias, 141
  'out-group' homogeneity effect, 141
compassionate care, 2, 94, 96, 212
communication, definition, 180
conscientisation, 197–8
critical reflection, 184–6
'the 6 C's', 212
cultural level
  oppression
    'acceptable' behaviour, 33
    active and empathic listening, patients/
      service users, 34
    analysis, 34–5
    definition, 33
    professional groups, 33
  Thompson's PCS model
    acts of resistance, 191–2
    anti-oppressive practice, 189–90
    language and terminology, 194–6
    openness, transparency and
      demystification, 196
    personal research, oppression and
      anti-oppression, 193–4
    shared team culture, 190–191
    working collectively, 192

Understanding Vulnerability: A Nursing and Healthcare Approach, First Edition. Edited by Vanessa Heaslip
and Julie Ryden.
© 2013 John Wiley & Sons, Ltd. Published 2013 by John Wiley & Sons, Ltd.

decision making power, 53
dehumanisation
    'community', 82
    definition, 81–2
    I-Thou and I-It concept, 84
    'moral exclusion', 83
dementia, 74
disciplinary gaze
    Foucault's three processes, 56–7
    medical surveillance, 57–8
disciplinary power, 56–7
discourses
    characteristics, 113
    definitions, 112, 113
    dominant discourse, 114, 115
    language, 114–16
'discrimination and oppression'
    definition, 28–31
    dehumanisation, 81–5
    infantilisation, 77–8
    invisibilisation, 74–6
    marginalisation, 72–4
    medicalisation, 78–81
    stereotyping, 66–9
    stigmatisation, 68–72
    trivialisation, 85–6
    welfarism, 81
dispersed power
    disciplinary power, 56–7
    discourse and power, 55–6
    'personal is the political', 54–5

elegant challenge, 186–7
empathy, 85, 92, 124, 125, 148, 164, 187, 194
environment infantilisation, 78
essentialism
    group membership, 122
    identity, 119–20
    and stereotyping, 120–122
etic and emic perspectives, *11,* 11–12
European Convention on Human Rights
        (ECHR), 199
exclusionary othering, 163
expert power, 48–9

Foucault's three processes of disciplinary gaze,
        56–7

gender exploitation
    equal pay, 160
    housework, 160
    material and physical exploitation, women,
        160

'pay gap', 160
gypsy/travelling community
    education, 17
    healthcare access, 17
    provision, caravan sites, 16
    social status, 16

hardy personality, 151
HCPC *see* Health and Care Professions
        Council (HCPC)
Health and Care Professions Council (HCPC),
        3, 179, 199, 210
health and social care services, 215–16
healthcare and vulnerability
    admission to hospital, 7–8
    Health Ombudsman Report, 8–9
    lack of choice, 9
    physiological and psychological effects,
        clients, 9–10, **10**
    unthinking and unquestioning practice, 8
Health Ombudsman Report, 8–9
Health Professions Council (HPC), 94, **95,** 98
heuristic availability
    description, 141
    incorrect judgements, 142
HPC *see* Health Professions Council (HPC)
Human Rights Act (HRA), 198, 199
hysteria, 112

inclusionary othering, 163–4, 166
infantilisation, 77–8
informational power, 48–9
intergroup relations, 147–8
internationally recruited nurse (IRN),
        121–2
'inter-personal' communication skills
    communication definition, 180
    vs. 'intra-personal', 180
    noise disruption, 181, 182
    non-verbal cues, 181
    vulnerability reduction, 182
invisibilisation
    coronary heart disease, 76
    cultural assumptions and discourses, 75
    definition, 74
IRN *see* internationally recruited nurse (IRN)

language and terminology, health care setting
    sensitivity and insensitivity, oppressive use,
        194, *195*
    term 'black', 195
law, health care settings
    anti-discriminatory legislation, 201, 202

law, health care settings (*cont'd*)
  disabled people, 201
  Equality Act, 198, 199–200, 202
  equality impact assessments, 201
  European Convention on Human Rights
    (ECHR), 199
  Human Rights Act (HRA), 198, 199
  Mental Health Act 1983, 203
  proactive use of law, 202
  protection, torture and mistreatment, 199,
    200
  'the Polo Mint effect', 203
learned helplessness
  definition, 149
  process, 149–50
legitimate power, 47
Liverpool Care Pathway, 2
Lukes' concept of power
  decision making, 53
  non-decision making, 53–4
  shaping desires, wants and needs, 54

marginalisation
  definition, 72
  dementia, 74
  learning disabilities, 73, 74
  MRSA, 73
  social attitudes, 73
  social exclusion, 72
Marxist and 'system' theories of power
  gender oppression 'patriarchy', 50
  hegemony, 51, 52
  ideology, 51
  institutional racism, 50–51
  position, social hierarchy, 49
  ruling ideology, 51
  structural and social class inequalities, 50
  structural disablism, 50
  time for reflection activity, 51, 52
ME *see* myalgic encephalomyelitis (ME)
medicalisation
  cancer, 79–80
  chronic leg ulcers, 80
  death and process of dying, 79
  disability, 79
  'normal' and 'natural' processes, women's
    lives, 79
Mental Health Act 1983, 203
Methicillin-resistant *Staphylococcus aureus*
  (MRSA), 73
Mid Staff NHS Trust review, 1
Mid Staffordshire NHS Trust enquiry, 1
minimal intervention, 187–8

MRSA *see* Methicillin-resistant
    Staphylococcus aureus (MRSA)
multiple identities, 124–5
mutual vulnerability, 19–20
myalgic encephalomyelitis (ME), 112

National Health Service (NHS)
  core values, 2–3
  definition, 3
  evidence-based standardised care, 2
  hospital and community settings, 96
  older people care, 96
  and private care organisations, 2
National Service Framework for Older
    People, 13
Neck of Femur Care Pathway, 2
NHS *see* National Health Service (NHS)
non-decision making power, 53–4
The *No Secrets* document, 14
Nursing and Midwifery Council (NMC), 35,
    36, 44, 94, **95**, 179, 189, 210

obedience and compliance
  Asch experiment, 170
  'lethal/near lethal shocks', 169–70
  Milgram experiment, 169
openness and demystification, 196
oppression
  'civilised oppression', 30
  definition, 29–30
  hardship and injustice, 29, 30
  inhuman/degrading treatment, individuals,
    29, 30
  negative and demeaning exercise, power,
    29, 31
  PCS model *see* personal, cultural and
    structural (PCS) model, oppression
  time for reflection, 29
'othering'
  description, 161
  exclusionary, 163
  on healthcare, 162
  homeless people, 165
  inclusionary, 163–4, 166
  respectful, 164
  scapegoating, 163
  'sleep out', 164
over attention, 85–6

'perceptual defence', 137
personal, cultural and structural (PCS) model
  oppression
    adaptation, 32, *32*

cultural level, 33–5
personal level, 32–3
structural level, 35–7
professional culture, 99–100
personality 'syndromes', 145
personal level
oppression, 32–3
Thompson's PCS model
challenging, 186–7
clear and explicit theory base, 189
critical reflection, introspection, and
self-awareness, 184–6
interpersonal communication skills,
180–182
minimal intervention, 187–8
'strength-based approach', 183–4
therapeutic relationship, 182–3
political correctness, 86
'the Polo Mint effect', 197, 203
power
abuse *see* abuse, power
definition, 38–9
description, 38
'dispersed power', 54–7
effect, 40–41
Marxist and 'system' theories of power,
49–52
older people, health service, 37–8
political view, 38
'power over', 39–41
'power to', 39–41
psychological, 39
sources
coercive power, 46–7
expert power, 48–9
legitimate power, 47
referent power, 47–8
reward power, 46
three faces of power *see* Lukes' concept of
power
traditional 'pluralist' theories, 45
types, 39–40
prejudice
definition, 144
The Nature of Prejudice, 143
as personality trait, 144–5
reduction, 148
professional culture and vulnerability
activity, 97, 98
and 'belongingness'
activity, 103
conformity and compliance, 101
development, nurse education, 103

rules, clinical practice guidance,
100–101
students' experience, 101, *102*
codes, 95
deficiencies, nursing, 96
health care course, 92
health care professionals, 94, 95
horizontal violence, 105–6
NHS, 96
personal values, 93–4
popular and unpopular patients, 98
ritual and routine work practices, 104
socialisation, 93
Thompson's PCS model, 99–100
professional socialisation, 93
psychological distance, 83
psychology
advocates and detractors, 133
availability heuristic, 141–2
definition, 132–3
discrimination and oppression, reduction,
134
intergroup relations, 147–8
judgements and attributions
attribution theory, 138, 139
'being rude', 140
lack of control, 149
learned helplessness, 149–50
prejudice *see* prejudice
resilience and hardy personality, 150–151
social categorisation, 145–6
stereotyping, 146–7
subjective perception, 134–8
psychosocial experience
definition, 154
exploitative nature, capitalism, 157–9
gender exploitation, 159–61
historical explanations, 156–7
institutional and structural racism, 157
organisational level, 166–71
'othering' *see* 'othering'
sociology, vulnerability and oppression,
155–6

Realistic Group Conflict Theory, 147
referent power, 47–8
resilience, definition, 150
respect and dignity, 2
reward power, 46

Safeguarding Vulnerable Groups
Act 2006, 14
shared team culture, 190–191

social construction
  Black and Minority ethnic (BME) societies,
    112, 121
  definition, 111
  discourses and vulnerability *see* discourses
  essentialist *see* essentialism
  identity
    activity, 116, 117
    fixed and static, 117
    groupings, 118
    oppression and power, 122–4
    and practice, 125–8
    'self-fulfilling prophecy', 118–19
  multiple identities, 124–5
social exclusion, 72
socialisation *see* Professional socialisation
sociology, definition, 155
speech infantilisation, 77
stereotypes
  'crabbit' old women/men, care
    environments, 68, 69
  features, 66–7
  filing system, 66
  learning disability, 68
  social categorization, 67, 68
  social information, 66
stigma, 68–9
stigmatisation
  activity, Lin and Phelan's process, 72
  'bed blocker', 70
  definition, 68–9
  overweight patients, 70
  worthy and unworthy patients, 70, 71
stressful work, 167–8
structural level
  oppression
    healthcare, 35, 36
    'institutional oppression', 35
    NMC requirements, 35
  Thompson's PCS model *see* Thompson's
    PCS model
subjective perceptions, psychology
  factors, perceptual set, 137
  'perceptual defence', 137
  Rubin's Vase, 135, 136
  schemas, 137
  sensation and, 134
  typing errors, 136

therapeutic relationship
  Carl Roger's core conditions, 183

'psychological contact', 182
Thompson's PCS model *see also* Personal,
    cultural and structural (PCS) model
  cultural level strategies *see* cultural level,
    Thompson's PCS model
  personal level strategies *see* personal level,
    Thompson's PCS model
  structural level strategies
    participation, democratic process,
      203–5
    politicisation and conscientisation,
      197–8
    'use the law', 198–203
  vulnerability reduction, 179–80

'unpopular patient', 46, 47, 73, 98, 137, 162,
    167

vulnerability
  advocacy and service user representative
    groups, 216–17
  definition, 6–7
  description, 3–4, 209
  as existential experience, 18–19
  health and social care services, 215–16
  and healthcare, 7–10
  healthcare professional regulators, 215
  help/advice from organisations, 214–15
  models
    care burden and coping capacity, 21
    dynamic continuum – balance, *21*
    environmental and personal resources,
      21, *21, 23,* 23–4
    environmental supports
      examination, 22
    personal resources examination, 22
  mutual vulnerability, 19–20
  positive dimensions, 20
  power *see* power
  professional definitions, 10–12
  reduction *see* 'anti-oppressive practice'
  as shifting experience, 18
  social groups
    identification, 14–15
    interaction, 15–18
  'the 6 C's', 212
  vulnerable populations identification, 12–13

Weber's concept of coercion, 40–41
welfarism, 81
Winterbourne View review, 1